easy dairy-free ketogenic recipes

200+ low-carb family favorites for weight loss and health

INTERNATIONAL BESTSELLING AUTHOR

Maria Emmerich

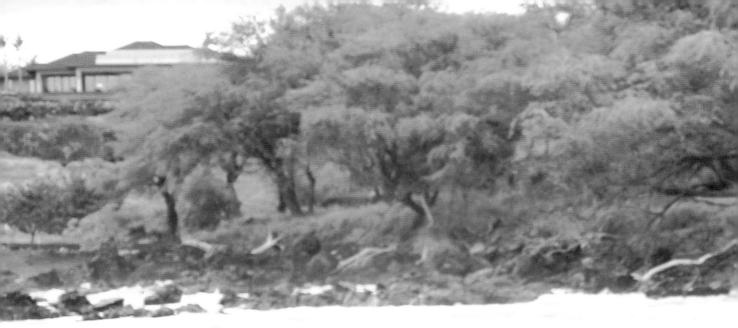

First Published in 2018 by Victory Belt Publishing Inc.

Copyright © 2018 Maria Emmerich

ISBN-13: 978-1-628602-66-1

Interior design by Justin-Aaron Velasco

Printed in Canada

TC 0318

Contents

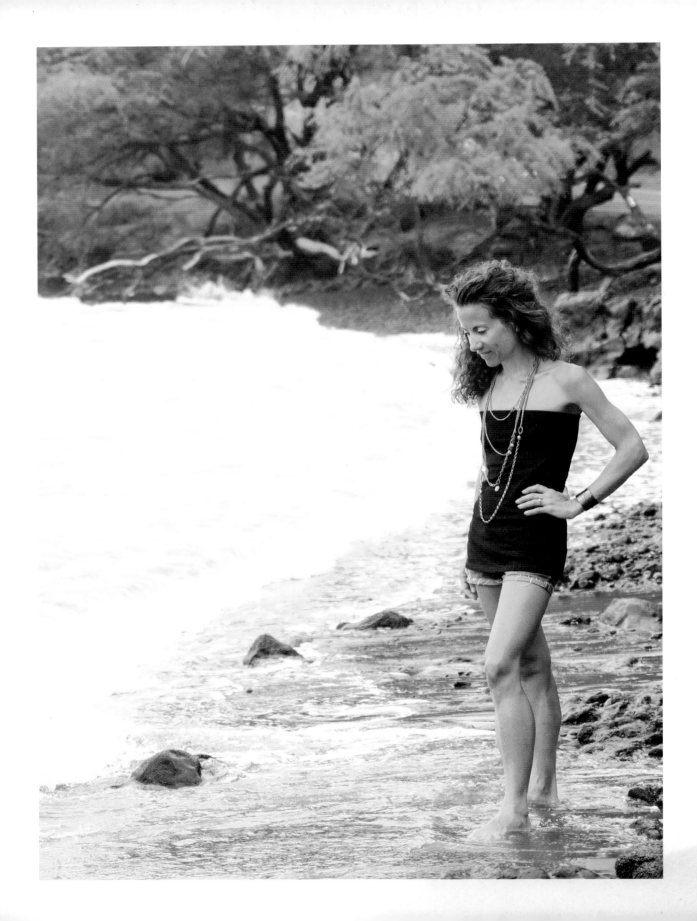

Introduction

What Is Keto?

For hundreds of thousands of years, human beings ate mostly meat and vegetables—the so-called caveman diet. With the onset of modern civilization and the development of agriculture, the human body was asked to digest and metabolize larger and larger amounts of starches and refined sugars. But our bodies are unable to utilize significant quantities of carbohydrates. Therefore, we develop symptoms. The good news is that the ketogenic diet offers a solution—a practical and healthy method for reversing the modern plague of poor health and obesity.

The ketogenic diet is a high-fat, moderate-protein, low-carb style of eating that has powerful health benefits. Originally developed in the 1920s to treat epileptic seizures, the diet fell out of favor once antiseizure medications became available. More than seventy years later, it was rediscovered as an effective alternative to pharmaceutical treatments. Since then, it has grown in popularity and has received increasing attention for the variety of maladies that it treats (see the illustration on the next page).

The ketogenic diet is too often viewed as simply a sugar-elimination diet. But really, it is a low-carb diet, and that is an important distinction. The keto diet eliminates or severely restricts all the foods that turn into sugar in the body, which include carbohydrates and even protein, as well as refined and natural sugars. After all, complex carbohydrates (including "healthy" whole grains and root vegetables) are just glucose molecules hooked together in a long chain. The digestive tract breaks them down into glucose . . . also known as sugar!

People tend to focus on calorie reduction for weight loss because they are told that metabolism comes down to calories in, calories out. But our bodies are much more complex than that. It's hard to lose weight simply by cutting calories. Eating less and losing excess body fat do not necessarily go hand in hand. A low-calorie, high-carbohydrate diet sets off a series of biochemical signals in your body that pull you out of balance, making it difficult to access stored body fat for energy. As a result, you reach a plateau beyond which you simply can't lose any more weight. Furthermore, diets based on limiting calories usually fail because people on these restrictive diets get tired of feeling hungry and deprived all the time. Unsatisfied, they go off their diets, put the weight back on, and then feel like failures for not having enough willpower or discipline to stay on track.

In reality, though, successful weight loss has little to do with discipline. It's more about focusing on *what* to eat than how much. On a ketogenic diet, you can eat enough food to feel satisfied and still lose body fat, without obsessively counting calories or fat grams.

Health Benefits of the Ketogenic Diet

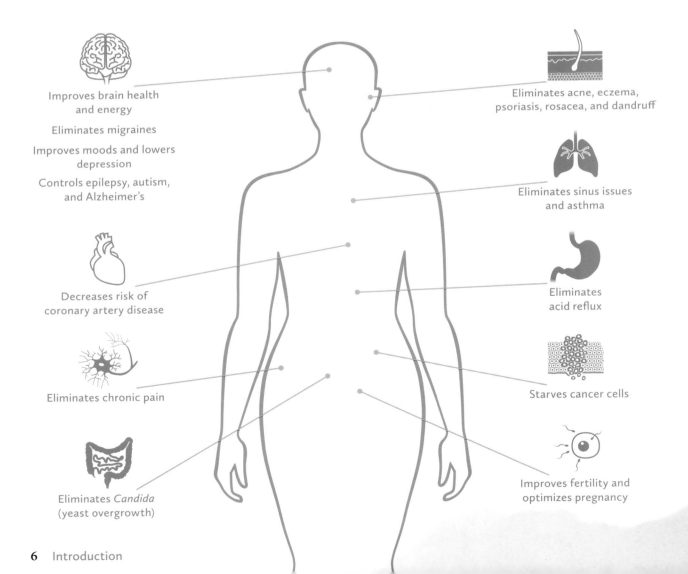

Improves brain health and energy

Eliminates migraines

Improves moods and lowers depression

Controls epilepsy, autism, and Alzheimer's

Decreases risk of coronary artery disease

Eliminates chronic pain

Eliminates *Candida* (yeast overgrowth)

Eliminates acne, eczema, psoriasis, rosacea, and dandruff

Eliminates sinus issues and asthma

Eliminates acid reflux

Starves cancer cells

Improves fertility and optimizes pregnancy

Why Go Dairy-Free?

I find that eliminating dairy helps many people reach their goal weight. For half of my clients, dairy spikes insulin and holds them back from losing any weight. Other problems can arise with dairy consumption as well: When your gut is damaged and inflamed, a phenomenon called "atrophy of the villi" occurs. Dairy is digested at the ends of the villi, which are little fingerlike pieces of tissue that line the intestinal wall. If your villi are damaged, you may not be able to absorb dairy well, leading to symptoms such as acid reflux, indigestion, gas, and/or bloating. Once you heal the intestinal wall with an anti-inflammatory ketogenic diet, you may be able to reincorporate dairy, in smaller amounts at first.

However, some clients are truly allergic to casein, a protein found in dairy, and can never consume dairy. In that case, replace the butter used in recipes with tasty keto fats like avocado oil, coconut oil, duck fat, lard, and tallow.

To reintroduce dairy, start with goat cheese and see if your weight loss stalls or your weight creeps up. If it doesn't, try ghee next. Then progress to butter and cheese made from cow's milk if your body tolerates them.

Establishing a Well-Formulated Ketogenic Diet

Fat, protein, and carbohydrate are the three macronutrients that human beings need for growth and health. A well-formulated ketogenic diet can be thought of as a distribution of these three macronutrients in that order, from high to low. Here is a good formula for most people to follow.

Step 1: Eliminate Sugar and High-Carbohydrate Foods

Sugar causes inflammation, and even complex carbohydrates such as brown rice, oatmeal, and potatoes are just glucose molecules hooked together in a long chain that the digestive system breaks down into glucose. So step one of your transition to the ketogenic diet is to cut out sugar and carbohydrates. Even the carbohydrates found in vegetables are broken down into sugar, so if you want to enter ketosis, limiting starchy vegetables—along with refined and natural sugars and grains, of course—is essential.

Focus on reducing your carbohydrate intake to 30 grams or less per day. For people with diabetes, this level may need to be even lower, about 20 grams per day or less, to counteract insulin resistance.

Step 2: Hit Your Protein Goal

Our Paleolithic ancestors thrived on animal proteins and the fat that came with them. This is what sustained them through the winter. Protein is essential for maintaining lean body mass, which includes muscles, organs, and bones. Getting adequate protein each day, or at least averaging it out over the course of a week, is very important for maintaining lean mass and strength as you age.

In general, it is better to eat too much protein than too little. Not hitting your daily protein goal will result in a loss of lean mass over time, which nobody wants. Also, protein has a high thermic effect of food (TEF), which is the amount of energy the body needs to expend in order to digest a particular food. Fat and carbohydrate have a low TEF (about 3 percent and 8 percent, respectively), whereas protein has a TEF of 25 percent. This means that for every 100 calories of protein you eat, only 75 of those calories really count. On top of that, protein is one of the most satiating macronutrients. It helps keep you feeling full longer.

A good goal is 0.8 times your lean body mass in grams of protein. Try to hit this target each day or average it out over the course of a week (some days can be lower, some higher). For example, if you weigh 143 pounds and have 30 percent body fat, your lean mass is about 100 pounds (143 x 0.7 = 100). So your protein goal would be 80 grams a day (100 x 0.8 = 80).

Step 3: Use Fat as a Lever

If you cut out sugar and carbohydrates and hit your protein goal, what's left? The f-word—yep, fat. It's a key macronutrient that has been wrongfully demonized for decades. When you are keto-adapted, healthy fat is your primary fuel source. Fat also helps make the hormones that keep you feeling satiated and keep cravings at bay.

The amount of fat you need to eat depends on your caloric needs. To lose weight, you want to consume fewer calories than you burn. Most of my clients find that 1,000 to 1,400 calories is a good range after they've become keto-adapted. Once you have hit your protein goal, the rest of your calories should come from fat, either from the meat you're eating or from fat added to your meals. For example, if you're eating 1,400 calories, 80 grams of protein, and 20 grams of carbs, you are left with 1,000 calories to consume in the form of fat:

80 grams + 20 grams = 100 grams x 4 calories per gram = 400 calories

1,400 total calories – 400 calories from protein & carbs =
1,000 calories from fat

One gram of fat has 9 calories, so that leaves you with 111 grams of fat to eat:

1,000 calories ÷ 9 calories per gram = 111 grams of fat

So, in this example, you would shoot for 111 grams of fat or less per day. Remember, the less fat you eat, the more stored body fat will be used for fuel (which leads to fat loss—exactly what you want when your goal is to lose weight).

Once you are keto-adapted, you'll feel full with fewer calories. There is no need to force extra fat into your diet to try to raise your ketone levels or correct your macronutrient ratios. In the first couple of weeks after switching to keto, you might need to turn up your intake of healthy fat to push yourself over the adaptation divide. But if weight loss is your goal, then reducing your fat intake will force your body to create ketones from stored fat.

As long as you limit your carb intake (to 30 grams or less per day, but ideally 20 grams or less) and don't exceed your protein goal, you will achieve ketosis, a state in which your body can use dietary fat and body fat equally well. If there isn't enough dietary fat coming in, your body will turn to stored fat for fuel— leading to weight loss!

So eat fat just until you are full or until you reach your calorie limit for the day, whichever comes first. I say "calorie limit" because early on, you *can* overeat fat and hold yourself back. If you have been following a high-carb diet, it's likely that you have leptin resistance, which means that leptin, the hormone that tells your body that you are full, isn't working as it should. As a result, you never feel full, even after a large meal. A ketogenic diet will heal your body, and your hormones will begin to fire properly. After leptin resistance is healed, it is hard to overeat fat when your carb and protein amounts are correct because you will feel full and satisfied.

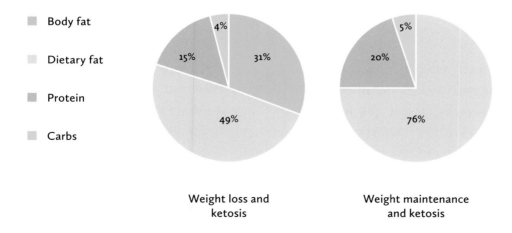

Weight loss and ketosis

Weight maintenance and ketosis

Choosing Healthy Fats

When it comes to which fats to consume, the more saturated fatty acids (SFAs) those fats contain, the better. Saturated fats like MCT oil, coconut oil, tallow, and lard are your best choices: they are stable, anti-inflammatory, and less prone to oxidation, which can cause inflammation in the body. Grass-fed and organic fat sources are preferred.

MCT stands for *medium-chain triglycerides,* which are chains of fatty acids. Consuming fats that contain an abundance of MCTs is particularly beneficial because, unlike long-chain triglycerides, MCTs are used quickly by the body and not stored in the fat cells. A bonus: any MCTs not immediately utilized are converted to ketones, which can be helpful when you are first becoming keto-adapted. Until your body is efficient at generating ketones from stored body fat, ketones from MCTs can help feed your brain.

MCTs are naturally found in coconut oil and palm oil. MCT oil is extracted from coconut oil or palm oil and has a higher concentration of MCTs. Another advantage is that unlike coconut oil, MCT oil remains liquid even when refrigerated.

Avoid polyunsaturated fatty acids (PUFAs), which are unstable fats found in products such as margarine, vegetable oil, and vegetable shortening—all of which you should steer clear of at all times! You should also avoid trans fats, which are created when hydrogen is added to unsaturated fats (causing them to become partially hydrogenated). The food industry uses trans fats because they are less expensive and extend the shelf life of foods, but trans fats are very detrimental to health.

Maintaining a Healthy Balance of Micronutrients

Macronutrients are the focus on a well-formulated ketogenic diet, but it's also important to get adequate amounts of certain *micronutrients*—the vitamins, minerals, and electrolytes that your body needs. Maintaining a healthy balance of these micronutrients can mean the difference between feeling great on your keto diet and feeling so awful that you want to give up.

At this point, you may be thinking, "How am I supposed to get my vitamins and minerals if I'm not eating a lot of fruits and vegetables?" You might think that "superfoods" like kale and blueberries are essential for meeting your body's nutritional needs. But take a look at this chart comparing the nutrient density of apples, blueberries, and kale to beef and beef liver.

(per 100 g)	APPLES	BLUEBERRIES	KALE	BEEF	BEEF LIVER
Calcium (mg)	5	6	72	11	11
Magnesium (mg)	4	6	17	19	18
Phosphorus (mg)	11	12	28	175	387
Potassium (mg)	90	77	228	370	380
Iron (mg)	0.1	0.3	0.9	3.3	8.8
Zinc (mg)	0.1	0.2	0.2	4.5	4
Selenium (mcg)	0	0.1	0.5	14.2	39.7
Vitamin A (IU)	0	0	0	40	53,400
Vitamin B6 (mg)	0	0.1	0.1	0.4	1.1
Vitamin B12 (mcg)	0	0	0	2	111
Vitamin C (mg)	4	9.7	41	2	27
Vitamin D (IU)	0	0	0	7	19
Vitamin E (mg)	0.1	0.6	0.9	1.7	0.63
Niacin (mg)	0.1	0.4	0.5	4.8	17
Folate (mcg)	0	6	13	6	145

As you can see, 100 grams of beef packs more nutrients than 100 grams of apples, blueberries, or kale, without all the inflammatory sugars. And organ meats like beef liver are even more nutrient-dense—they are the *real* superfoods! A ketogenic diet based primarily on animal proteins is a very micronutrient-rich diet, especially if you include organ meats on a regular basis.

Water, sodium, and electrolytes

When you adopt a ketogenic lifestyle, one of the first effects you experience is a rapid improvement in sensitivity to the hormone insulin. Low-carb eating causes insulin levels to fall quickly. As insulin levels fall, your kidneys begin to release fluid. A common complaint I hear from clients who are just getting started on keto is that they have to urinate more often than usual in the middle of the night. If this happens to you, too, know that this effect will go away eventually.

The good news is that when your kidneys release excess fluid, it becomes easier for your body to burn fat. The bad news is that as the water goes, essential sodium and other electrolytes go along with it. When sodium falls below a certain level (which can happen quickly), undesirable side effects, such as headaches, dizziness, cramping, and low energy, can occur. Soon after you start keto, you might notice that if you stand up quickly, you feel faint. This is because you are dehydrated! Just drinking water isn't going to work, though; you need more sodium, too. Salt is not the evil that your doctors may have warned you about; you have to start thinking differently. A well-formulated ketogenic diet requires a lot more sodium.

Even if you don't experience any obvious side effects when you switch to keto, you need extra water and sodium. Eliminating packaged foods removes a lot of sodium from your diet, and most keto foods don't contain a lot of liquid, so you need to drink at least half of your body weight in ounces of water each day. If you get the fierce headaches that some people get when starting out, add sodium. Try to get about 6 grams of sodium per day. My favorite way to get more sodium (as well as electrolytes and a ton of minerals) is to consume homemade bone broth. It is so easy to make—you can even do it in a slow cooker! I often make a huge batch in the pot that Craig used to use for home brewing (yes, we have come a long way in our journey!). I freeze the broth in small containers, and it keeps for a long time. If you really don't want to make your own bone broth, you can use store-bought bouillon: it contains a lot of sodium, tastes good as a hot drink, and can eliminate carbohydrate cravings. Watch out for MSG and gluten, though; not all brands of bouillon are healthy.

In addition to drinking bone broth, I suggest that you replace your table salt with real salts, such as Celtic sea salt and Himalayan rock salt. These salts are either harvested from ancient seabeds or made by evaporating seawater that has a high mineral content. They contain about 70 percent of the sodium found in regular table salt (which has been refined, bleached, and processed until it is pretty much pure sodium chloride, often with anticaking agents added). The other 30 percent consists of minerals and micronutrients (including iodine) found in mineral-rich seas. I greatly prefer the taste of real salts to table salt; they are well worth the extra bucks. Do not make the mistake of using a brand of sea salt that adds dextrose (a form of sugar) as an anticaking agent and is devoid of iodine and other nutrients.

Potassium

If you don't want to lose muscle, pay attention here! Because a ketogenic diet (even a well-formulated one) causes you to excrete a lot of sodium, you will eventually lose a lot of potassium as well. Keeping your potassium level up safeguards your lean mass as you lose weight. Just like sodium, adequate potassium prevents cramping and fatigue. A deficiency in potassium can cause low energy, heavy legs, and dizziness, and you might cry easily.

I often teach nutrition classes, and at the end of each class, I answer participants' questions. One question I frequently hear, especially from people who have high blood pressure, is, "How do you recommend getting potassium if you don't recommend eating bananas or potatoes?" It's interesting that doctors often recommend bananas and potatoes to their patients with high blood pressure. Sure, those foods taste great, but in reality, they are *causing* the blood pressure problem, not fixing it! As your insulin levels increase, so does your blood pressure. And there are foods that are much higher in potassium than the insulin-spiking banana and potato. Dried herbs, for example, contain a lot of potassium, without any of the sugar or starch.

To ensure that you are getting adequate potassium, start adding potassium-rich foods like dried basil, chervil, dill, oregano, parsley, saffron, tarragon, and turmeric to your diet. You can also supplement with 99 milligrams of potassium twice a day. Keeping your sodium and magnesium intake up will help preserve your potassium, too.

Magnesium

A main source of magnesium for many people is fortified whole grains ("fortified" just means that a supplement containing magnesium has been added). So if you remove grains from your diet, you are eliminating a major source of magnesium. Taking calcium supplements also increases your chance of a magnesium deficiency, as calcium competes with magnesium for uptake. That being said, a well-formulated ketogenic diet doesn't cause a massive depletion of magnesium like a high-carb diet does. Your body uses 54 milligrams of magnesium to process just 1 gram of sugar or starch! That creates a high demand for magnesium. No wonder it is one of the most common deficiencies that I see in clients.

Most people who have high blood pressure and/or are overweight, insulin resistant, or diabetic are deficient in magnesium. Insulin stores magnesium, but if your insulin receptors are blunted and your cells grow resistant to insulin, you can't store magnesium; therefore, it passes out of your body through urination. Magnesium in your cells relaxes your muscles. If your magnesium level is too low, your blood vessels will constrict rather than relax, which raises your blood pressure and decreases your energy level.

It is not entirely necessary to get a blood test to see if you are deficient in magnesium; the fact is that most people don't get enough magnesium. About 70 percent of people don't get the minimum recommended amount.

You may be wondering why we need to supplement with minerals like magnesium if our ancestors never did. Well, most of the magnesium they ingested was found in the water they drank from streams and wells. Today, most people drink treated, softened, or bottled water, which is devoid of magnesium. Magnesium salts present in untreated water leave deposits in pipes and make it difficult to get a decent lather with soap. These problems were solved with the development of water softeners, but the softening process created a new problem by getting rid of the magnesium that our bodies need.

Because our water is now depleted of magnesium and adequate amounts are not found in foods, I suggest taking at least 400 milligrams of a quality chelated magnesium supplement each day. It helps repair muscles, naturally relaxes blood vessels and tight muscles, and is a miracle cure for migraines and many other ailments. Most people find magnesium relaxing, so taking it at bedtime may help you sleep. On rare occasions, magnesium is energizing, so if you find yourself unable to sleep after taking it, I suggest taking 400 milligrams at breakfast and, if needed, another dose at lunch. Everyone has a different tolerance. You can also try topical magnesium gels and lotions, which are readily absorbed through the skin.

Chelated magnesium is combined with an amino acid agent to promote absorption. So if the dosage is 1,000 milligrams of magnesium citrate, the amount of magnesium in the supplement isn't 1,000 milligrams. The amino acid is heavier than magnesium; only about 15 percent of the total weight is magnesium. The only way to know for sure how much magnesium you're getting from a particular supplement is to look at the Recommended Daily Intake (RDI). The RDI for magnesium is 400 milligrams, so if you see that a dose of the supplement contains 50 percent of the RDI, then you know that each dose contains 200 milligrams of magnesium, and you should take two doses to reach the recommended 400-milligram amount.

The only problematic side effect of magnesium is loose stool. This is more likely to occur if you purchase magnesium oxide, which is a nonabsorbable form. Instead, look for magnesium glycinate (I have only been able to find it online). If you are taking a small dose and still have issues with loose stool, try using topical magnesium or Epsom salts in a bath as an alternative.

Testing for Ketones

Testing for ketones can help you determine whether you have achieved ketosis. To understand the different methods of testing for ketones, you need to know a little bit about ketone bodies. Functionally, there are three types of ketone bodies:

- Acetone
- Acetoacetate
- Beta-hydroxybutyrate (BHB)

Each of the three kinds of ketone tests looks for one of these three ketone bodies. Acetone is tested in the breath, acetoacetate in the urine, and BHB in the blood. Each method has its advantages and disadvantages.

- **Urine test strips (Ketostix):** If you test your urine for ketones using urine test strips, your results in the early stages of switching to keto will typically reflect higher levels of ketones because your body hasn't started using ketones for fuel yet. After you are fully keto-adapted, you will see fewer and fewer ketones in your urine because your body will be using those ketones for fuel instead of excreting them. Urine test strips are also susceptible to changes in your state of hydration. The more hydrated you are (remember, you should be drinking lots of water!), the lower the ketone level on the urine test strip will be. So urine test strips are not a particularly accurate method of testing.
- **Breath testing (Ketonix breath analyzer):** Your breath acetone level gives you a good idea of how much fat your body is turning into fuel, but it doesn't directly correlate to the amount of BHB in your blood.
- **Blood ketone testing:** Blood ketone testing is the best indicator of your true state of ketosis. Within a BHB range of 0.5 to 5.0 millimoles per liter of blood, your body is in ketosis and using ketones as its primary fuel source. I like the Precision Xtra Blood Glucose & Ketone Monitoring System best.

More is not better when it comes to ketones. Many studies have shown that ketone levels have no correlation to weight loss. If you are metabolically damaged (or insulin resistant), you won't be able to utilize ketones for fuel as efficiently, which can result in higher ketone levels. Your focus should be on hitting your protein goal and restricting total carbs to 30 grams or less (or, ideally, 20 grams or less). If you do those two things, your body will get into ketosis regardless of your blood ketone measurements.

Meal Planning: The Key to Success

Now that you've got a little background in the science behind the ketogenic diet, let's talk about food!

I have a wonderful mother who loves to cook, but when I was little, she worked full-time. On many nights when she came home from work, she would often say in a flustered tone, "I have no idea what to make for dinner!" Even at the young age of five, I could feel her stress.

Planning is the key to success in anything, including healthy eating. But if meal planning seems like too difficult an approach or your schedule is already jam-packed, see if you can commit a block of time one day a week, such as on a Sunday afternoon, to meal prep. With already-prepared meals stashed away in the fridge or freezer, you can look forward to stress-free lunches and dinners during the week, not to mention that you will save time that you would normally use to prepare weekday meals.

For a quick start, you can use a trick that my husband, Craig, and I often employ. While he cleans up after dinner, I prepare dinner for the next night. So, if I want to make Slow Cooker Philly Steak Sandwiches (page 204), I fill the insert of my slow cooker with the ingredients and store the insert in the fridge. I also take some premade waffles out of the freezer and transfer them to the fridge to thaw. All I have to do the next morning is take the slow cooker insert out of the fridge, place it in the slow cooker, and turn it on. When I get home in the evening, I take the waffles out of the fridge to toast and dinner is ready—a complete meal in about five minutes!

If you're looking for really easy dinners that you can toss in the slow cooker, try one of these recipes.

Top 7 Slow Cooker Dinners

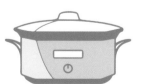

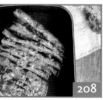
204
Slow Cooker Philly
Steak Sandwiches

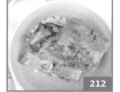
208
Easy BBQ
Brisket

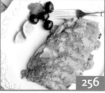
212
Curry Short Ribs

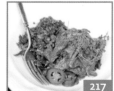
217
Jamaican Jerk
Pot Roast

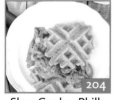
224
Chinese Five-Spice
Roast Beef

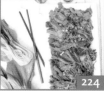
238
Easy Barbecue Ribs

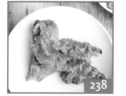
256
Cilantro Lime
Slow Cooker Ribs

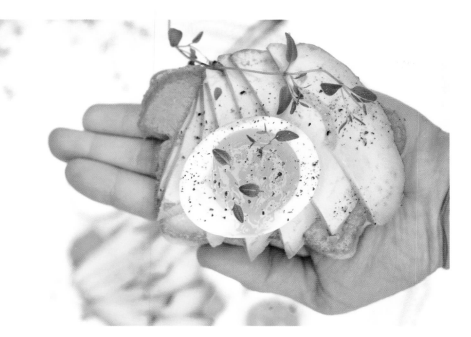

Make Your Own Keto Convenience Food

Who doesn't like convenience? If you come home from a long day at work extremely hungry but have nothing prepared, you are more likely to grab something unhealthy to eat. Here are some suggestions that will make meal planning a snap:

- Double or triple a recipe to make a larger batch. Divide and freeze the leftovers in either family-sized or individual servings, so all you have to do is grab a container from the freezer to reheat. (If you find that the microwave dries out your leftovers, try reheating them in your toaster oven!)

- Make larger batches so you can take the leftovers for lunch. Leftover chili and soups are great options for easy lunches. Remember to transfer the container from the freezer to the fridge the night before.

- Freeze the ingredients for slow cooker recipes in gallon-sized plastic storage bags; fill three to five different bags so you have multiple options. Then all you have to do is drop the contents of the bag into the slow cooker before you leave for the day.

- Cook an extra batch of keto waffles (see page 204) to freeze for later. Separate the waffles with sheets of wax paper to prevent them from sticking together in the freezer. The waffles can be eaten for breakfast or used to make sandwiches for any meal.

- Keep hard-boiled eggs (see page 81) and other grab-and-go keto foods in the fridge. And always have keto brioche in the freezer for easy sandwiches!

- Thaw steaks or ground beef in the refrigerator for easy dinners during the week; it doesn't take long to pan-fry a steak in a skillet or brown ground beef for taco night.

7 Meals in 6 Minutes or Less

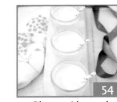 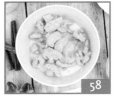 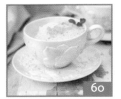 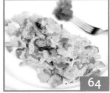

54

58

60

64

Cherry Almond
Breakfast Shake

French Toast Cereal

Lemon
Minute Muffins

Loaded
Scrambled Eggs

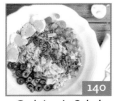 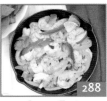

140

141

288

Crab Louie Salad

Salad Kabobs

Super Fast
Shrimp Fajitas

Top 12 No-Cook Meals and Snacks

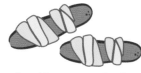 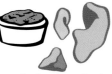

Dill pickles wrapped in ham

Handful of olives

Pork clouds and salsa

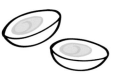 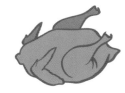 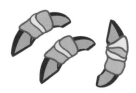

Hard-boiled eggs
(you can even purchase
them premade and peeled)

Organic rotisserie chicken

Turkey-wrapped
avocado slices

 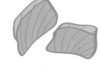

Gluten-free jerky or
beef sticks

Smoked salmon or marlin

Packet of tuna or salmon
with keto mustard or mayo
(Primal Kitchen is a good brand)

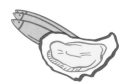

Canned anchovies, sardines,
or smoked oysters

Precooked shrimp cocktail

Canned crabmeat in lettuce
wraps, topped with mayo

Dinner in 10

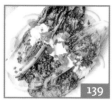
BLT Grilled Romaine

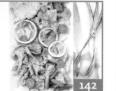
Chef's Salad

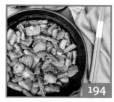
Tender
Chicken Livers

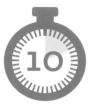

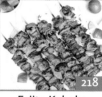
Easy Chicken and
Asparagus Stir-Fry

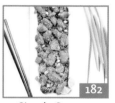
Simple Sesame
Chicken

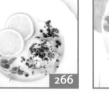
Spanish Spiced
Lamb Chops

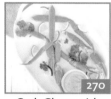
Saucy BBQ Wraps

Fajita Kabobs

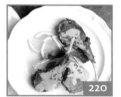
Simple Lamb Chops with
Lemon Mustard Gravy

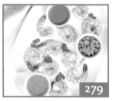
Cowboy Steak
for Two

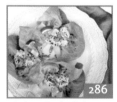
Pan-Fried Fish with
Tartar Sauce

Crab Claws with
Spicy Mustard Sauce

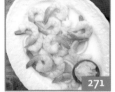
Easy Pickled Shrimp
with Curry Mayo

Ahi Poke

Garlic Lime
Broiled Shrimp

Asian-Style Salmon
Lettuce Cups

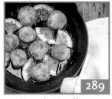
Simple Scallops
in Garlic Sauce

4 Fabulous Desserts in 6 Minutes

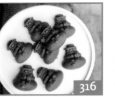

316

Grand Marnier
Chocolate Candies

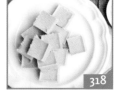

318

Snickerdoodle Bites

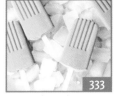

333

Chocolate
Pudding Pops

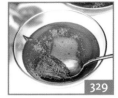

329

Mexican
Chocolate Mousse

Single-Serving Meals

Are you looking for simple meals for one? Although I suggest making large batches, you can store extra servings in individual portions in the refrigerator or freezer for easy lunches and dinners. You can also try these scrumptious recipes that serve one person:

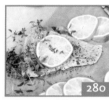

280

Personal Salmon
en Papillote

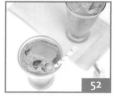

52

Iced Green Tea
Latte

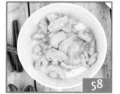

58

French Toast Cereal

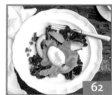

62

Smoked Salmon,
Egg, and Avocado

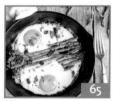

65

Breakfast Asparagus

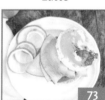

73

Easy Breakfast
Sandwich

Top Ten Tips for Success on a Ketogenic Diet

1. Plan Ahead

As discussed in the previous section, meal planning is the number-one key to success. Always having easy meal options at the ready is how I avoid overeating or eating the wrong kinds of food. Preparing meals in advance or batch cooking and freezing means that I have lots of delicious homemade meals to choose from.

2. Add More Flavor to Your Meals

Do not skimp on seasoning! Most people use too little seasoning because we have been pressured to reduce our intake of salt. But salt is not the evil nutrient we have been taught to fear, and on a ketogenic diet, you need more of it. Adding some textured salt, fresh herbs, or a little acid at the end of cooking can boost flavor. A hit of lime juice at the end of cooking really steps up the taste of a dish. And although it may smell funky, fish sauce, with its umami flavor, can make everything from chicken to beef to fish taste extra-special.

3. Make Conscious Choices

If you are wishy-washy and unsure, you are likely going to cheat. Make good, thoughtful choices. I'm a stubborn German. When I decided to change my lifestyle with eating and exercise, I stuck with it even when I didn't want to. I used my stubbornness, which is often thought of as a bad trait, for good.

4. Keep a Food Journal

If you don't prepare your meals for the week ahead of time, try writing down what you are going to eat the next day and preparing those foods in advance. Or, if you are a visual person like me, take pictures of your food. Better yet, find a keto buddy who can help you stay accountable and send your buddy photos of what you're eating.

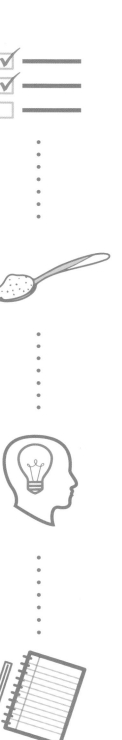

5. Let Cooking Be Your Therapy After a Stressful Day

Cooking is very therapeutic. It also can be a great time to bond with your children and other family members. Try turning on some relaxing music or choose music based on what you're cooking for dinner.

6. Eat Before Social Events

There were times in the past when I wouldn't remember what I ate because I had chatted away at an event. Eating at home before the event means that you can walk away from the buffet table to focus on quality conversation. Since you won't be hungry, you won't be tempted by unhealthy choices. But if you think you'll be tempted by the dessert table, try keeping a stash of treats in your freezer like I do. That way, I know I can enjoy a tasty keto dessert at home later, which helps me not reach for sugary treats when I'm away from home. See page 20 for a list of desserts that can be prepared in 6 minutes or less.

7. Bring a Dish to Pass at a Social Gathering

As a host, I always appreciate it when people bring food, but I don't assume that there will be keto-friendly options at every social event or potluck I attend. Below is a list of fast and easy appetizers to take with you to a party.

6 Scrumptious Appetizers in 6 Minutes

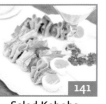

Salad Kabobs
141

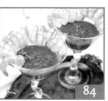

Spicy
Shrimp Cocktail
84

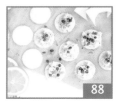

Tuna Salad
Crostini
88

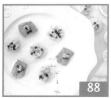

Smoked Salmon
Crostini
88

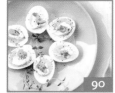

Almost Deviled Eggs
90

Amazing
Marinated Olives
92

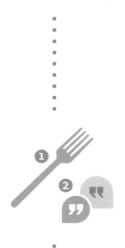

8. Limit the Food Options on Your Plate

Our brains get bored of the same flavors, but if you have a lot of different flavors on your plate, it is easy to overeat. We experience something called "habituation" to the smell and taste of food as we eat, in which our sensory neurons become less receptive with constant exposure to a stimulus. This is why we overeat at a potluck or buffet—lots of choices keep stimulating the senses. But if you have one food on your plate or limit your choices during a meal, your brain will get bored and send a signal to stop eating. So don't fill your plate with three or four options; stick to one or two, or a main dish and a side.

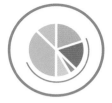

9. Get Enough Sleep

I know this advice sounds simple, but it really isn't. With work, family, and leisure activities, sleep is often the first thing we cut back on. How does a lack of sleep interfere with a ketogenic diet? It has to do with the cravings for sugar and carbohydrates that occur in the wake of sleep deprivation, which can tempt you to stray from the keto way of eating. And you can become so tired that the last thing you want to do is cook.

10. Avoid Eating During Stressful Events

Do you find that you sometimes get indigestion or diarrhea after eating in a stressful situation? While under stress, your heart rate goes up, your blood pressure rises, and blood is forced away from your digestive system and moved to your head for quick thinking and to your arms and legs in preparation for a fight-or-flight response. There can be as much as four times less blood flowing to your digestive system, which means that your body cannot burn calories as effectively, and that causes a sluggish metabolism.

The issue with eating while you are under stress is that even if you are eating the most nutritious food in the world, your body won't be able to break down and absorb those nutrients properly because there is a decreased enzymatic output in your intestines (which can be as much as 20,000-fold). You're also more susceptible to acid reflux or heartburn.

My suggestion is to avoid eating during meetings at work and to enjoy a peaceful little break for lunch instead. Also, try not to eat while stressed after an argument. Instead, do some yoga; the blood is flowing to your extremities anyway!

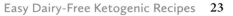

My Top Ten Keto Kitchen Tools

If it were up to my husband, we would have every gadget there is, but I enjoy simplicity and do not like clutter. You can make a small investment in a few items, and you'll save time and money in the long run. Here are my top choices.

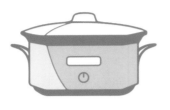

Slow Cooker

What it's useful for: Making meals while you're away from home. If you don't have a lot of time to cook, this is a great tool that can be used daily.

What to look for: 5- or 6-quart capacity with a removable insert

Price: $20–$180

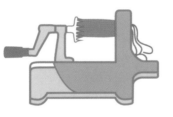

Spiral Slicer

What it's useful for: Making zucchini and broccoli noodles

What to look for: A quality spiral slicer that will stay in place as you use it; I like the Joyce Chen Saladacco model

Price: Under $20

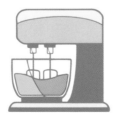

Stand Mixer

What it's useful for: Whipping egg whites, making cheesecakes and other baked goods

What to look for: Buy the best-quality mixer you can afford, preferably one for which you can purchase optional attachments

Price: $150–$500

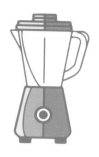

High-Quality Blender

What it's useful for: Making smoothies, salad dressings, and dips

What to look for: A high-speed blender such as Blendtec or Vitamix

Price: $150–$700

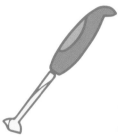

Immersion Blender

What it's useful for: Making shakes and mayonnaise (pages 34 and 35), pureeing soups

What to look for: A small handheld blender that takes up minimal storage space

Price: Under $30

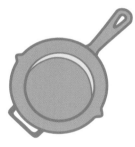

Large Cast-Iron Skillet

What it's useful for: Frying eggs and other foods, stovetop-to-oven preparations

What to look for: At least a 10-inch skillet with a high rim for deep frying; preseasoned skillets are more expensive, but you might be able to find a used cast-iron skillet at a thrift store

Price: Under $20

Quality Knife

What it's useful for: Chopping vegetables and herbs, slicing meats and bread

What to look for: A good sharp knife with a comfortable handle

Price: $100–$300

Ice Cream Maker

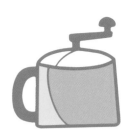

What it's useful for: Making dairy-free ice creams, sherbets, and sorbets

What to look for: I prefer a model that has a churning bucket that can be stored in the freezer; I make keto ice cream treats weekly, so I love that I can store the bucket in the freezer so it's frozen when I need it

Price: $45–$100

Toaster Oven

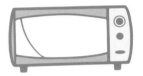

What it's useful for: Reheating leftovers, cooking single-serving recipes, and keeping the kitchen cool in summer, when you don't want to turn on the oven

What to look for: A quality toaster oven that goes up to at least 400°F

Price: $25 and up

Radio/Music

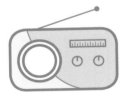

What it's useful for: Making your time in the kitchen fun!

What to look for: Don't wait until the holiday season to play music while you cook. Let your meals determine your music selections; try cooking to Italian opera, reggae, or ranchera. Turn on your favorite local or online radio station or listen to music from your own collection.

Price: Free

A Few Optional Items

Smoker

What it's useful for: Smoking ribs, salmon, and even cauliflower steaks

What to look for: A heavy-gauge model with a thermostat. This is the best cooking vessel we own!

Price: $100–$150

Whipped Cream Canister

What it's useful for: Making frozen fat bombs, whipping coconut cream as a garnish for dairy-free keto desserts

What to look for: I prefer a canister with a handheld pump, such as the one sold by Pampered Chef; they make a safe canister that doesn't have too much pressure that could harm you.

Price: $20–$99

Baking Stone

What it's useful for: Making pizza and cookies

What to look for: A large rectangular baking stone will give you more options than a round stone. Be sure to preheat the stone in the oven, which will create a nice crispy crust, and use a piece of unbleached parchment so grease does not seep into the stone. This will also prevent smoke from filling your kitchen due to heating the grease in the stone.

Price: $10–$40

Multi-Cooker

What it's useful for: Pressure cooking, slow cooking, steaming, and sautéing; some models have additional functions, such as yogurt making

What to look for: A programmable or Bluetooth model. The Instant Pot is a popular brand of multi-cooker.

Price: $80–$160

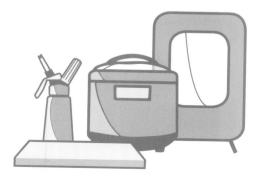

Using the Recipes in This Book

This book's nearly 200 delicious dairy-free keto recipes include some handy features to help you along on your keto journey.

Icons

I've marked the recipes with a number of icons, as applicable. First, there are icons highlighting those recipes that are free of nuts and/or eggs, which are problematic for some people:

If a recipe isn't free of a particular allergen but a substitution or an omission will make it free of that allergen, you will see the word OPTION below the icon, like this:

OPTION   OPTION

Nutritional Information

I've also included nutritional information for each recipe, listing the total calories along with the fat, protein, carbohydrate, and fiber counts in grams, along with keto ratings of low, medium, or high. You'll find this information helpful as you fine-tune your personal targets for these macronutrients.

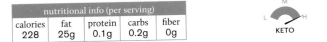

nutritional info (per serving)				
calories	fat	protein	carbs	fiber
228	25g	0.1g	0.2g	0g

When it comes to ingredients, I give the easiest option first because I want to make the ketogenic lifestyle approachable even for novice cooks. Some of the simpler ingredients may not be ideal (boxed broth versus homemade bone broth, for example), but if those ingredients help people start to enjoy cooking, I am happy that they are trying and I do not judge. If you are a more advanced cook, you are welcome and encouraged to use the more advanced ingredients.

The following is a list of my favorite "shortcut" keto products. Even those of us who love to cook need to rely on shortcuts once in a while!

If you are a visual learner like me or you want more information, I offer many Skype and online video classes at MariaMindBodyHealth.com/video-classes/

Top Ten Food Products That Make My Life Easier

1. Primal Kitchen brand mayonnaise and salad dressings
2. Organic rotisserie chickens from Whole Foods
3. Kettle & Fire brand bone broth
4. Grass-fed beef delivery from ButcherBox
5. Simple Girl sauces (use stevia to sweeten)
6. Pork rinds
7. Quality seafood delivery from Sizzlefish
8. Ketoned Bodies frozen keto meals
9. Maria's Keto Kitchen Spices
10. Everly Drink Mix

In Conclusion

With all this information in hand, I wish you luck on your keto journey. I know that this lifestyle can seem overwhelming, but try one new thing each week; this week maybe change your breakfast from cereal to eggs, and next week start walking after dinner. Baby steps are what worked for me. Instead of feeling overwhelmed, feel empowered by having the tools you need for success. Move away from deprivation diets that are centered around fat-free, man-made foods; a ketogenic diet means real food, real satisfaction, and a healthy metabolism. Here's to happy and healthy dairy-free cooking and eating!

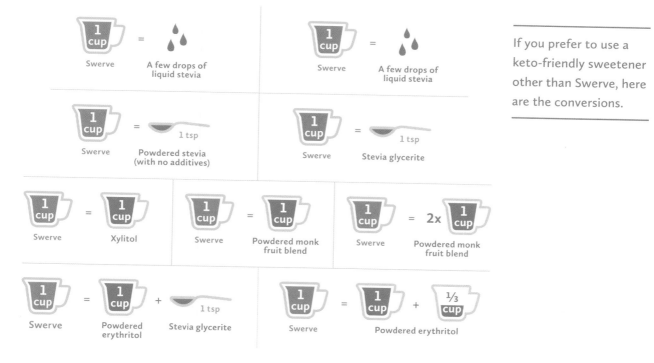

If you prefer to use a keto-friendly sweetener other than Swerve, here are the conversions.

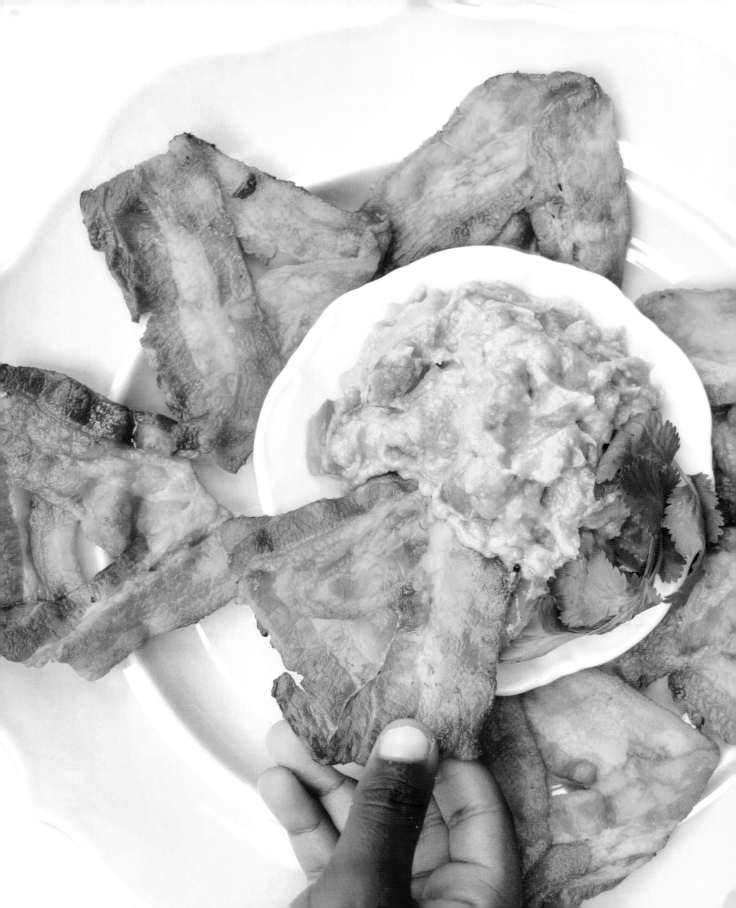

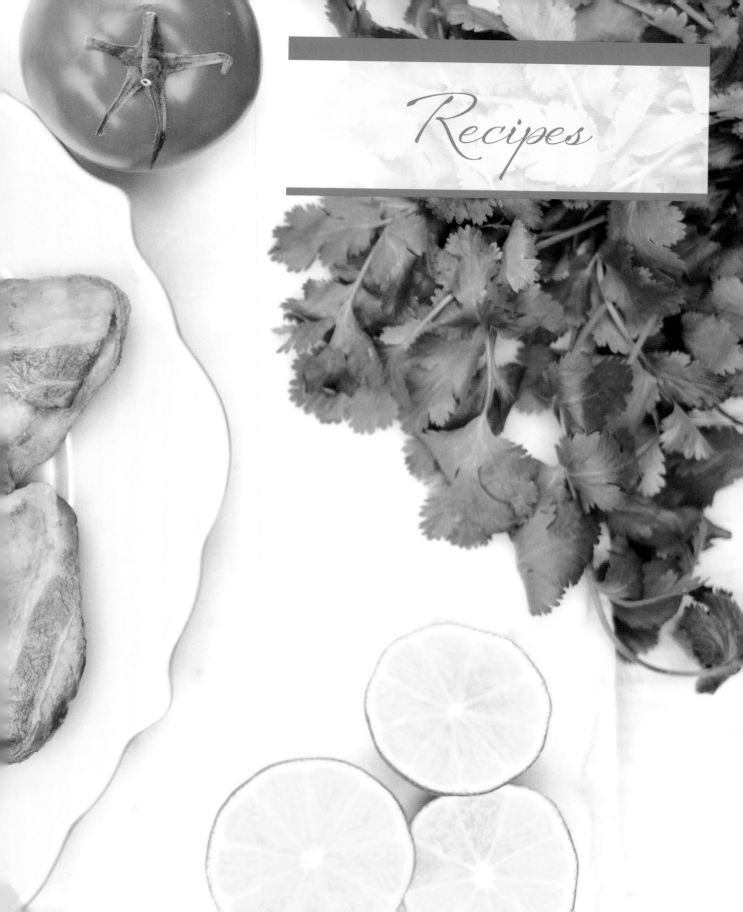

Recipes

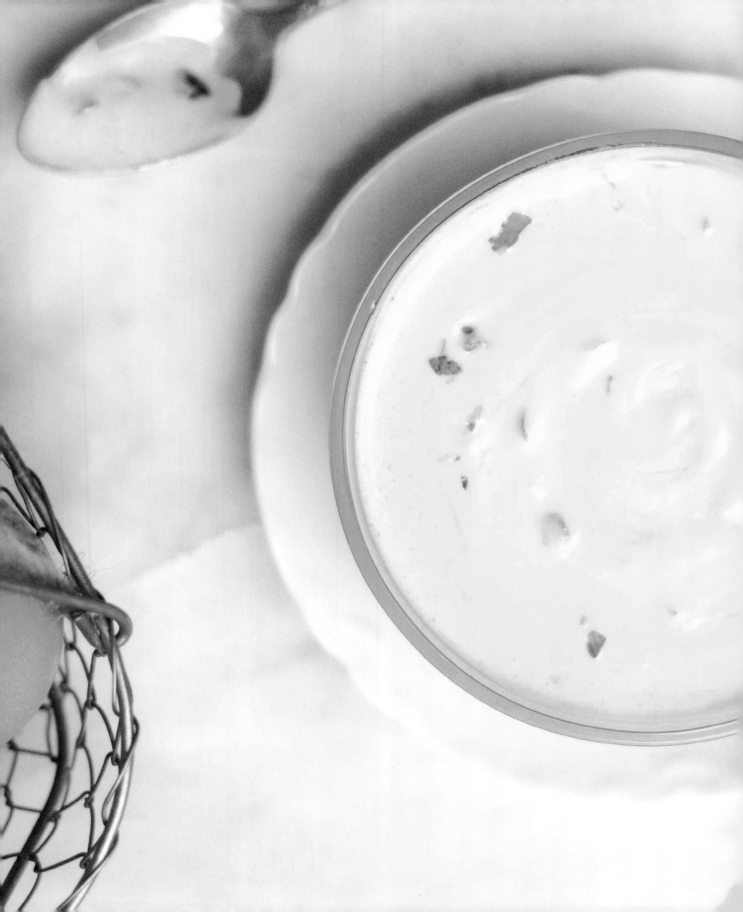

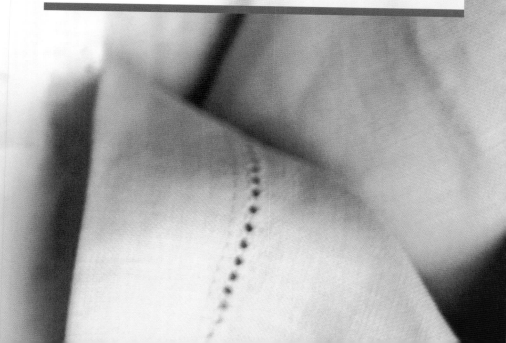

Chapter 1:
Basics

MAYONNAISE

KETO   OPTION

Homemade mayonnaise is so much tastier and healthier than store-bought! You can also use this recipe to make Baconnaise by simply swapping out the oil for bacon fat.

prep time: 5 minutes *yield:* 1½ cups (about 1 tablespoon per serving)

2 large egg yolks

2 teaspoons lemon juice

1 cup MCT oil or other neutral-flavored oil, such as macadamia nut oil or avocado oil

1 tablespoon Dijon mustard

½ teaspoon fine sea salt

Special Equipment:

Immersion blender

1. Put the ingredients in the order listed in a wide-mouth pint-sized jar. Place an immersion blender at the bottom of the jar. Turn the blender on and very slowly move it to the top of the jar. Be patient! It should take you about a minute to reach the top. Moving the blender slowly is the key to getting the mayonnaise to emulsify.

2. Store in a jar in the refrigerator for up to 5 days.

Note: **To make this mayo nut-free, don't use a nut-based oil.**

Variation: *Baconnaise. Replace the MCT oil with melted, but not hot, bacon fat. Taste and add salt, if needed. (It may be salty enough from the bacon fat.)*

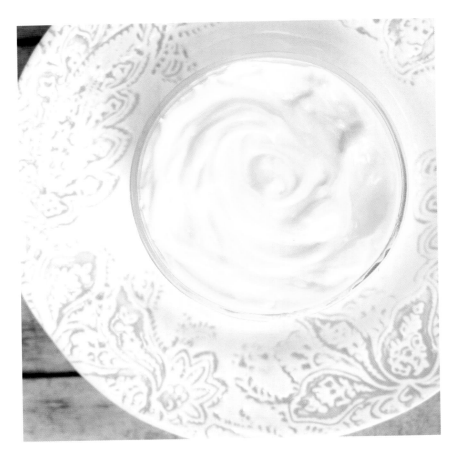

nutritional info (per serving of mayonnaise)				
calories	fat	protein	carbs	fiber
92	10g	0.3g	0.1g	0g

nutritional info (per serving of baconnaise)				
calories	fat	protein	carbs	fiber
123	13g	0.3g	0.2g	0g

EGG-FREE MAYO

3 tablespoons lemon juice

2 tablespoons coconut vinegar or apple cider vinegar

1 tablespoon Swerve confectioners'-style sweetener or equivalent amount of liquid or powdered sweetener (see page 29)

1½ teaspoons Dijon mustard

1¼ teaspoons fine sea salt

½ cup extra-virgin olive oil

½ cup expeller-pressed coconut oil, softened but not melted (see Note)

1. Place the lemon juice, vinegar, sweetener, mustard, and salt in a blender or food processor and blend to combine well.

2. Turn the blender to low speed and slowly drizzle in the olive oil drop by drop at first; once ¼ cup of the oil has been incorporated, you can increase the rate of the drizzle. Add the softened coconut oil to the blender and puree just until combined. Place in a jar that has a lid.

3. Store in an airtight container in the refrigerator for up to a week.

Note: *Expeller-pressed coconut oil has the least coconut-y taste of all the coconut oils, so it's a good choice when you want a more neutral flavor, as you do here. If you'd like an even more neutral taste, palm oil is a good alternative.*

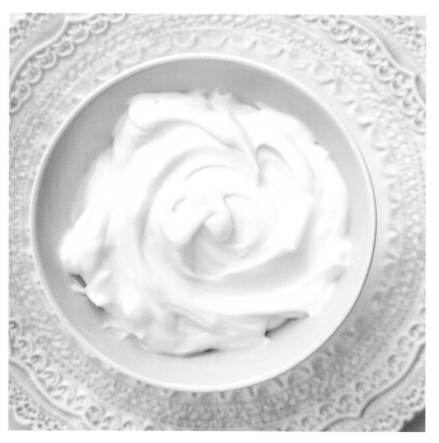

nutritional info (per serving)				
calories	fat	protein	carbs	fiber
228	25g	0.1g	0.2g	0g

STEAK SAUCE

prep time: 3 minutes yield: 1½ cups (2 tablespoons per serving)

1 cup tomato sauce

2 to 3 tablespoons Swerve confectioners'-style sweetener or equivalent amount of liquid or powdered sweetener (see page 29)

2 tablespoons prepared yellow mustard

1½ tablespoons apple cider vinegar

1½ teaspoons wheat-free tamari, or 2 tablespoons coconut aminos

¼ teaspoon fish sauce (optional)

2 drops Tabasco sauce

¼ teaspoon fine sea salt

¼ teaspoon ground black pepper

Place all of the ingredients in a small bowl and stir well to combine. Taste and adjust the seasoning and sweetness to your liking. Store in an airtight container in the refrigerator for up to a week.

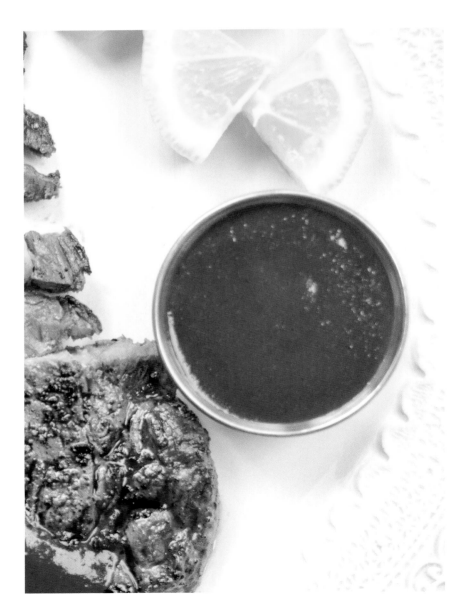

nutritional info (per serving)				
calories	fat	protein	carbs	fiber
11	0.2g	0.2g	2g	1g

COMEBACK SAUCE

Comeback sauce is a classic in Mississippi. The name literally means that the sauce is so good, you will come back for more! It tastes great on greens, coleslaw, or anything fried. In the South, they use chili sauce in this sauce, but since chili sauce often contains corn syrup, I use chili powder instead. Serve this sauce with Lemon Pepper Chicken Tenders (page 176) or Tender Chicken Livers (page 188).

prep time: **4 minutes** *yield:* **1½ cups (2 tablespoons per serving)**

1 cup mayonnaise, homemade (page 34 or 35) or store-bought, or Baconnaise (page 34)

¼ cup tomato sauce

¼ cup Swerve confectioners'-style sweetener or equivalent amount of liquid or powdered sweetener (see page 29)

1 tablespoon lemon juice

1 teaspoon Frank's RedHot sauce (more or less depending on how hot you like it)

½ teaspoon wheat-free tamari, or 2 teaspoons coconut aminos

1 teaspoon smoked paprika

½ teaspoon fine sea salt

½ teaspoon chili powder

½ teaspoon garlic powder

½ teaspoon onion powder

¼ teaspoon ground allspice

¼ teaspoon ground black pepper

Place all of the ingredients in a small bowl and stir until well combined. Store in an airtight container in the refrigerator for up to 5 days.

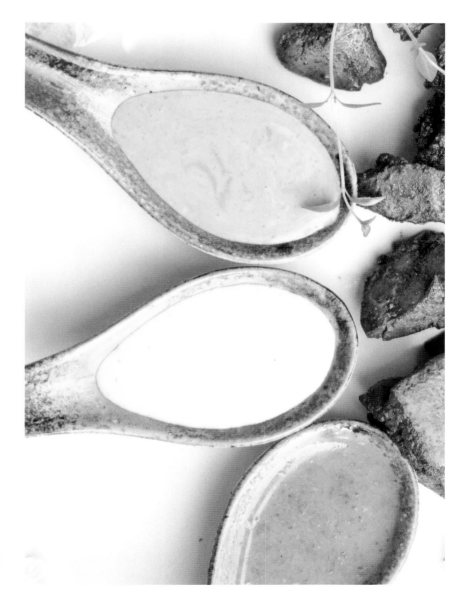

nutritional info (per serving)				
calories	fat	protein	carbs	fiber
124	13g	0.1g	1g	0.3g

CREAMY LIME SAUCE

½ cup mayonnaise, homemade (page 34 or 35) or store-bought

2 tablespoons lime juice

1 tablespoon paprika

1 clove garlic, smashed to a paste

Fine sea salt, to taste

Place all of the ingredients in a small bowl and stir well to combine. Taste and adjust the seasoning to your liking. Store in an airtight container in the refrigerator for up to 5 days.

Note: *This sauce tastes great on fish.*

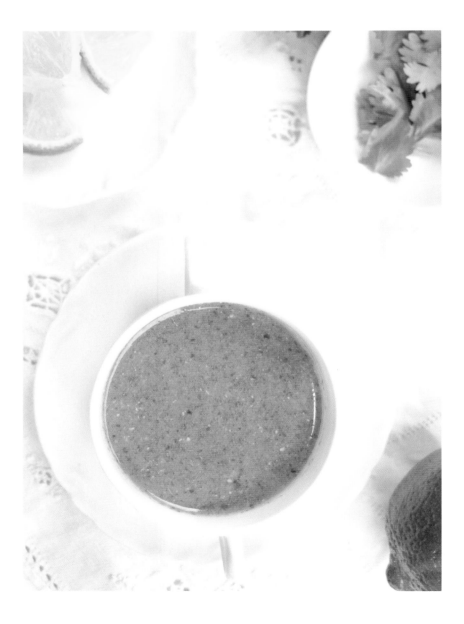

nutritional info (per serving)				
calories	fat	protein	carbs	fiber
138	15g	0.1g	1g	0g

CILANTRO LIME DRESSING

prep time: 3 minutes *yield:* 1½ cups (2 tablespoons per serving)

1 cup chopped fresh cilantro

3 tablespoons lime juice

3 tablespoons avocado oil or extra-virgin olive oil

2 cloves garlic, smashed, or 1 clove pressed from a head of roasted garlic

⅛ teaspoon fine sea salt

Place all of the ingredients in a small food processor and puree until smooth. Taste and adjust the seasoning to your liking. Store in an airtight container in the refrigerator for up to 5 days.

Note: *This sauce pairs well with Garlic Lime Broiled Shrimp (page 279).*

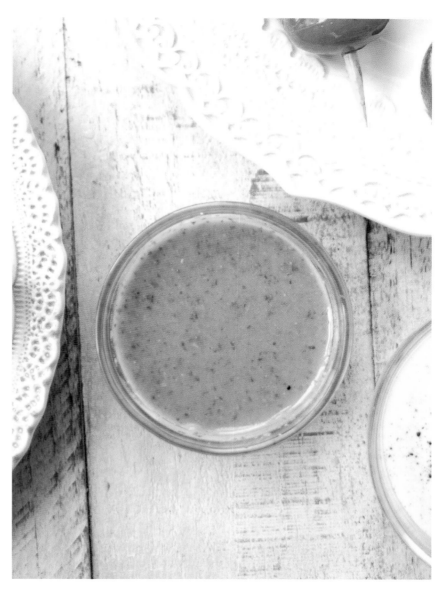

nutritional info (per serving)				
calories	fat	protein	carbs	fiber
8	1g	0.2g	1g	0.3g

TARTAR SAUCE

prep. time: **3 minutes** *yield:* **1½ cups (3 tablespoons per serving)**

1 cup mayonnaise, homemade (page 34 or 35) or store-bought

¼ cup diced dill pickles

¼ cup dill pickle juice

2 tablespoons Swerve confectioners'-style sweetener or equivalent amount of liquid or powdered sweetener (see page 29) (optional)

Pinch of fine sea salt

Place all of the ingredients in a small bowl and stir well to combine. Taste and adjust the sweetness and salt to your liking. Store in an air-tight container in the refrigerator for up to 5 days.

Tip: *Serve with Bacon-Wrapped Cod (page 272) or Salt-Crusted Fish (page 282).*

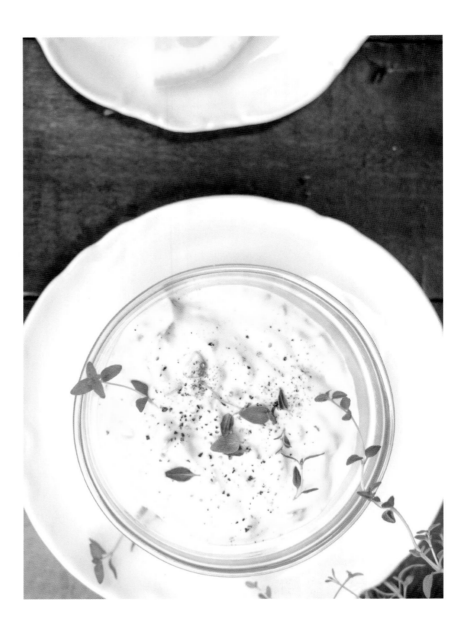

nutritional info (per serving)				
calories	fat	protein	carbs	fiber
180	20g	0g	0g	0g

BÉARNAISE SAUCE

I am a sauce lover. That is almost an understatement. In my former life, I would dredge my steaks in ketchup or steak sauce, but there is a ton of sugar in those common staples. I still need my sauces, though, so now I make my own. Use this as a dipping sauce for Herby Broth Fondue (page 210) or on a juicy steak; it tastes amazing that way!

prep time: 5 minutes *cook time:* 15 minutes
yield: 1 cup (about 3 tablespoons per serving)

¼ cup lard or butter-flavored coconut oil

2 tablespoons chopped fresh tarragon leaves

1 shallot, minced

2 tablespoons coconut vinegar or white wine vinegar

6 large egg yolks

Fine sea salt

1. Melt the lard in a medium-sized saucepan over medium heat. Add the tarragon, shallot, and vinegar and simmer for 15 minutes. Remove the pan from the heat and allow the mixture to cool a bit.

2. Place the egg yolks in a blender and turn it to low speed. Slowly pour in the warm (not hot) lard mixture in a very slow, steady stream while the blender is running. If you add it too fast, the sauce will break. Taste the sauce and add salt to your liking. Set aside at the back of the stove or in another warm spot to keep warm until ready to serve.

3. Store in an airtight container in the refrigerator for up to 3 days. Reheat gently in a double boiler so the sauce doesn't separate.

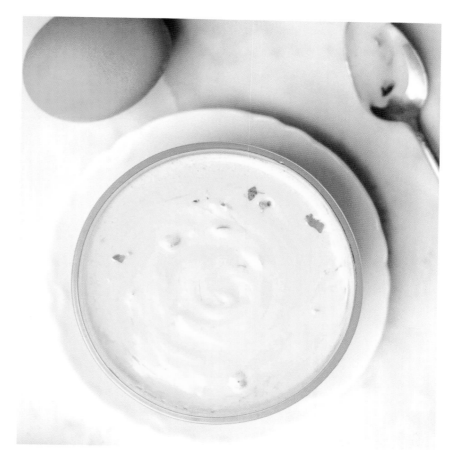

nutritional info (per serving)				
calories	fat	protein	carbs	fiber
152	14g	4g	2g	0.1g

ROMANESCO SAUCE

I love this sauce with steak (see page 206) or as a dipping sauce for fondue (see page 210). But the ways to use it are nearly limitless—try it drizzled over scrambled or fried eggs or slathered on grilled chicken or fish.

prep time: **5 minutes** *yield:* **1 cup (¼ cup per serving)**

½ (12-ounce) jar roasted red peppers, drained (about ½ cup)

½ cup Kite Hill brand cream cheese style spread

2 tablespoons chopped fresh basil leaves, or 1½ teaspoons dried basil

2 cloves garlic, chopped

½ teaspoon fine sea salt

Place all of the ingredients in a blender or food processor and pulse until smooth. Adjust the seasoning to your liking. Refrigerate the sauce until you're ready to use it; it will keep for up to 5 days.

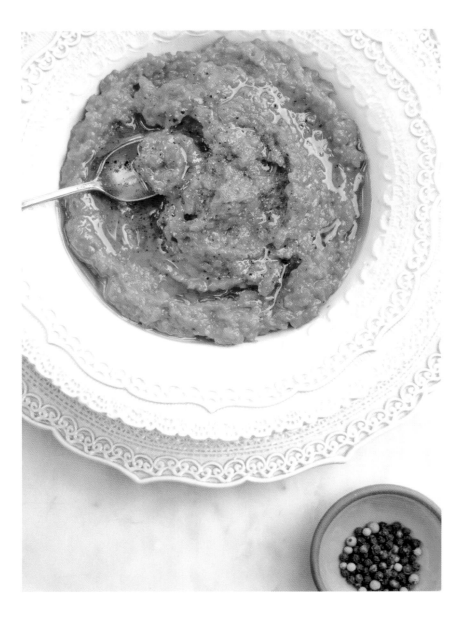

nutritional info (per serving)				
calories	fat	protein	carbs	fiber
70	5g	1g	3g	1g

SIMPLE BBQ SAUCE

prep time: **2 minutes** *yield:* **2 cups (2 tablespoons per serving)**

1½ cups tomato sauce

½ cup beef or chicken bone broth, homemade (page 106) or store-bought

1 tablespoon Swerve confectioners'-style sweetener or equivalent amount of liquid or powdered sweetener (see page 29), or more to taste

1 teaspoon liquid smoke

1 teaspoon garlic powder

1 teaspoon onion powder

¼ teaspoon fine sea salt

Place all of the ingredients in a medium-sized bowl and stir well to combine. Taste and adjust the sweetness and seasoning to your liking. Store in an airtight container in the refrigerator for up to 2 weeks.

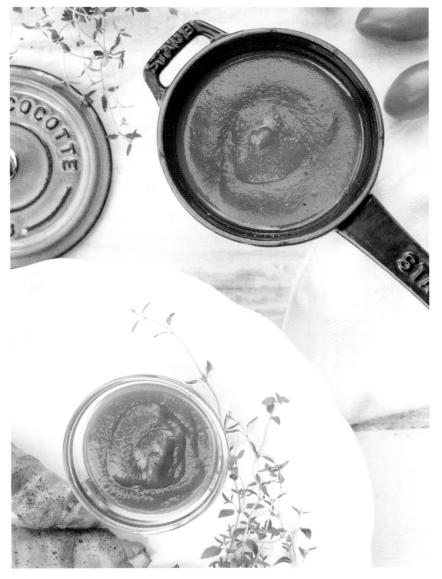

nutritional info (per serving)				
calories	fat	protein	carbs	fiber
7	0.2g	0.2g	1g	0.2g

CRAB LOUIE DRESSING

2 cups mayonnaise, homemade
(page 34 or 35) or store-bought

1 cup tomato sauce

½ cup finely diced dill pickles

3 tablespoons dill pickle juice
(from the jar of pickles)

Place all of the ingredients in a medium-sized bowl and stir to combine.
Store in an airtight container in the refrigerator for up to 5 days.

Note: *Crab Louie dressing is often made with sweet pickle relish. If you'd
like to add some sweetness, feel free to add ⅛ teaspoon of stevia glycerite
or a pinch of Swerve confectioners'-style sweetener.*

Tip: *This dressing is the classic choice for Crab Louie Salad (page 140),
but it also tastes great drizzled over grilled seafood or chicken.*

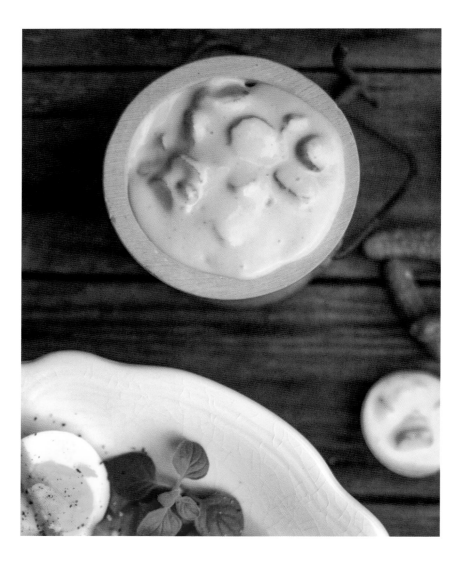

nutritional info (per serving)				
calories	fat	protein	carbs	fiber
184	20g	0.1g	1g	0.1g

CREAMY RANCH DRESSING

prep time: 5 minutes, plus 2 hours to chill

yield: 1½ cups (2 tablespoons per serving or 12 servings)

1 cup mayonnaise, homemade (page 34 or 35) or store-bought

½ cup chicken or beef bone broth, homemade (page 106) or store-bought

½ teaspoon dried chives

½ teaspoon dried dill weed

½ teaspoon dried parsley

¼ teaspoon garlic powder

¼ teaspoon onion powder

⅛ teaspoon fine sea salt

⅛ teaspoon ground black pepper

Place all of the ingredients in a blender or large bowl and pulse or stir to combine. Cover and refrigerate for 2 hours before serving. Store in an airtight container in the refrigerator for up to 2 weeks.

Busy Family Tip: *For an even easier way to make this dressing, try my ranch seasoning mix. All you have to do is add mayo and broth to the spice mix and you're done!*

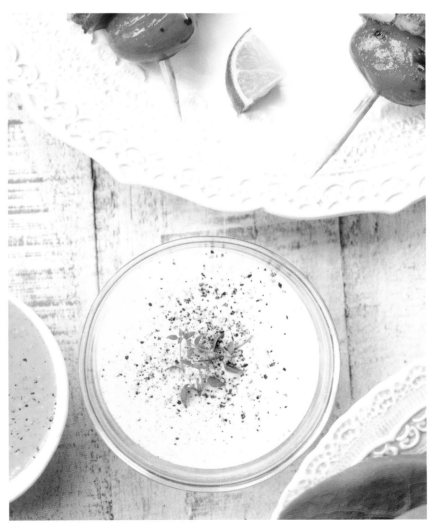

nutritional info (per serving)				
calories	fat	protein	carbs	fiber
66	7g	0.2g	0.1g	0g

GREEK VINAIGRETTE

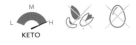

prep time: **4 minutes**   *yield:* **1 cup (2 tablespoons per serving)**

½ cup avocado oil or extra-virgin olive oil

5 tablespoons red wine vinegar or apple cider vinegar

2 tablespoons lime or lemon juice

2 teaspoons chopped garlic

2 teaspoons Dijon mustard

½ teaspoon dried basil leaves

½ teaspoon dried oregano leaves

¼ teaspoon fine sea salt

Place all of the ingredients in a blender and puree until smooth. Store in an airtight container in the refrigerator for up to 2 weeks.

Tip: *Serve with Greek Chicken Thighs (page 186) or Lamb Chops with Gyro Salad (page 228).*

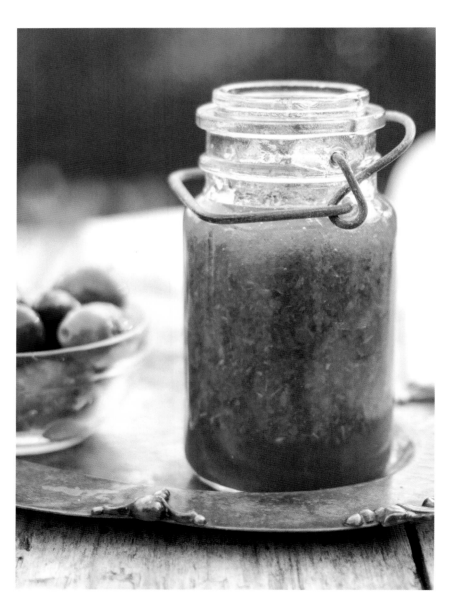

nutritional info (per serving)				
calories	fat	protein	carbs	fiber
126	14g	0g	1g	0g

CINNAMON SYRUP

prep time: **3 minutes**   cook time: **2 minutes**
yield: **¾ cup (2 tablespoons per serving)**

½ cup coconut oil

¼ cup Swerve confectioners'-style sweetener or equivalent amount of liquid or powdered sweetener (see page 29)

1 to 2 teaspoons ground cinnamon, to taste

1 teaspoon maple or vanilla extract

Pinch of fine sea salt

Tip: *This syrup is great over Super Keto Pancakes (page 79).*

1. Place all of the ingredients in a saucepan, starting with 1 teaspoon of cinnamon, and heat over medium heat until the coconut oil is melted (or place in a microwave-safe bowl and microwave for 30 seconds or until completely melted). Stir well and taste; add up to 1 teaspoon more cinnamon, if desired.

2. Store in an airtight container in the refrigerator for up to 2 weeks. If the syrup hardens, reheat until liquefied.

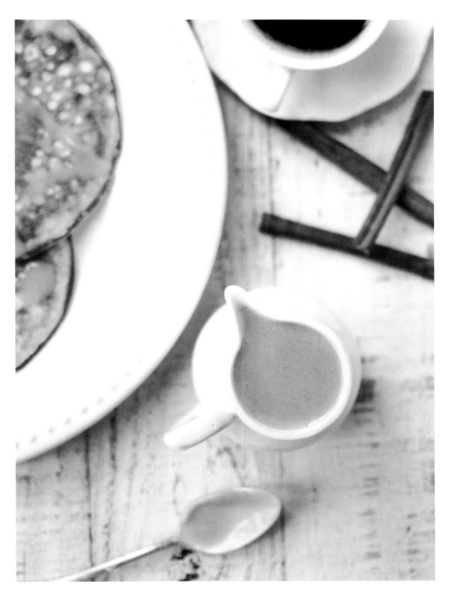

nutritional info (per serving)				
calories	fat	protein	carbs	fiber
156	18g	0g	1g	0.4g

LEMON SYRUP

KETO

prep time: **5 minutes**   *cook time:* **2 minutes**   *yield:* **1 cup (2 tablespoons per serving)**

½ cup coconut oil

¼ cup Swerve confectioners'-style sweetener or equivalent amount of liquid or powdered sweetener (see page 29)

3 tablespoons lemon juice

1 teaspoon lemon extract, or 7 drops lemon oil

⅛ teaspoon fine sea salt

1. Place all of the ingredients in a saucepan and heat over medium heat until the coconut oil is melted (or place in a microwave-safe bowl and heat in the microwave for 30 seconds or until completely melted). Stir well and use over waffles or pancakes. If the syrup hardens, reheat until liquefied.

2. Store in an airtight container in the refrigerator for up to 2 weeks.

nutritional info (per serving)				
calories	fat	protein	carbs	fiber
116	14g	0g	0.4g	0g

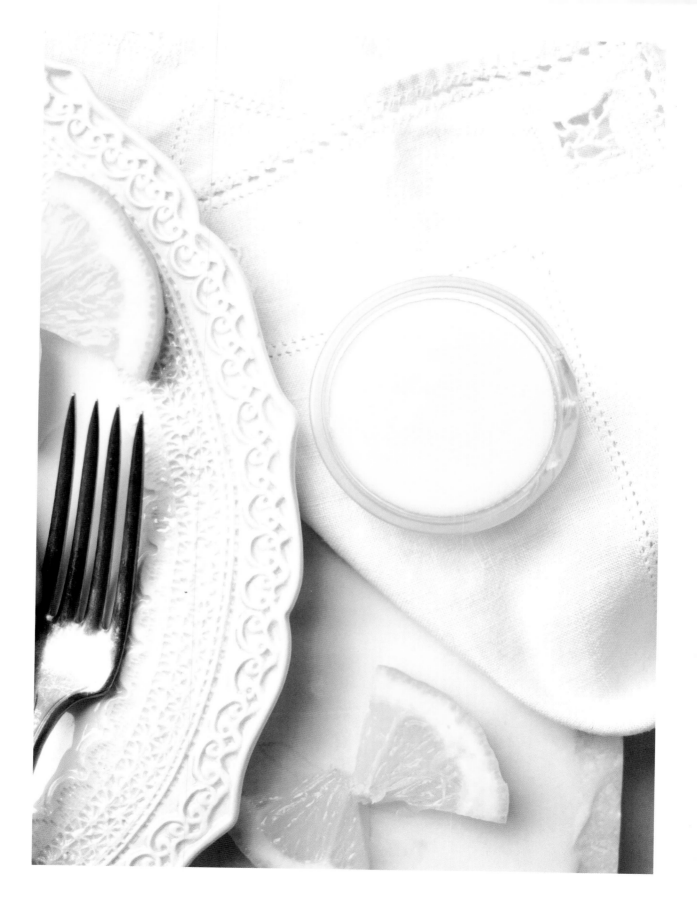

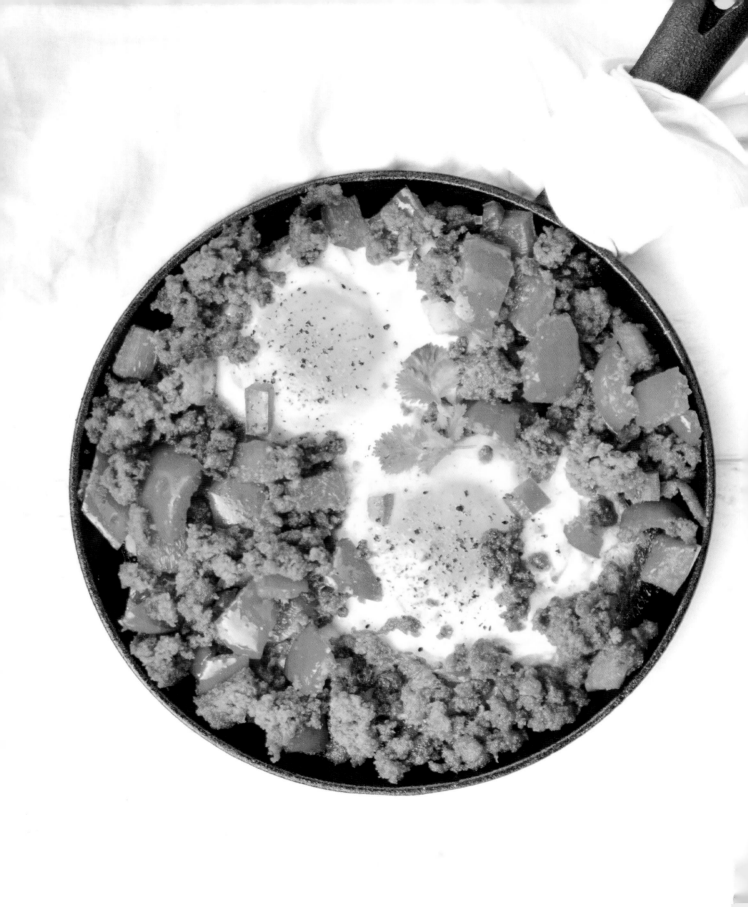

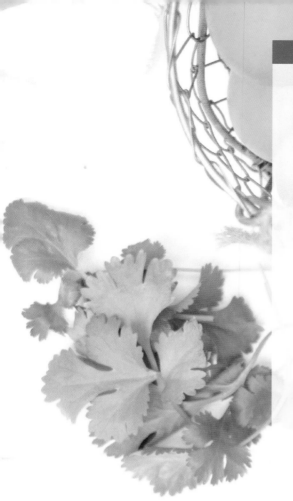

Chapter 2:
Break-Your-Fast

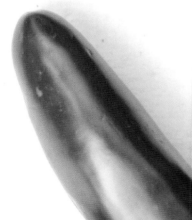

ICED GREEN TEA LATTE

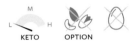

KETO   OPTION

I have a client who told me that her downfall was a Starbucks green tea latte with skim milk. After we broke down how much sugar and calories she would eliminate if she made my version instead, she was sold! Not to mention that she saved a lot of money and time by making her drinks at home.

prep time: **3 minutes**   *yield:* **1 serving**

½ cup hot (not boiling) water

1 tablespoon matcha powder

8 ounces cold unsweetened cashew milk (or hemp milk if nut-free)

2 teaspoons Swerve confectioners'-style sweetener or equivalent amount of liquid or powdered sweetener (see page 29), or 5 drops vanilla-flavored liquid stevia

Ice

Place the hot water and matcha powder in a blender and pulse until smooth. Add the milk and sweetener and blend well. Pour into a glass over ice. This latte is best served fresh.

nutritional info (per serving)				
calories	fat	protein	carbs	fiber
38	1g	1g	7g	0g

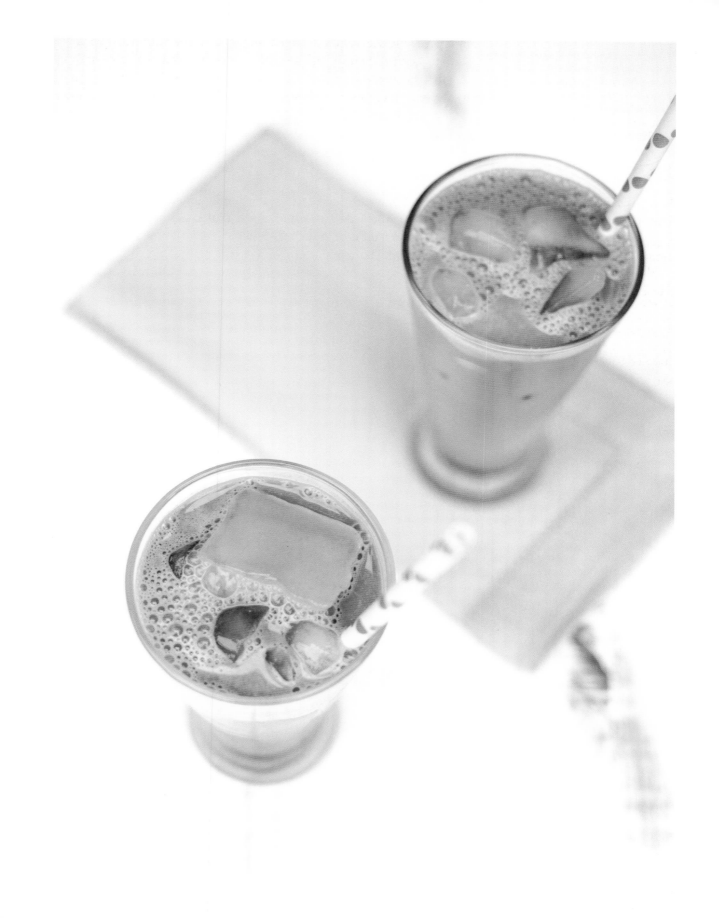

CHERRY ALMOND BREAKFAST SHAKE

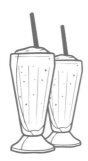

This shake includes a pinch of salt, which may seem odd since salt is probably the last thing that comes to mind when you think of sweets (unless you once accidentally used salt in place of sugar!). As contradictory as it may sound, salt truly changes a sweet recipe from tasty to jaw-dropping and can make your treats taste sweeter. It adds complexity to the entire dish by balancing and elevating flavors and conveying tones that you didn't even know were in the dish. For example, salt makes spices more fragrant and citrus more vibrant.

The major offense would be to use iodized table salt. First, sugar is often added to table salt as a binding agent. Second, you want the salt to complement the components in the dish instead of making it taste chemically, which table salt can do. For this shake, I suggest using a salt that dissolves well, such as very finely ground sea salt or flaked sea salt.

Many pastry chefs say that you should double the salt in any classic dessert recipe and cut back on the sugar. The takeaway here is that salt is a flavor enhancer, not a flavor replacer. Even fast-food restaurants understand this! A small milkshake has more sodium than a small order of french fries!

prep time: **4 minutes**   *yield:* **2 servings**

1 cup unsweetened cashew milk or almond milk (or coconut milk for a thicker drink)

1 cup strong brewed cherry or hibiscus tea, chilled (or more cashew milk)

¼ cup almond butter or Kite Hill brand cream cheese style spread

1 teaspoon cherry extract

½ teaspoon almond extract

¼ cup Swerve confectioners'-style sweetener or equivalent amount of liquid or powdered sweetener (see page 29), or more to taste

Pinch of fine sea salt

Crushed ice

1. Place all of the ingredients, except the ice, in a blender and blend until smooth. Just before serving, add the crushed ice and puree again until smooth. Pour into 2 glasses and serve.

2. Store in an airtight container in the refrigerator for up to 3 days.

nutritional info (per serving)				
calories	fat	protein	carbs	fiber
203	18g	9g	7g	3g

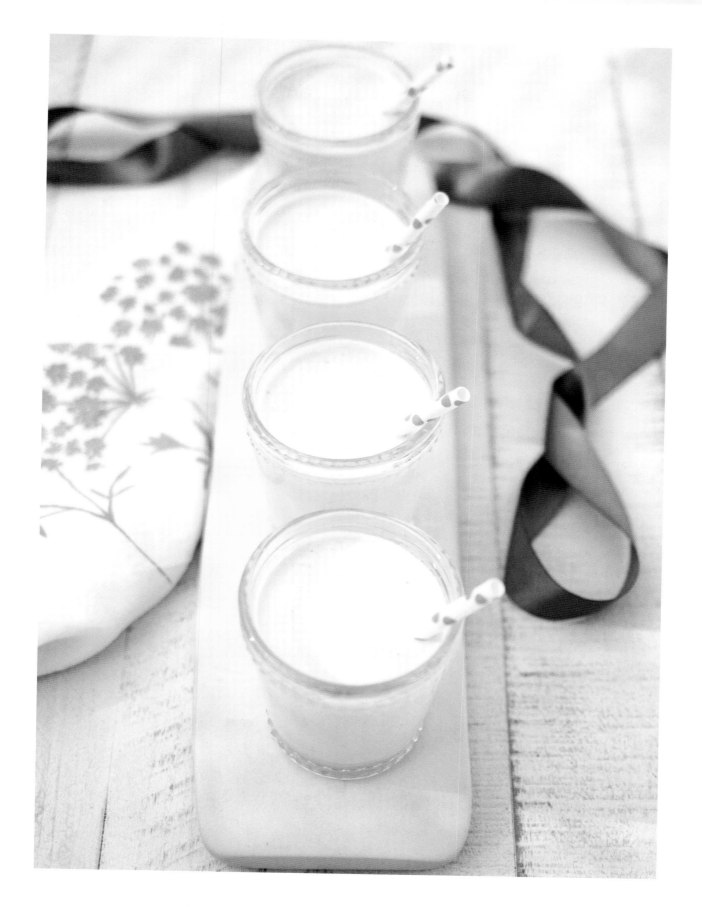

AMAZING PROTEIN SHAKE

KETO   OPTION

prep time: 5 minutes (not including time to cook eggs)
yield: 4 servings (1 cup per serving)

4 hard-boiled eggs (see page 81), peeled (see Note)

1 (13½-ounce) can full-fat coconut milk

1 cup unsweetened almond milk (or hemp milk if nut-free)

½ cup Swerve confectioners'-style sweetener or equivalent amount of liquid or powdered sweetener (see page 29)

1 teaspoon stevia glycerite, plus more to taste

Seeds scraped from 2 vanilla beans (about 8 inches long), or 2 teaspoons vanilla extract

¼ cup unsweetened cocoa powder, plus more to taste

1 teaspoon ground cinnamon

⅛ teaspoon fine sea salt

1. Place all of the ingredients in a blender and puree until very smooth. Taste and add up to an additional teaspoon of stevia glycerite and more cocoa powder, if desired.

2. Store in an airtight container in the refrigerator for up to 4 days. The flavor of this shake is best after it sits for a day in the fridge.

Note: *If you're making this shake for a child under the age of one, use only the egg yolks.*

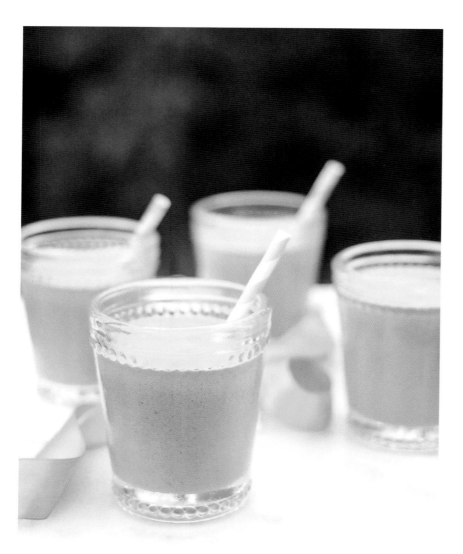

nutritional info (per serving)				
calories	fat	protein	carbs	fiber
234	21g	8g	4g	2g

BAKED EGGS AND HAM

4 large eggs, beaten

4 slices ham, diced

½ teaspoon fine sea salt

Pinch of ground black pepper

Fresh herbs of choice, for garnish (optional)

I love to use mini cocottes for this recipe, but ramekins work just as well.

prep time: **3 minutes**   *cook time:* **12 to 14 minutes**   *yield:* **2 servings**

1. Preheat the oven to 350°F. Grease two 4-ounce ramekins.

2. In a large bowl, whisk the eggs, ham, salt, and pepper until combined. Divide equally between the ramekins.

3. Place the ramekins in the oven and bake until the eggs are puffed and set in the center, 12 to 14 minutes. Garnish with fresh herbs, if desired.

4. Store in an airtight container in the refrigerator for up to 3 days. To reheat, place in a preheated 350°F oven for 5 minutes or until warmed through.

Busy Family Tip: You can make the egg and ham mixture up to 4 days ahead. Simply pour it into the ramekins, cover, and store in the refrigerator until ready to bake.

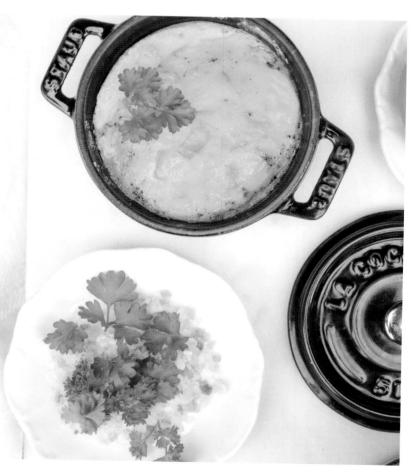

nutritional info (per serving)				
calories	fat	protein	carbs	fiber
285	19g	25g	1g	0.1g

FRENCH TOAST CEREAL

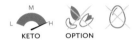

KETO · OPTION

prep time: 4 minutes, plus 10 minutes to chill *yield:* 1 serving

2 tablespoons melted coconut oil

2 tablespoons Swerve confectioners'-style sweetener or equivalent amount of liquid or powdered sweetener (see page 29)

1 teaspoon ground cinnamon

½ teaspoon maple or vanilla extract

1 ounce pork rinds, crumbled into ¼- to ½-inch pieces

1 cup unsweetened cashew milk or almond milk (or hemp milk if nut-free), for serving

1. Place the melted coconut oil, sweetener, cinnamon, and extract in a small bowl. Stir well to combine. Add the crumbled pork rinds and stir well to coat.

2. Cover and place the bowl in the refrigerator to chill for at least 10 minutes or until ready to eat (it will keep in an airtight container in the refrigerator for up to 3 days).

3. When ready to eat, uncover and break up the cereal a bit with a spoon. Just before serving, pour in the milk.

Busy Family Tip: *I like to make a quadruple batch of this cereal for easy breakfasts throughout the week.*

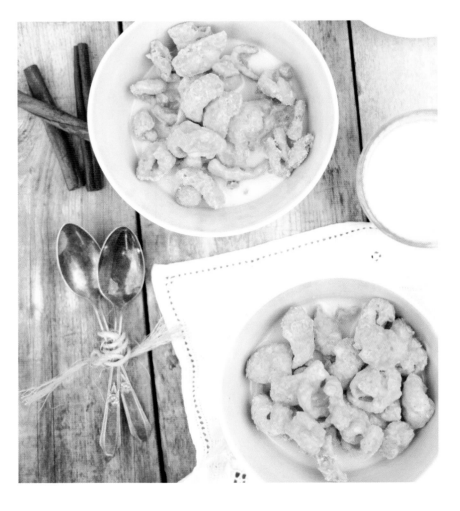

nutritional info (per serving)				
calories	fat	protein	carbs	fiber
426	42g	15g	2g	1g

BREAKFAST BACON FAT BOMBS

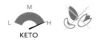

prep time: **7 minutes (not including time to cook eggs or bacon)** *yield:* **4 servings**

6 hard-boiled eggs (see page 81), peeled and halved

3 tablespoons mayonnaise, homemade (page 34) or store-bought

1 teaspoon fine sea salt

½ teaspoon dried chives

1 cup diced bacon, cooked until crispy

1. Remove the egg yolks from the whites and place the yolks in a bowl. Dice the whites and set aside.

2. To the bowl with the egg yolks, add the mayo, salt, and chives. Combine until smooth. Add the diced egg whites and gently stir to combine.

3. Take 2 tablespoons of the egg mixture and roll it into a golf ball–sized ball. Roll the ball in the cooked bacon. Repeat with the remaining egg mixture and bacon and serve.

4. Store in an airtight container in the refrigerator for up to 4 days.

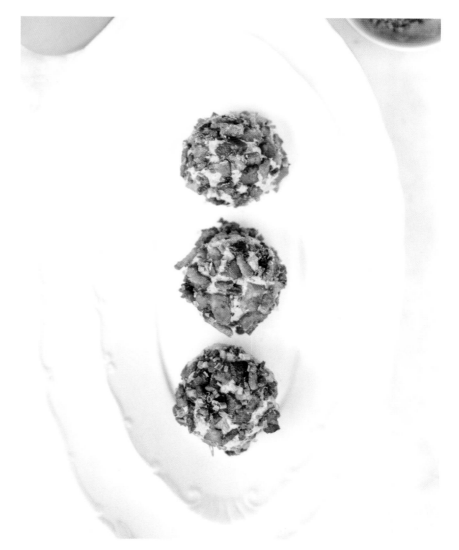

nutritional info (per serving)				
calories	fat	protein	carbs	fiber
274	24g	16g	0g	0g

LEMON MINUTE MUFFINS

½ cup coconut flour

¼ cup Swerve confectioners'-style sweetener or equivalent amount powdered sweetener (see page 29)

1 teaspoon baking soda

Pinch of fine sea salt

4 large eggs

¼ cup coconut oil, melted but not hot

½ cup lemon juice

1 teaspoon lemon or vanilla extract

Glaze (optional):

3 tablespoons coconut oil, melted

3 tablespoons Swerve confectioners'-style sweetener or equivalent amount of powdered sweetener (see page 29)

¾ teaspoon lemon extract

For Garnish (optional):

Grated lemon zest

Fresh mint sprigs

1. Grease five 4-ounce microwave-safe cups or ramekins (use ramekins if baking the muffins in the oven). If using the oven, preheat the oven to 350°F.

2. In a medium-sized bowl, whisk together the coconut flour, sweetener, baking soda, and salt. Stir in the eggs, melted coconut oil, lemon juice, and extract.

3. Divide the batter among the greased cups or ramekins, filling each about three-quarters full.

4. To make in the microwave, place each cup or ramekin in the microwave and cook on high for about 1 minute 30 seconds, until a toothpick inserted in the middle comes out clean. To make in the oven, bake for 8 to 12 minutes, until a toothpick inserted in the middle comes out clean.

5. Meanwhile, stir together the ingredients for the glaze, if using.

6. Remove the muffins from the microwave or oven and top each with 1 tablespoon of the glaze, if desired. Garnish with grated lemon zest and a small sprig of fresh mint, if desired. Eat warm right out of the cup or ramekin. Best consumed when fresh.

Busy Family Tip: *Fill the cups or ramekins with the batter and store covered in the refrigerator for easy on-the-go breakfasts that can be cooked as needed. The batter will keep in the refrigerator for 3 days.*

nutritional info (per serving)				
calories	fat	protein	carbs	fiber
265	25g	7g	9g	4g

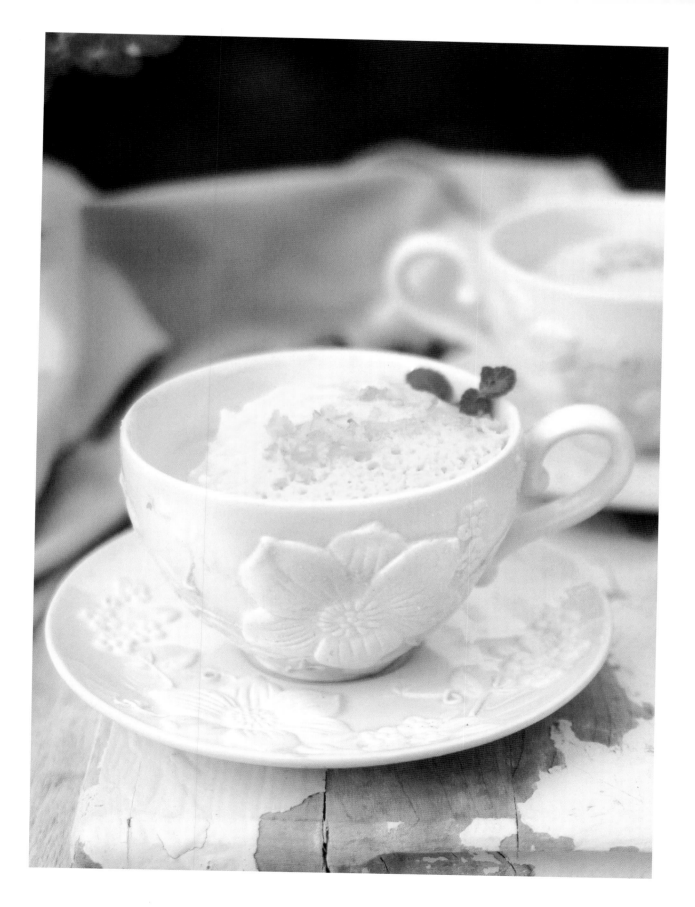

SMOKED SALMON, EGG, AND AVOCADO

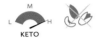

I adore a breakfast salad. If you're wondering what to do with the rest of the avocado, I like to freeze it, which keeps it bright green. All you have to do is sprinkle the peeled avocado with a teaspoon of lemon juice and wrap it tightly in plastic wrap. Place in the freezer for up to a month. When you are ready to consume it, simply allow it to thaw. Another way to freeze avocados, such as to avoid wasting them if you buy too many at once, is to place them in the freezer unpeeled for up to a month.

prep time: 5 minutes *cook time:* 3 minutes *yield:* 1 serving

1 large egg

1 tablespoon distilled white vinegar

1 cup torn leafy lettuce

1 tablespoon Greek Vinaigrette (page 46) or Cilantro Lime Dressing (page 39)

¼ avocado, sliced

2 ounces smoked salmon

Fine sea salt and ground black pepper

1. To poach the egg, bring a pot of water to a simmer. Add the vinegar, which will help the egg white hold together. Break the egg into a ramekin or small bowl. Rapidly swirl the water with a spoon. Gently slide the egg into the simmering water and poach for about 3 minutes for just-set white and still-runny yolk (or cook the egg to your liking). Remove the poached egg with a slotted spoon and place on a paper towel to drain.

2. Place the lettuce on a plate and drizzle with the dressing. Top the lettuce with the sliced avocado, smoked salmon, and poached egg. Season with salt and pepper to taste.

Busy Family Tips: Here's another easy way to make a perfect poached egg: Put ½ cup of water in a mug. Add an egg and cover the mug with a saucer. Microwave on high for 1 minute. Poached eggs can be made ahead and kept in the refrigerator for up to 3 days. Reheat in barely simmering water for 30 seconds to 1 minute.

You can find amazing wild-caught smoked salmon at Trader Joe's.

I store tasty keto salad dressings in the refrigerator for easy additions to meals like this one.

nutritional info (per serving)				
calories	fat	protein	carbs	fiber
283	21g	18g	6g	4g

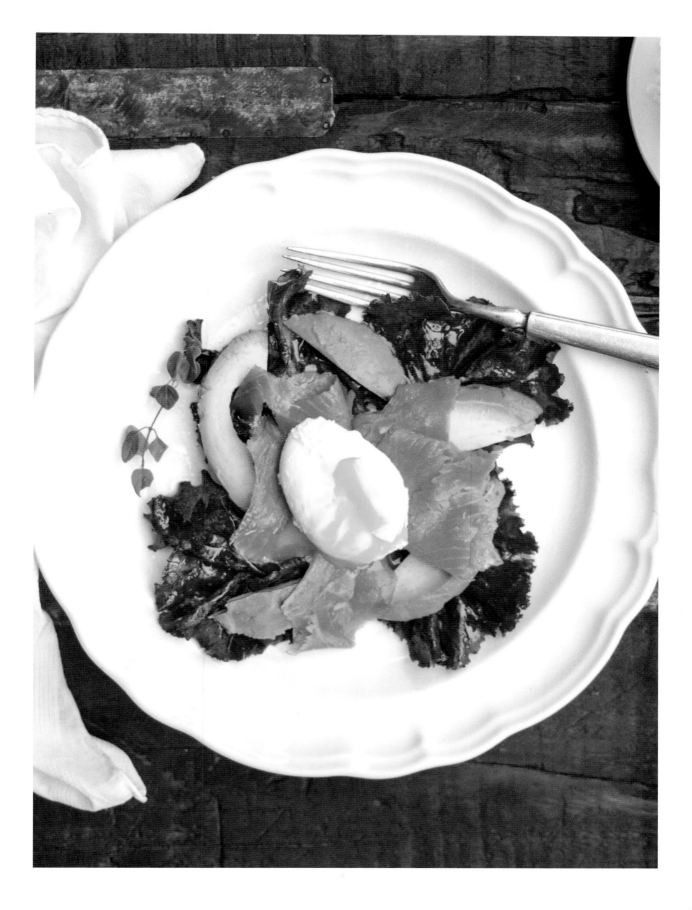

LOADED SCRAMBLED EGGS

1 tablespoon butter-flavored coconut oil or bacon fat

¼ cup sliced mushrooms

¼ cup diced red bell peppers

2 tablespoons diced onions

4 large eggs, beaten

¼ teaspoon fine sea salt

⅛ teaspoon ground black pepper

¼ cup diced ham

For Garnish:

Sliced scallions

Fresh parsley leaves

1. Heat the coconut oil in a skillet over medium heat. Add the mushrooms, peppers, and onions and sauté for 5 minutes or until the mushrooms turn golden.

2. Meanwhile, whisk the eggs in a bowl with the salt, pepper, and 2 tablespoons of water. Add the ham and stir to combine.

3. Pour the egg and ham mixture into the skillet with the mushroom mixture. Scramble over medium heat until the eggs are cooked to your liking. Serve garnished with sliced scallions and parsley.

4. Store in an airtight container in the refrigerator for up to 3 days. To reheat, place the eggs in a greased skillet over medium heat for a few minutes, until warmed to your liking.

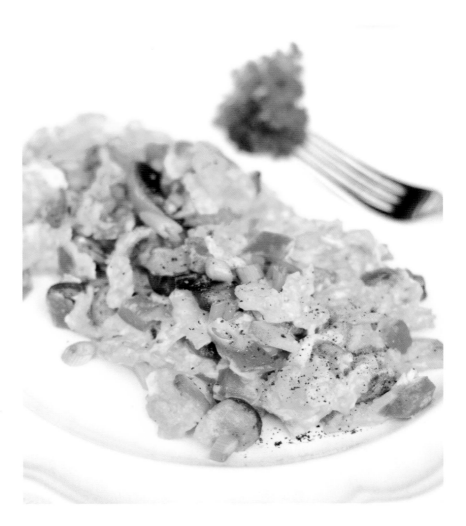

nutritional info (per serving)				
calories	fat	protein	carbs	fiber
281	22g	19g	2g	0.3g

BREAKFAST ASPARAGUS

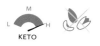
KETO

6 asparagus spears

2 strips bacon, diced

2 large eggs

1½ teaspoons chopped fresh chives

¼ teaspoon fine sea salt

⅛ teaspoon ground black pepper

1. Trim the woody ends off the asparagus.

2. Cook the bacon in a cast-iron skillet over medium heat until crispy, about 5 minutes. Remove the bacon from the skillet, leaving the drippings in the pan.

3. Add the asparagus to the hot pan and cook until crisp-tender, 5 to 6 minutes (depending on the thickness of the asparagus). Crack the eggs into the pan, over the asparagus. Sprinkle with the chives, salt, and pepper.

4. Lower the heat to medium-low and cook just until the egg whites are set and the yolks are still runny. Garnish with the reserved bacon.

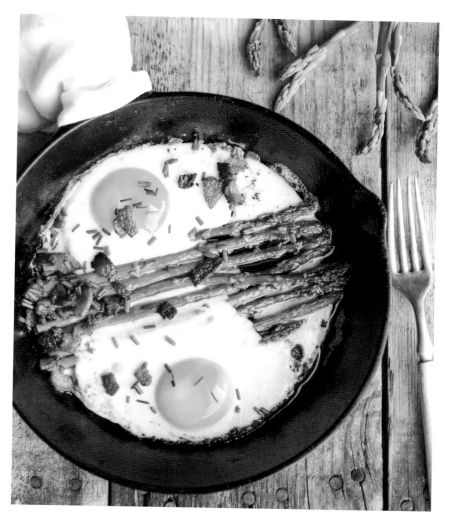

nutritional info (per serving)				
calories	fat	protein	carbs	fiber
335	24g	25g	5g	2g

SPICY FRIED EGGS WITH CHORIZO

prep time: **4 minutes**   *cook time:* **12 minutes**   *yield:* **2 servings**

1 tablespoon lard or coconut oil, plus more if needed

¼ cup diced red bell peppers

2 tablespoons diced onions

1 small jalapeño pepper, seeded and finely diced (optional)

4 ounces Mexican-style fresh (raw) chorizo, removed from casings

4 large eggs

¼ teaspoon fine sea salt

⅛ teaspoon ground black pepper

Fresh cilantro leaves, for garnish

1. Heat the lard in a cast-iron skillet or nonstick pan over medium heat. Add the red bell peppers, onions, and jalapeño, if using. Sauté until the onions are soft, about 4 minutes. Add the chorizo and cook while crumbling for 3 minutes or until cooked through. Remove from the pan and set aside.

2. Add another teaspoon of coconut oil to the pan, if needed. Crack the eggs into the skillet. Season with the salt and pepper. Cover and cook until the whites are cooked and the yolks are done to your liking, about 4 minutes for still-runny yolks. Divide the eggs between 2 serving plates. Place the chorizo mixture over the eggs and enjoy!

3. Store in an airtight container in the refrigerator for up to 3 days. To reheat, place in a greased skillet over medium heat for a few minutes, until warmed to your liking.

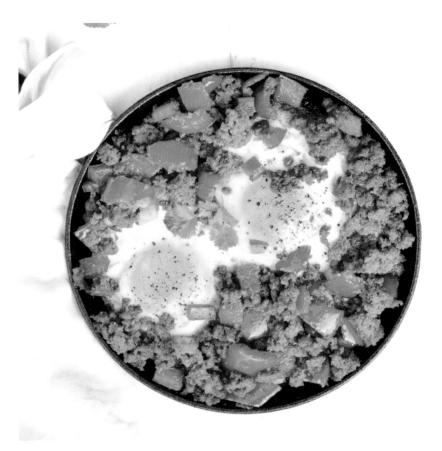

nutritional info (per serving)				
calories	fat	protein	carbs	fiber
379	31g	19g	4g	1g

LEMON POPPYSEED WAFFLES

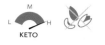

Waffles may sound like a difficult breakfast to make, but I make a quadruple batch and store them in the freezer. All I have to do is throw one in the toaster, like an Eggo waffle! It's so easy even my kids can make a healthy keto breakfast.

prep time: **4 minutes** (not including time to cook eggs)
cook time: **4 minutes per waffle** *yield:* **4 waffles** (1 per serving)

4 large eggs

4 hard-boiled eggs (see page 81), peeled

¼ cup coconut oil

¼ cup Swerve confectioners'-style sweetener or equivalent amount of liquid or powdered sweetener (see page 29)

2 tablespoons unflavored or vanilla-flavored egg white or beef protein powder

2 tablespoons lemon juice

2 tablespoons poppy seeds

2 teaspoons lemon extract, or 6 drops lemon oil

¾ teaspoon baking powder

¼ teaspoon fine sea salt

¼ cup Lemon Syrup (page 48), for serving

1. Heat a waffle iron to high heat.

2. Place the raw eggs, hard-boiled eggs, coconut oil, sweetener, protein powder, lemon juice, poppy seeds, extract, baking powder, and salt in a blender or food processor and pulse until smooth and thick.

3. Grease the hot waffle iron. Place 3 tablespoons of the batter in the center of the iron and close. Cook for 3 to 4 minutes, until the waffle is golden brown and crisp. Repeat with the remaining batter, regreasing the waffle iron as needed. Serve with the syrup.

4. Store in an airtight container in the refrigerator for up to 3 days or in the freezer for up to a month. To reheat, place in a toaster oven or in a preheated 375°F oven for 3 minutes or until warmed to your liking.

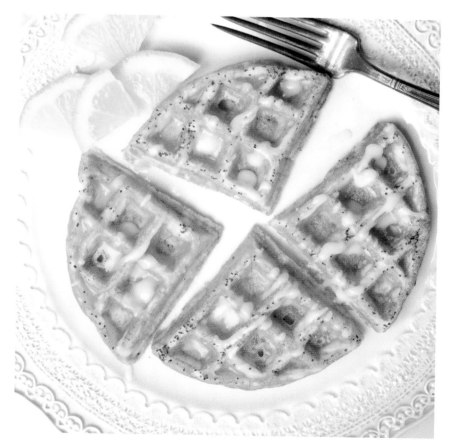

nutritional info (per serving)				
calories	fat	protein	carbs	fiber
268	24g	15g	2g	0.5g

BREAKFAST SAUSAGE SOUP
with Soft-Boiled Eggs

KETO   OPTION

I learned to make soft-boiled eggs using the boil-and-rest method: the eggs are placed in a pot and covered with cold water, then brought to a boil, covered, and removed from the heat to rest for 3½ minutes. Much to my mother's dismay, I found a better way to make soft-boiled egg that creates perfectly cooked eggs without fail. Instead of putting the eggs in cold water, you put them directly into simmering (not boiling!) water, as described below. When the eggs are boiled, the whites coagulate and become rubbery. To make perfect, ready-to-eat soft-boiled eggs with just-set yolks, simmer the eggs for a full 6 minutes.

prep time: **15 minutes**   *cook time:* **15 minutes**   *yield:* **6 servings**

1 tablespoon avocado oil

1 pound bulk breakfast sausage

½ cup diced onions

2 large cloves garlic, minced

1 teaspoon minced fresh sage

3 cups chicken bone broth, homemade (page 106) or store-bought, divided

1 cup tomato sauce

½ teaspoon fine sea salt

½ teaspoon ground black pepper

6 large eggs (omit for egg-free)

For Garnish (optional):

Diced avocado

Fresh herbs, such as thyme

1. Heat the oil in a Dutch oven or stockpot over medium heat. Add the sausage, onions, garlic, and sage and cook for about 6 minutes, breaking up the sausage into small chunks as it browns.

2. Add ¼ cup of the chicken broth to the pot and scrape the bottom to deglaze.

3. Add the remaining chicken broth, tomato sauce, salt, and pepper and simmer over medium heat for 8 minutes. Taste and adjust the seasoning.

4. Meanwhile, make the soft-boiled eggs: Fill a medium-sized saucepan halfway with water and bring the water just to a simmer. Gently place the eggs in the simmering water one at a time. Cook the eggs for 5 to 6 minutes, depending on how runny you prefer the yolks: 5 minutes will give you runny yolks and 6 minutes will give you yolks that are just set. Make sure to hold the water at a simmer; don't let it come to a boil. Remove the eggs and run under cool water for 30 seconds. Once cool, carefully peel the eggs and slice them in half.

5. Ladle the soup into bowls, then top each bowl with the eggs. Garnish with diced avocado and fresh herbs, if desired.

6. Store in an airtight container in the refrigerator for up to 3 days. To reheat, place the soup in a saucepan over medium heat for 3 minutes or until warmed through.

nutritional info (per serving)				
calories	fat	protein	carbs	fiber
379	31g	20g	5g	1g

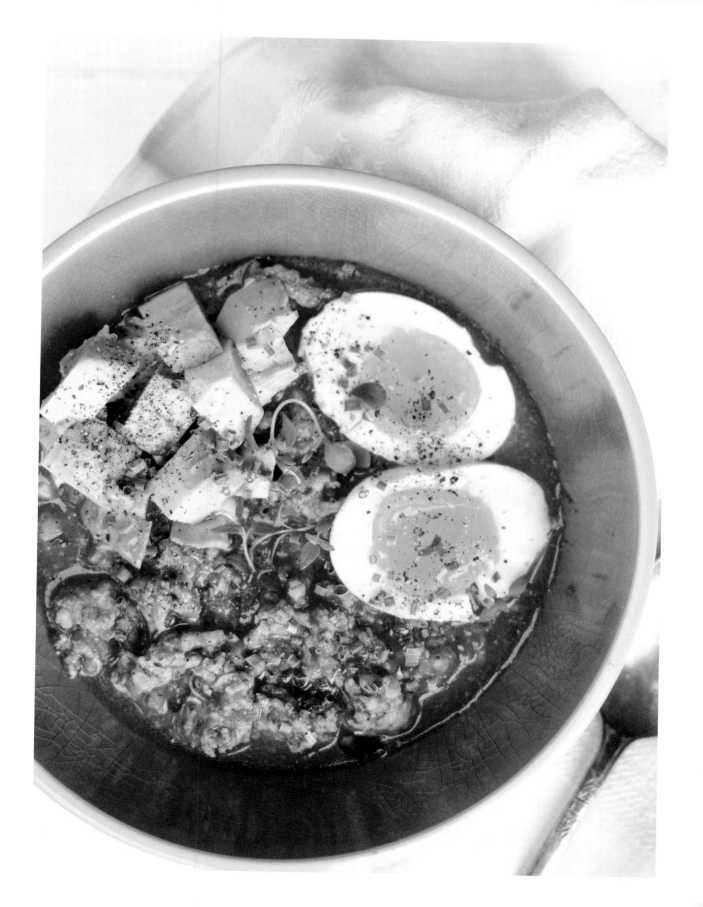

SILKY EGG BREAKFAST SOUP

In many countries, such as Thailand, savory soups for breakfast are quite common. The more I thought about it, the more I realized how comforting a warm bowl of soup on a cold winter morning would be!

prep time: **5 minutes**   *cook time:* **5 minutes**   *yield:* **2 servings**

2 cups chicken bone broth, homemade (page 106) or store-bought

5 large eggs, beaten

2½ tablespoons fish sauce

2 cups diced leftover cooked chicken (see Note)

Fine sea salt (optional)

Juice of 1 lime

For Garnish:

Fresh cilantro leaves

Sliced scallions (sliced on the bias)

Lime wedges

Freshly ground black pepper

1. Bring the broth to a boil in a large pot over medium-high heat. Slowly add the beaten eggs while whisking the broth. Reduce the heat to low and cook for 2 more minutes. Add the fish sauce and leftover chicken and continue cooking until the chicken is heated through. Taste and add salt, if needed. Add the lime juice and stir well.

2. Pour the soup into bowls and garnish with cilantro, scallions, lime wedges, and freshly ground pepper.

3. Store in an airtight container in the refrigerator for up to 3 days. Reheat the soup in a pot over medium heat for 5 minutes or until warmed through.

Note: *I often make this soup with leftover roasted chicken. An organic rotisserie chicken from the supermarket also works well.*

nutritional info (per serving)				
calories	fat	protein	carbs	fiber
521	28g	60g	5g	1g

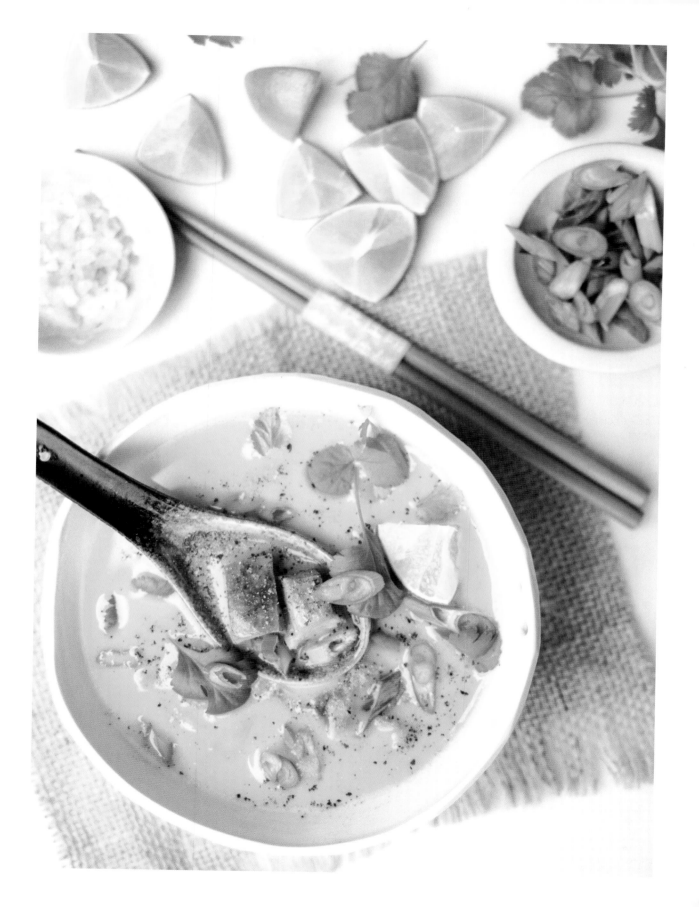

SNICKERDOODLE MINI MUFFINS

prep time: 5 minutes (not including time to cook eggs) cook time: 15 minutes
yield: 24 mini muffins (4 per serving)

4 large eggs

4 hard-boiled eggs (see page 81), peeled

½ cup Swerve confectioners'-style sweetener or equivalent amount of liquid or powdered sweetener (see page 29)

¼ cup vanilla-flavored egg white or beef protein powder

2 tablespoons ground cinnamon

1 teaspoon baking powder

¼ teaspoon fine sea salt

¼ cup coconut oil, melted

1 tablespoon vanilla extract

Glaze:

½ cup coconut oil

½ cup Swerve confectioners'-style sweetener or equivalent amount of powdered sweetener (see page 29)

1 teaspoon ground cinnamon

1 teaspoon vanilla extract

1. Preheat the oven to 325°F. Grease a 24-well mini muffin pan or line it with parchment paper liners.

2. Place the raw eggs, hard-boiled eggs, sweetener, protein powder, cinnamon, baking powder, and salt in a blender or food processor and pulse until smooth and thick. Add the coconut oil and extract and pulse to combine well.

3. Pour the mixture into the prepared muffin pan, filling each well about two-thirds full. Bake for 12 to 15 minutes, until a toothpick comes out clean when inserted in the center.

4. Meanwhile, make the glaze: Melt the coconut oil in a saucepan over medium heat with the sweetener, cinnamon, and extract. Drizzle the glaze over the muffins or dunk the tops of the muffins into the glaze.

5. Store in an airtight container in the refrigerator for up to 5 days or freeze for up to a month.

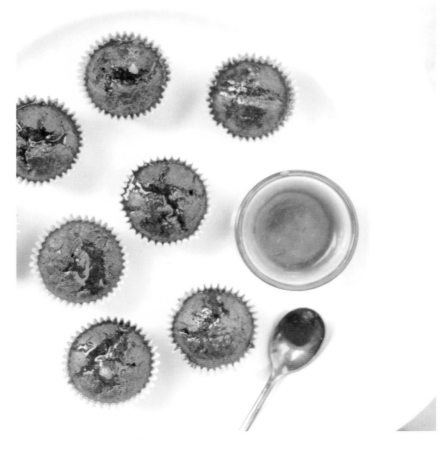

nutritional info (per serving)				
calories	fat	protein	carbs	fiber
348	34g	11g	2g	1g

EASY BREAKFAST SANDWICH

KETO

I love to make this sandwich for an on-the-go breakfast. Simply wrap it in parchment paper and take it with you for an easy portable meal!

prep time: **4 minutes**   *cook time:* **4 minutes**   *yield:* **1 serving**

1 teaspoon coconut oil, avocado oil, or bacon fat

2 large eggs

¼ teaspoon fine sea salt

⅛ teaspoon ground black pepper

2 ounces shaved ham

1 slice tomato

¼ avocado, sliced

1 slice red onion

1. Heat the oil in a cast-iron skillet over medium heat. Place 2 mason jar rings facedown in the skillet. Crack an egg into each ring to form a perfect circle for the "bun" of your sandwich. Season the eggs with the salt and pepper. Use a fork to scramble the eggs a little and break up the yolks. Cover and cook until the eggs are cooked through, about 4 minutes. Meanwhile, place the ham in the skillet to warm through.

2. Remove the eggs from the skillet. Place an egg on a plate. Top with the tomato slice, warm ham, and slices of avocado and red onion. Top with the other egg "bun."

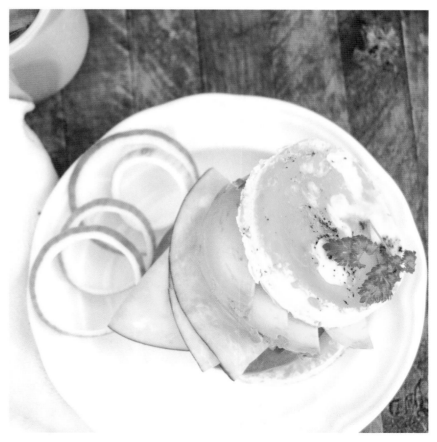

nutritional info (per serving)				
calories	fat	protein	carbs	fiber
455	35g	31g	5g	3g

IRISH BREAKFAST

I made this twist on the classic Irish breakfast on St. Patrick's Day to celebrate the holiday keto style. It was a hit with the whole family!

prep time: **8 minutes** *cook time:* **15 minutes** *yield:* **4 servings**

4 strips bacon

4 breakfast sausage links (precooked)

2 tablespoons lard or bacon fat, or more if needed

1 cup sliced button mushrooms

Fine sea salt

4 large eggs

Ground black pepper

1 small tomato, quartered

1 Keto Brioche (page 144)

Chopped fresh parsley or other herb of choice, for garnish

1. Cook the bacon in a large cast-iron skillet over medium-high heat until crispy, about 5 minutes. Remove to a platter, leaving the fat in the skillet. Add the sausages and cook, turning occasionally, until browned, about 3 minutes. Remove from the skillet and set on the platter with the bacon, leaving the drippings in the pan.

2. Add the lard to the skillet and heat until melted. Add the mushrooms and season with salt. Sauté until the mushrooms are golden, about 3 minutes. Remove the mushrooms and set on the platter with the meat.

3. Crack the eggs into the skillet. Season with salt and pepper. Cover and cook until the whites are set and the yolks are cooked to your liking. Remove to the platter with the meat and mushrooms.

4. If the skillet is dry, add a little more lard. Add the tomato quarters to the hot skillet and season with salt and pepper. Slice the brioche into ¼-inch-thick slices and place in the skillet with the tomatoes. Fry the tomatoes and brioche for 2 minutes per side. Remove from the skillet and place on the platter. Garnish with fresh herbs and serve.

nutritional info (per serving)				
calories	fat	protein	carbs	fiber
305	26g	16g	2g	1g

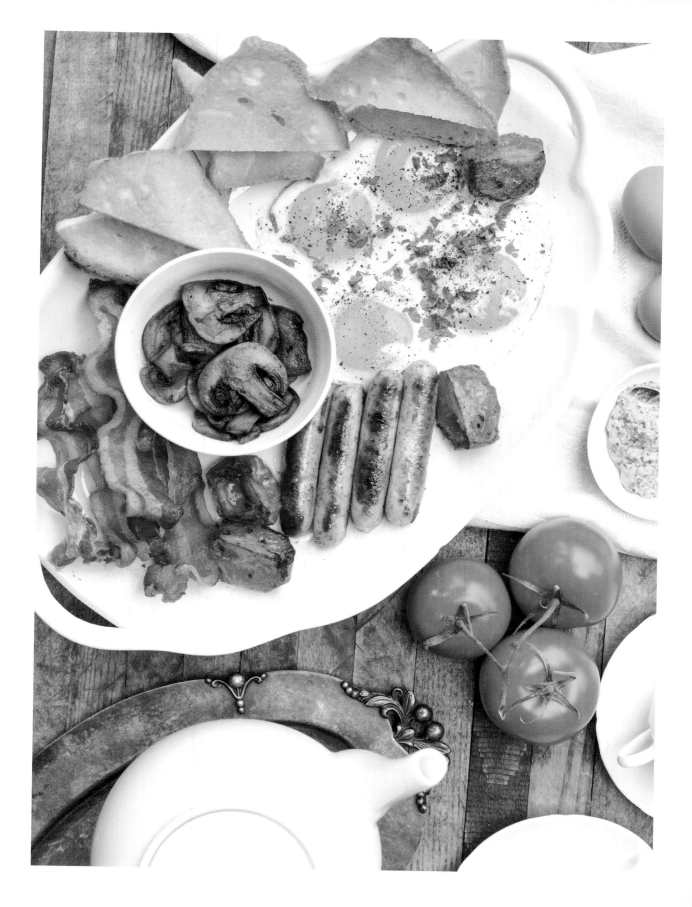

SOFT-BOILED EGGS
with Bacon-Wrapped Asparagus Dunkers

These bacon-wrapped asparagus dunkers are the ketogenic answer to breadsticks, the usual dunking device for soft-boiled eggs. If you want to make this breakfast even faster and easier to prepare, follow the variation at right, which uses cooked ham in place of the bacon and has you cook everything in the same pot.

prep time: **5 minutes** *cook time:* **15 minutes** *yield:* **2 servings**

8 asparagus spears

4 strips bacon

2 large eggs

2 teaspoons bacon fat

Fine sea salt and ground black pepper

Chopped fresh thyme leaves, for garnish

1. Preheat the oven to 400°F.

2. Make the dunkers: Trim the woody ends off the asparagus. Cut the bacon strips in half lengthwise to make 8 thin strips. Wrap a bacon strip diagonally around an asparagus spear to cover most of the spear; tuck in the end of the bacon to keep it from curling while baking. Place on a rimmed baking sheet and repeat with the rest of the bacon and asparagus. Bake for 12 to 15 minutes, until the bacon is almost crispy or cooked to your liking.

3. Meanwhile, soft-boil the eggs: Fill a medium-sized saucepan about halfway with water and bring just to a simmer. Gently place the eggs one at a time in the simmering water. Cook for 5 to 6 minutes, depending on how runny you prefer the yolks: 5 minutes will give you runny yolks and 6 minutes will give you yolks that are just set. Make sure to hold the water at a simmer; don't let it come to a boil. Remove the eggs and run under cold water for 30 seconds.

4. To serve, use a knife to take the cap off the tip of each egg and dot each of the warm yolks with 1 teaspoon of bacon fat. Sprinkle with salt, pepper, and thyme leaves and enjoy straight from the eggshell with the dunkers.

5. The eggs and dunkers are best served fresh; however, leftover dunkers can be stored in an airtight container in the refrigerator for up to 3 days. To reheat, place the dunkers on a rimmed baking sheet in a preheated 400°F oven for 4 minutes or until warmed through. Make the soft-boiled eggs just before serving or the yolks will harden in the refrigerator.

nutritional info (per serving)				
calories	fat	protein	carbs	fiber
231	17g	16g	2g	1g

Variation: *Ham-Wrapped Asparagus Dunkers.* To make this shortcut version, replace the bacon with 8 slices of ham. Fill a medium-sized saucepan about halfway with water and bring to a boil. After trimming the woody ends off the asparagus, place the asparagus in the boiling water and boil for 5 to 7 minutes, until crisp-tender. (The cook time will depend on how thick your asparagus spears are.) Using tongs, remove the asparagus from the boiling water and set aside.

Reduce the heat under the saucepan to keep the water at a simmer. Place the eggs in the simmering water and soft-boil them, following the instructions in Step 3, opposite.

While the eggs are cooking, wrap a slice of ham around each asparagus spear. To serve, follow Step 4, opposite.

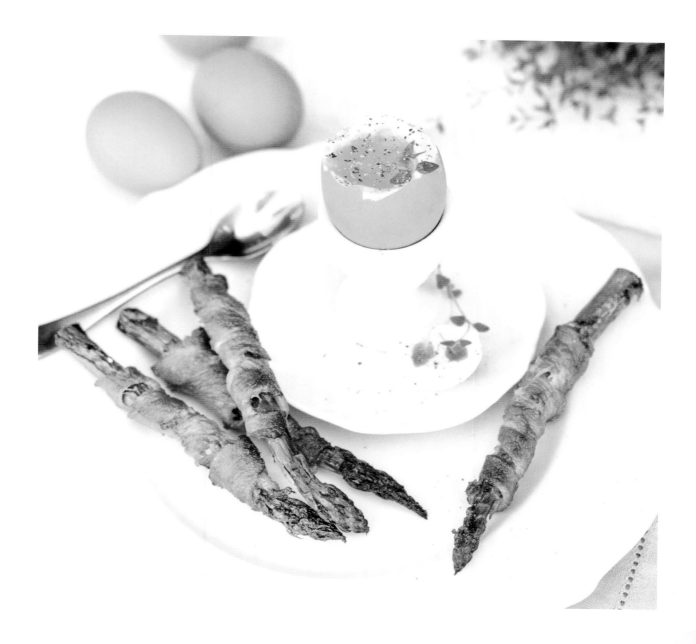

REUBEN EGGS BENEDICT

1 Keto Brioche (page 144)

1½ teaspoons coconut oil or lard, for frying

4 large eggs

8 slices corned beef

¼ cup fermented sauerkraut

Thousand Island Dressing:

3 tablespoons mayonnaise, homemade (page 34) or store-bought, or Baconnaise (page 34)

1 tablespoon chopped dill pickles

1 tablespoon tomato sauce

Pinch of fine sea salt

1. Cut the brioche into four ½-inch-thick slices. Fry in a skillet with the coconut oil until golden brown and toasted.

2. Meanwhile, poach the eggs following the method described on page 62.

3. While the eggs are poaching, prepare the dressing: Place the mayo, pickles, tomato sauce, and salt in a small dish and stir well to combine.

4. Place 2 slices of corned beef on each brioche slice. Top each with 1 tablespoon sauerkraut, a poached egg, and 1 tablespoon of dressing.

5. Store in an airtight container in the refrigerator for up to 3 days. To reheat, place on a rimmed baking sheet in a 400°F oven for 4 minutes or until warmed through.

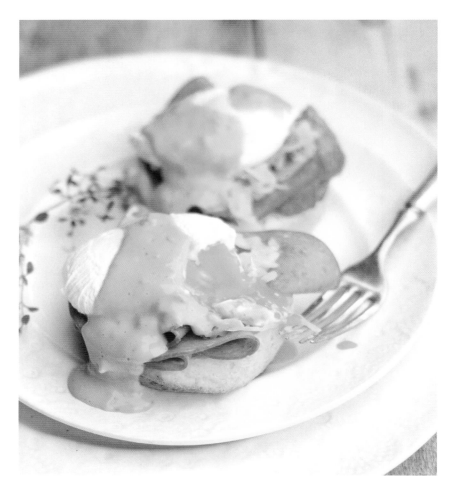

nutritional info (per serving)				
calories	fat	protein	carbs	fiber
546	40g	45g	2g	0.1g

SUPER KETO PANCAKES

When I was a little girl, my parents would take me to dairy breakfasts at farms in central Wisconsin on Saturday mornings in June. Hundreds of families would gather to enjoy a buffet-style breakfast that included pancakes, bacon, breakfast sausages, and eggs to celebrate dairy month. Here is my take on a June dairy breakfast with keto-style pancakes!

prep time: 3 minutes (not including time to cook eggs) *cook time:* 4 minutes
yield: 4 pancakes (2 per serving)

2 large eggs

2 hard-boiled eggs (see page 81), peeled

2 tablespoons Swerve confectioners'-style sweetener or equivalent amount of liquid or powdered sweetener (see page 29)

1 teaspoon ground cinnamon

1 teaspoon vanilla extract

¼ teaspoon fine sea salt

¼ teaspoon baking powder

Coconut oil, for the skillet

¼ cup Cinnamon Syrup (page 47), for serving

1. Place all of the ingredients, except the coconut oil and syrup, in a blender and combine until very smooth.

2. Heat 1½ teaspoons of coconut oil in a skillet over medium heat. Once hot, pour one-quarter of the batter into the skillet. Cook until golden brown, about 2 minutes, then flip and cook until done, another 1 to 2 minutes. Remove from the skillet and repeat with additional coconut oil and batter. Serve with the syrup.

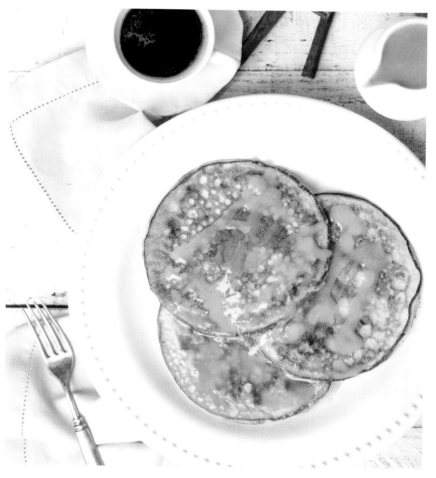

nutritional info (per serving)				
calories	fat	protein	carbs	fiber
186	14g	12g	3g	1g

FRENCH TOAST PUDDING

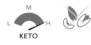

prep time: **5 minutes** *(not including time to cook eggs)*

yield: **4 servings (1 cup per serving)**

10 hard-boiled eggs (see page 81), peeled

1 (13½-ounce) can full-fat coconut milk

½ cup Swerve confectioners'-style sweetener or equivalent amount of liquid or powdered sweetener (see page 29), plus 1 to 2 teaspoons stevia glycerite (or to desired sweetness)

2½ teaspoons maple extract

2 teaspoons ground cinnamon

⅛ teaspoon fine sea salt

1. Place all of the ingredients in a blender and puree until very smooth. Taste and add more stevia glycerite, if desired.

2. Store in an airtight container in the refrigerator for up to 4 days.

Note: *If you're making this pudding for a baby one year old or younger, omit the egg whites. (The whites, which contain more protein than the yolks, can increase the chance of developing egg allergies if introduced before the age of one.) I made this pudding with just the egg yolks for my son Kai's breakfasts all week long when he was a baby, and he loved it!*

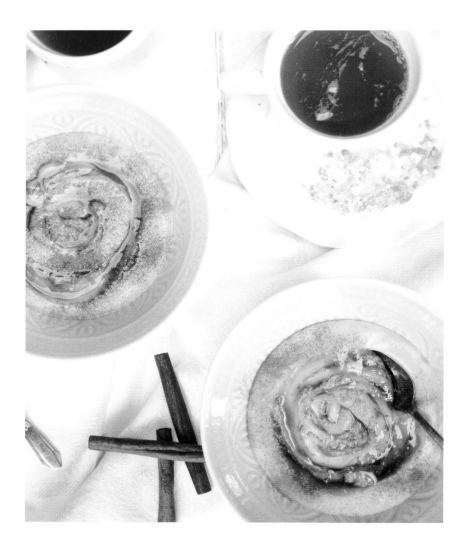

nutritional info (per serving)				
calories	fat	protein	carbs	fiber
300	26g	16g	3g	1g

PERFECT HARD-BOILED EGGS

Do you ever get frustrated by hard-boiled eggs that don't peel easily? Using a pressure cooker makes the eggs a snap to peel—and it takes only 3 minutes! If you don't own a pressure cooker, I've got you covered. See the variation below for making hard-boiled eggs on the stovetop.

prep time: 1 minute   *cook time:* 3 minutes, plus time to release pressure
yield: 6 servings (3 eggs per serving)

18 large eggs

Special Equipment:

Pressure cooker (I use my Instant Pot)

1. Place the eggs in a pressure cooker and cover completely with water. Seal. Turn to high pressure for 3 minutes. After 3 minutes, do a quick pressure release. Remove the eggs and run cold water over them to stop the cooking. Peel the number of eggs you plan to eat or use in a recipe right away.

2. Store unpeeled eggs in an airtight container in the refrigerator for up to 5 days.

Variation: *Stovetop Hard-Boiled Eggs. Place the eggs in a saucepan and cover with cold water. (Tip: Older eggs are easier to peel than super fresh eggs.) Bring to a boil and immediately remove the pan from the heat. Cover and let the eggs cook in the hot water for 11 minutes. Remove the eggs from the hot water, rinse with very cold water to stop the cooking, and then peel.*

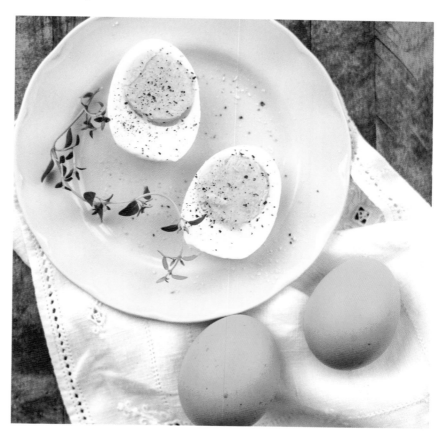

nutritional info (per serving)				
calories	fat	protein	carbs	fiber
180	14g	18g	0g	0g

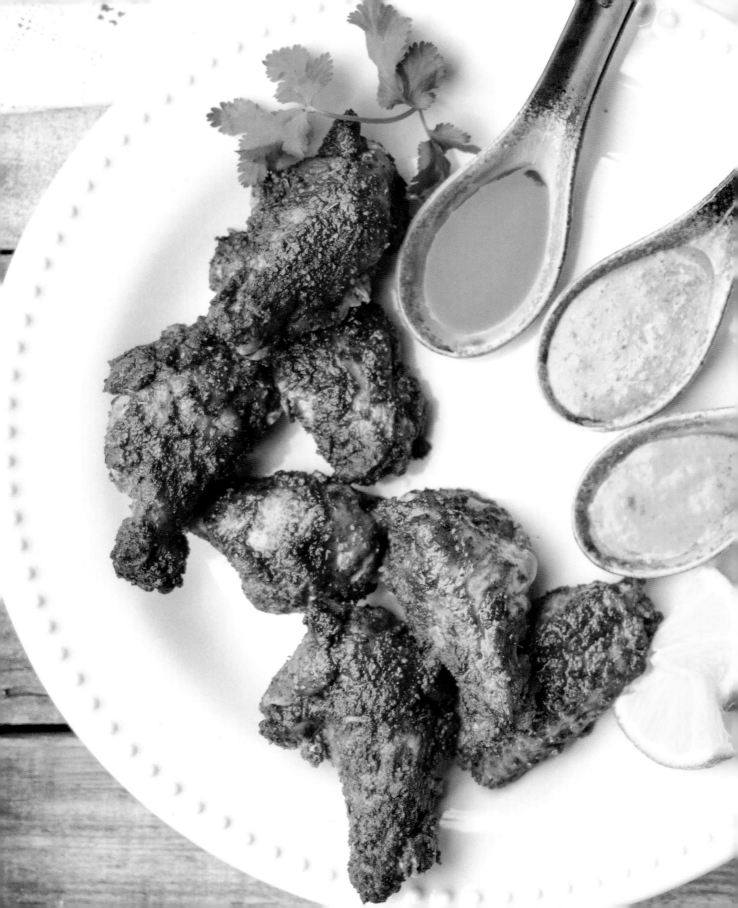

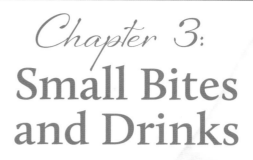

Chapter 3:
Small Bites and Drinks

SHRIMP COCKTAIL

Keto Cocktail Sauce:

¾ cup tomato sauce

1 tablespoon prepared horseradish, or more to taste

1 tablespoon lemon juice

1 to 2 teaspoons Swerve confectioners'-style sweetener or equivalent amount of liquid or powdered sweetener (see page 29)

½ teaspoon onion powder

½ teaspoon fine sea salt

1 pound precooked large shrimp

1 lemon, sliced into wedges, for serving (optional)

I love shrimp cocktail! My keto cocktail sauce makes it easy to enjoy this classic appetizer at home. You can make the sauce ahead; it tastes great with crab, too.

prep time: 5 minutes   *yield:* 8 servings as an appetizer, 4 servings as a meal

1. Make the sauce: Place the sauce ingredients in a small bowl and stir well to combine. Adjust the seasoning to taste.

2. Serve the shrimp with the cocktail sauce, with lemon wedges on the side, if desired.

3. Store in an airtight container in the refrigerator for up to 3 days.

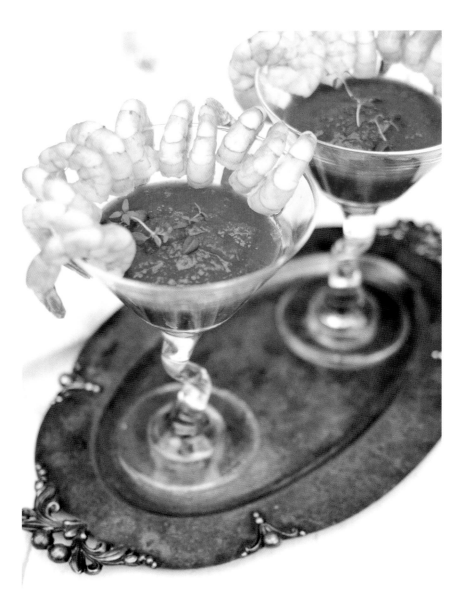

nutritional info (per serving)				
calories	fat	protein	carbs	fiber
76	1g	14g	2g	0.5g

PICO DE GALLO

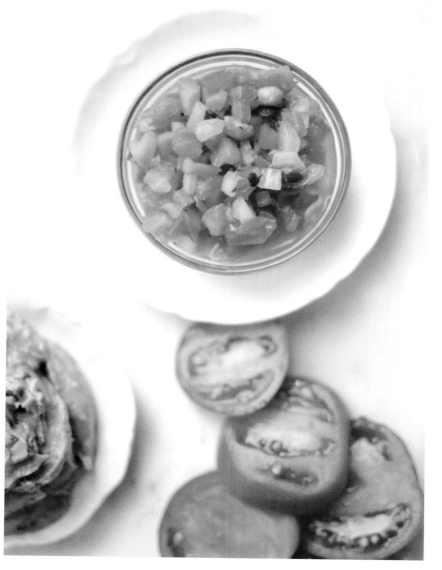

L ⌐ M ⌐ H
KETO

1 large tomato, diced (about 1½ cups)

½ cup chopped white onions (about 1 medium)

2 cloves garlic, minced

2 tablespoons lime juice

2 tablespoons chopped fresh cilantro

1 jalapeño pepper, seeded and finely diced

½ teaspoon fine sea salt

Pico de gallo is a great dipping option for Bacon Chips (page 91). It also can be served with my South of the Border Steak (page 200) or over scrambled eggs.

prep time: **7 minutes**   *yield:* **2¼ cups (about ½ cup per serving)**

Place all of the ingredients in a small bowl and stir until well combined. Store in an airtight container in the refrigerator for up to 5 days.

nutritional info (per serving)				
calories	fat	protein	carbs	fiber
32	0.1g	1g	6g	1g

CITRUS AVOCADO SALSA

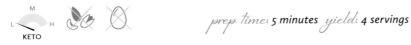

KETO

prep time: **5 minutes** *yield:* **4 servings**

1 cup diced tomatoes

1 small avocado, pitted and diced

¼ cup chopped fresh cilantro leaves

2 tablespoons avocado oil, MCT oil, or extra-virgin olive oil

4 drops orange oil, or 1 teaspoon orange extract

Juice of 1 lime

Fine sea salt and ground black pepper

1. Place the tomatoes, avocado, and cilantro in a small bowl. Add the avocado oil, orange oil, and lime juice and stir. Season to taste with salt and pepper.

2. Store in an airtight container in the refrigerator for up to 4 days.

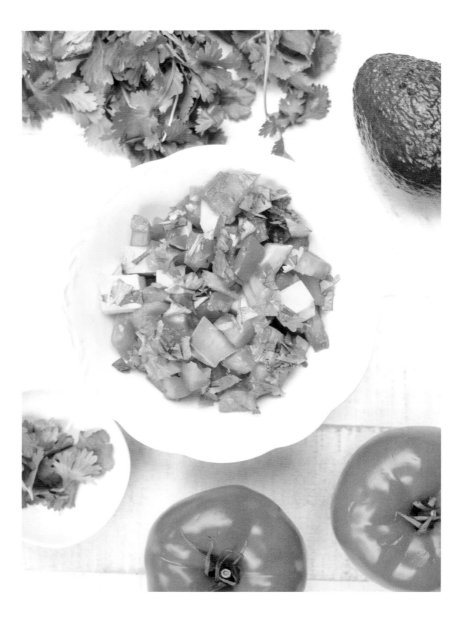

nutritional info (per serving)				
calories	fat	protein	carbs	fiber
140	13g	1g	7g	3g

GUACAMOLE

This tastes great with Bacon Chips (page 91), smothered over hamburgers, stuffed into chicken (see page 164), or dolloped over scrambled eggs.

prep time: **15 minutes**   *yield:* **3 cups (½ cup per serving)**

3 avocados, peeled and pitted

3 to 4 tablespoons lime juice

½ cup finely diced onions

2 plum tomatoes, diced

2 cloves garlic, smashed to a paste

3 tablespoons chopped fresh cilantro

1 teaspoon fine sea salt

½ teaspoon ground cumin

1. Place the avocados and 3 tablespoons of lime juice in a large bowl and mash to the desired consistency.

2. Add the rest of the ingredients and stir until well combined. Taste and add more lime juice, if desired.

3. For the best flavor, cover tightly and refrigerate for 1 hour, or serve immediately.

4. To store, transfer the guacamole to a large resealable plastic bag, squeeze out as much air as you can, and seal the bag shut. It will keep in the refrigerator for up to 3 days when stored this way.

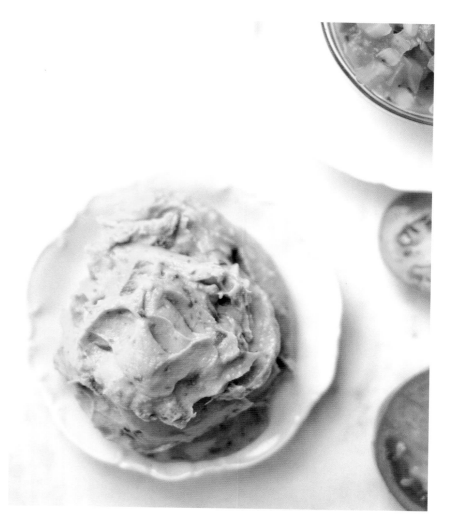

nutritional info (per serving)				
calories	fat	protein	carbs	fiber
313	26g	11g	13g	7g

JICAMA CROSTINI—
Two Ways

KETO   OPTION

These crostini make an elegant appetizer. If you'd like to make both types—the tuna salad and the smoked salmon—you'll have enough crostini for a party. Just remember to double the amount of jicama and salt for the base.

prep time: 5 minutes *yield:* 12 servings of each type (2 crostini per serving)

Crostini Base:

(makes enough for 24 crostini)

1 medium jicama

⅛ teaspoon fine sea salt

Tuna Salad Crostini:

1 (2-ounce) can tuna packed in water, drained

3 tablespoons mayonnaise, homemade (page 34 or 35) or store-bought, or Baconnaise (page 34)

¼ teaspoon fine sea salt

Pinch of ground black pepper

3 tablespoons capers, for garnish

1 teaspoon fresh thyme leaves or other herb, such as parsley or chives, for garnish

Freshly ground black pepper, for garnish

Smoked Salmon Crostini:

24 (1-inch) pieces smoked salmon

3 tablespoons stone-ground mustard

3 tablespoons capers, for garnish

1 teaspoon fresh dill or thyme leaves, for garnish

1. Make the crostini base: Peel the jicama and cut crosswise into very thin slices. Stop when you have 24 slices. Using a round cookie cutter or the lid of a mason jar, cut a 1½-inch round from each slice. Discard the scraps.

2. Place the jicama rounds on a platter. Season with the salt.

3. If making the tuna salad crostini, place the tuna in a small bowl. Add the mayo, stir well, and season with the salt and pepper. Place 1½ teaspoons of the tuna salad on each jicama round and garnish with 3 or 4 capers, a few thyme leaves, and some freshly ground pepper.

4. If making the smoked salmon crostini, place a piece of smoked salmon on each jicama round. Top with ½ to 1 teaspoon of mustard and garnish with 3 or 4 capers and a few dill or thyme leaves.

5. Store in separate airtight containers in the refrigerator for up to 3 days.

nutritional info for tuna salad crostini (per serving)				
calories	fat	protein	carbs	fiber
31	3g	0.2g	2g	1g

nutritional info for smoked salmon crostini (per serving)				
calories	fat	protein	carbs	fiber
27	0.4g	2g	3g	2g

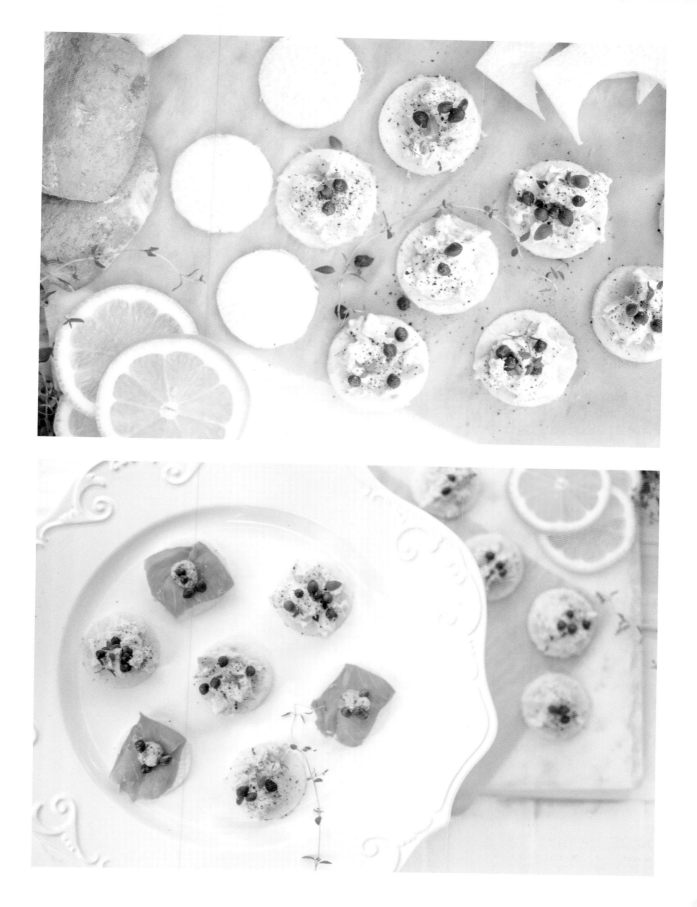

ALMOST DEVILED EGGS

KETO

To make deviled eggs even easier, pick up already boiled and peeled eggs from your local grocery store. Even I get pressed for time, and peeling eggs can take forever. The convenience of precooked and peeled eggs makes recipes like this one super easy!

prep time: 5 minutes (*not including time to cook eggs*)
yield: 12 servings (2 halves per serving)

1. Spread a little mayo on each egg half. Top with a squirt of mustard. Sprinkle with salt and garnish with thyme leaves and some freshly ground pepper.

2. Store in an airtight container in the refrigerator for up to 3 days.

12 hard-boiled eggs (see page 81), peeled and halved

¼ cup mayonnaise, homemade (page 34) or store-bought

About 2 teaspoons prepared yellow mustard

½ teaspoon fine sea salt

For Garnish:

Fresh thyme leaves

Freshly ground black pepper

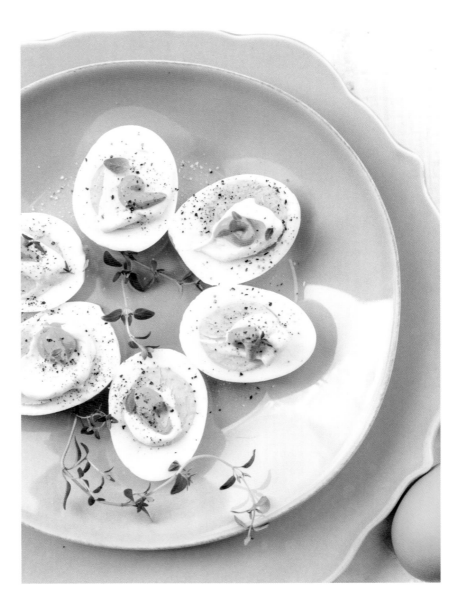

nutritional info (per serving)				
calories	fat	protein	carbs	fiber
94	8g	6g	0g	0g

BACON CHIPS WITH DIPS

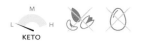

prep time: 5 minutes (not including time to make dips)   cook time: 12 minutes
yield: 6 servings

12 strips thin-cut bacon, cut into 2-inch pieces

1 batch Citrus Avocado Salsa (page 86), for serving

1 batch Guacamole (page 87), for serving

1. Preheat the oven to 400°F. Line a baking sheet with parchment paper.

2. To form the bacon pieces into triangle shapes, or "chips," fold them in thirds and place on the lined baking sheet. Place another baking sheet on top of the chips, then place a heavy object such as a cast-iron skillet on top of the second baking sheet to help keep the bacon flat. Bake for 6 to 12 minutes, until the bacon is crispy.

3. Transfer the bacon chips to a platter with a bowl of each dip. These chips are best served fresh.

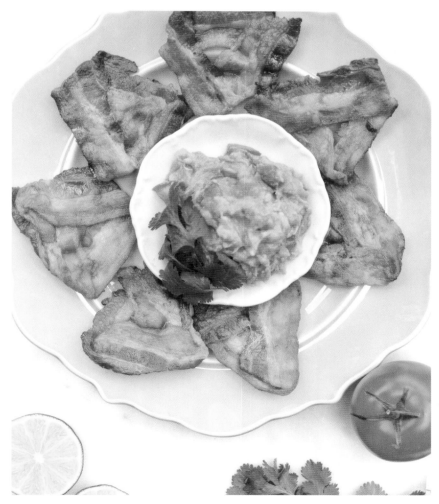

nutritional info (per serving)				
calories	fat	protein	carbs	fiber
402	34g	11g	18g	9g

AMAZING MARINATED OLIVES

prep time: **5 minutes**   *yield:* **8 servings (¼ cup per serving)**

1 cup pitted black olives

1 cup pitted green olives

½ cup extra-virgin olive oil

¼ cup lemon juice

2 tablespoons chopped fresh cilantro

4 drops orange oil

2 cloves garlic, minced

1. Place all of the ingredients in a medium-sized bowl. Stir well to combine. For the best flavor, cover and refrigerate overnight before serving.

2. Store in an airtight container in the refrigerator for up to a week.

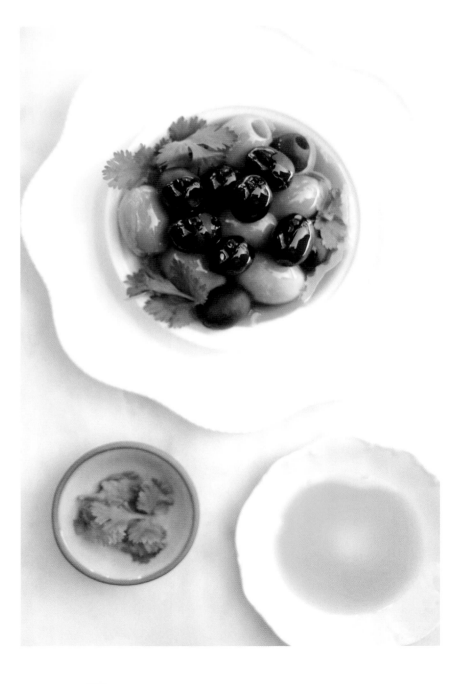

nutritional info (per serving)				
calories	fat	protein	carbs	fiber
173	19g	0.3g	2g	1g

SIMPLE SHRIMP PARFAIT

prep time: **10 minutes** *yield:* **8 servings**

1 cup pitted green olives

4 cherry tomatoes, quartered

2 tablespoons avocado oil or extra-virgin olive oil

1 tablespoon lime juice

Fine sea salt and ground black pepper

1 pound precooked, peeled, and deveined medium shrimp

Fresh basil or cilantro leaves, for garnish

1. Place the olives and tomatoes in a bowl. Add the oil and lime juice and season to taste with salt and pepper. Stir well and divide among 8 stemmed glasses.

2. Top each glass with 3 to 4 shrimp, then sprinkle the shrimp with a little salt and pepper. Garnish each parfait with basil. Cover and refrigerate until ready to serve.

3. Store in an airtight container in the refrigerator for up to 3 days.

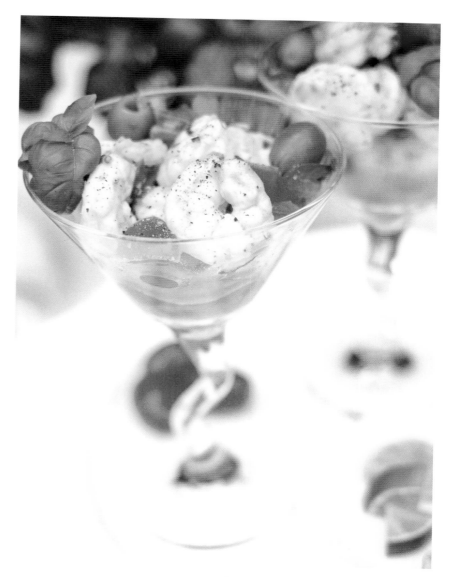

nutritional info (per serving)				
calories	fat	protein	carbs	fiber
141	9g	14g	2g	1g

DRY-RUBBED BAKED WINGS

prep time: **7 minutes**   *cook time:* **20 to 25 minutes**   *yield:* **4 servings**

3 teaspoons Italian seasoning

1½ teaspoons fine sea salt

1½ teaspoons paprika

1 teaspoon chili powder

½ teaspoon garlic powder

½ teaspoon onion powder

30 chicken wings or drumettes

3 tablespoons melted coconut oil or bacon fat

For Serving:

¼ cup Comeback Sauce (page 37)

¼ cup Creamy Ranch Dressing (page 45)

¼ cup Cilantro Lime Dressing (page 39)

Lime wedges

1. Preheat the oven to 450°F.

2. Place the Italian seasoning, salt, paprika, chili powder, garlic powder, and onion powder in a small bowl and stir to combine well.

3. Place the chicken wings in a large bowl. Pour the melted coconut oil over them and turn to coat. Then sprinkle the seasoning on all sides and turn to coat. Place the wings on a rimmed baking sheet.

4. Bake for 20 to 25 minutes, until the wings are cooked through and no longer pink inside. Serve with the sauces and lime wedges.

5. Store in an airtight container in the refrigerator for up to 4 days. To reheat, place the wings on a rimmed baking sheet in a 400°F oven for 5 minutes or until warmed through.

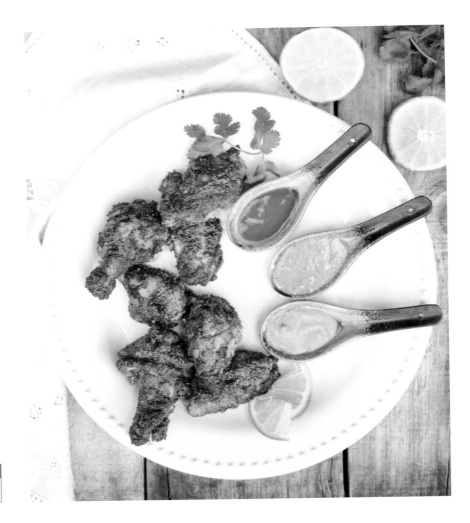

nutritional info (per serving)				
calories	fat	protein	carbs	fiber
391	29g	32g	0.5g	0.2g

DEVILISH DEVILED EGGS

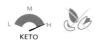

prep time: 15 minutes (not including time to cook eggs)
yield: 12 servings (2 halves per serving)

12 hard-boiled eggs (see page 81), peeled and halved

½ cup mashed avocado

1 tablespoon Baconnaise (page 34) or mayonnaise, homemade (page 34) or store-bought

1 teaspoon lime juice

½ teaspoon fine sea salt

½ teaspoon onion powder

1 large baby red bell pepper, cut into 48 small triangles

1. Remove the egg yolks and place them in a bowl (or a food processor). Mash the yolks with a fork (or pulse in the food processor) until they have the texture of very fine crumbles.

2. Add the mashed avocado, Baconnaise, lime juice, salt, and onion powder to the egg yolks and mix until smooth. Fill the egg white halves with the yolk mixture.

3. Garnish with the red bell pepper triangles for "horns."

4. Store leftovers in an airtight container in the refrigerator for up to 3 days.

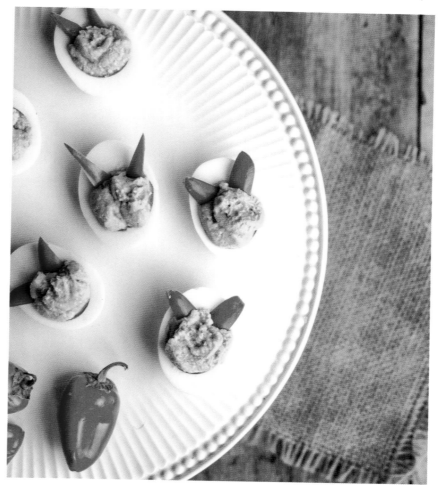

nutritional info (per serving)				
calories	fat	protein	carbs	fiber
83	7g	6g	1g	1g

DEVILED GREEN EGGS AND HAM

This twist on deviled eggs makes for a hearty snack. Given the ham and egg theme of these deviled eggs, I often serve them for breakfast (in that case, give each person a double serving). I am such a superfan of Dr. Seuss that I include a *Green Eggs and Ham*–themed recipe in each of my cookbooks!

Before I started working as a nutritionist, I worked at a camp where we had a puppet show based on Dr. Seuss's *The Lorax;* it taught the kids the importance of taking care of Mother Nature. I have amazing memories of working at this camp, and my children now get to experience the same camp once a month with their homeschool program. Anyway, if you are a fan of Dr. Seuss like I am, you must try these Green Deviled Eggs and Ham!

prep time: 8 minutes *(not including time to cook eggs and bacon or make mayo)*
yield: 12 servings *(2 egg halves and 2 slices of ham per serving)*

12 hard-boiled eggs (see page 81), peeled and halved

½ small avocado, pureed, or ½ cup Guacamole (page 87)

¼ cup mayonnaise, homemade (page 34) or store-bought

1 teaspoon coconut vinegar

½ teaspoon fine sea salt

4 strips bacon, cut into ¼-inch dice and fried until crispy

Sliced scallions, for garnish

Dried chives, for garnish

24 very thin slices ham, rolled

1. Remove the egg yolks and place them in a bowl (or a food processor). Mash the yolks with a fork (or pulse in the food processor) until they have the texture of very fine crumbles. Add the avocado, mayonnaise, vinegar, and salt and mix until smooth.

2. Fill the egg white halves with the egg yolk mixture and set them on a serving plate. Sprinkle with the bacon and garnish with scallions and chives. Place a slice of rolled-up ham between each pair of deviled eggs.

3. Store in an airtight container in the refrigerator for up to 3 days.

Busy Family Tip: *I keep a dozen hard-boiled eggs in my refrigerator at all times. My boys love to help me in the kitchen, and peeling eggs is one of the things they can do without my constant attention, freeing me to prepare other food.*

nutritional info (per serving)				
calories	fat	protein	carbs	fiber
489	38g	34g	2g	1g

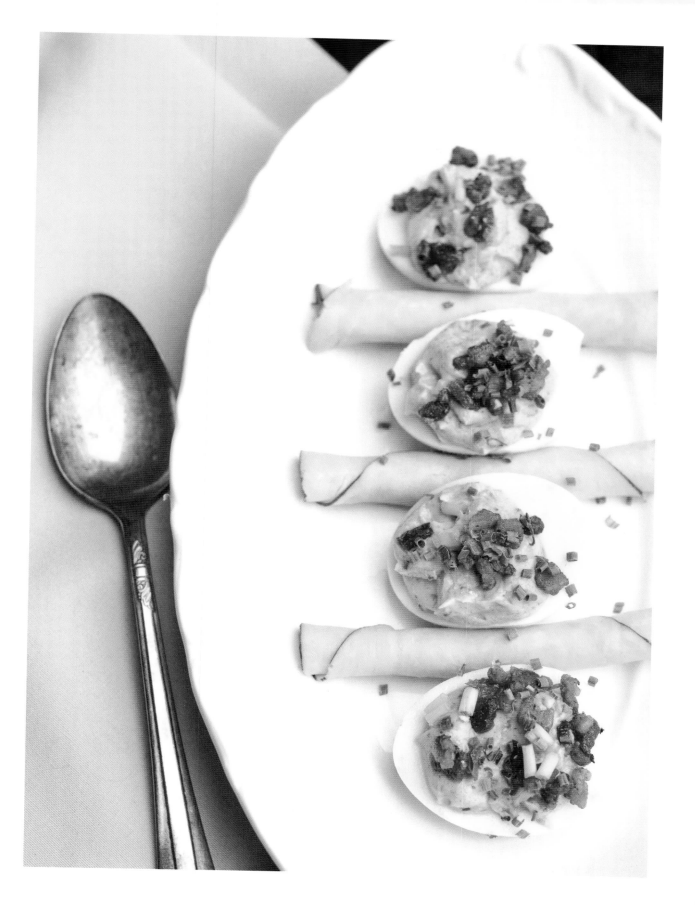

CUTE KITTY DEVILED EGGS

prep time: 15 minutes (not including time to cook eggs)
yield: 12 servings (2 halves per serving)

12 hard-boiled eggs (see page 81), peeled and halved

1 cup mayonnaise, homemade (page 34) or store-bought

1 teaspoon prepared yellow mustard

1 teaspoon fine sea salt

2 ounces cold-smoked salmon, such as Nova lox, cut into 48 small triangles

144 (½-inch-long) chive pieces (about 10 fresh chives)

48 black peppercorns

24 capers

1. Remove the egg yolks and place them in a bowl (or a food processor). Mash the egg yolks with a fork (or pulse in the food processor) until they have the texture of very fine crumbles. Add the mayonnaise, mustard, and salt and mix until smooth. Add more salt to taste.

2. Fill the egg white halves with the egg yolk mixture. Garnish each egg with 2 triangles at the top for ears, 6 pieces of chives for whiskers (3 on each side), 2 peppercorns for eyes, and a caper for a nose. Store in the refrigerator for up to 2 days.

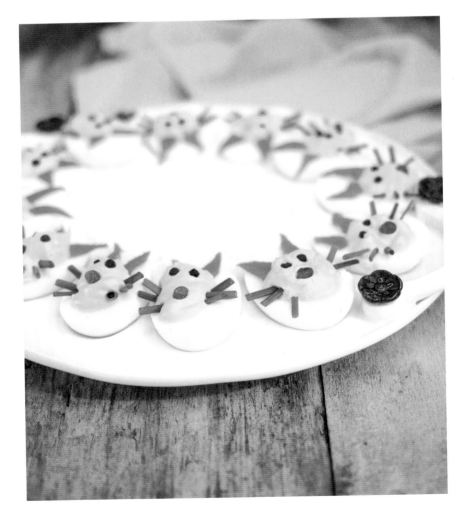

nutritional info (per serving)				
calories	fat	protein	carbs	fiber
204	20g	7g	0.3g	0.2g

MOROCCAN DEVILED EGGS

12 hard-boiled eggs (see page 81), peeled and halved

¼ cup mayonnaise, homemade (page 34) or store-bought

3 tablespoons harissa paste

½ teaspoon fine sea salt

For Garnish:

Chopped fresh chives

Chopped fresh cilantro

1. Remove the egg yolks and place them in a bowl (or a food processor). Mash the yolks with a fork (or pulse in the food processor) until they have the texture of very fine crumbles. Add the mayonnaise, harissa paste, and salt and mix until smooth.

2. Fill the egg whites with the egg yolk mixture. Garnish with the chives and cilantro.

3. Store in an airtight container in the refrigerator for up to 4 days.

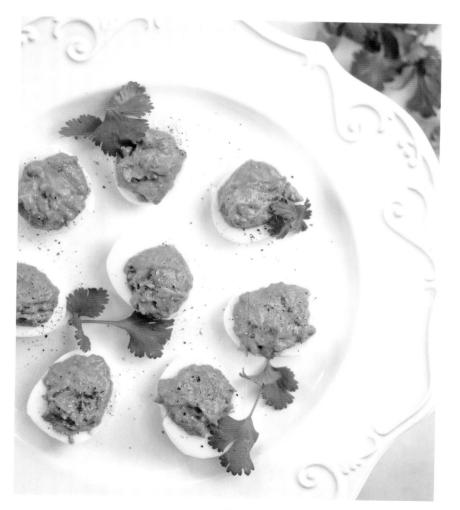

nutritional info (per serving)				
calories	fat	protein	carbs	fiber
90	8g	6g	0.1g	0g

HOMEMADE GINGER ALE

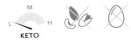

prep time: 5 minutes   cook time: 30 minutes   yield: 32 ounces concentrated ginger ale base (2 tablespoons per serving), enough for 16 ginger ales

Ginger Ale Base:

1 pound fresh ginger, unpeeled, cut into small dice

Peeled zest and juice of 2 lemons

1 quart unflavored sparkling water or seltzer water

1½ cups Swerve confectioners'-style sweetener or equivalent amount of liquid or powdered sweetener (see page 29), plus 1 to 2 teaspoons stevia glycerite (or to desired sweetness)

For Serving:

Ice

Unflavored sparkling water or seltzer water

Lime or lemon wedges

Special Equipment:

Pressure cooker (see Tip)

1. Combine the ginger and lemon juice in a food processor and process until minced, stopping the machine periodically to scrape down the sides, if necessary.

2. Place the puree in a pressure cooker along with the sparkling water, sweetener, and lemon zest. Seal and cook on high pressure for 30 minutes. Slowly release the pressure. Let cool slightly, then strain and chill.

3. To serve, place about 2 tablespoons of the ginger ale base in a glass filled with ice. Fill the glass with sparkling water and stir well to combine. Taste and add more ginger ale base, if desired. Garnish with a lime or lemon wedge and serve.

4. Store the ginger ale base in an airtight container in the refrigerator for up to 5 days or in the freezer for up to a month.

Tip: *If you don't have a pressure cooker, you can make the ginger ale base in a slow cooker. Place the ingredients for the base in the slow cooker and cook on low for 8 hours, then strain and chill.*

nutritional info (per serving)				
calories	fat	protein	carbs	fiber
31	0.3g	1g	6g	0.2g

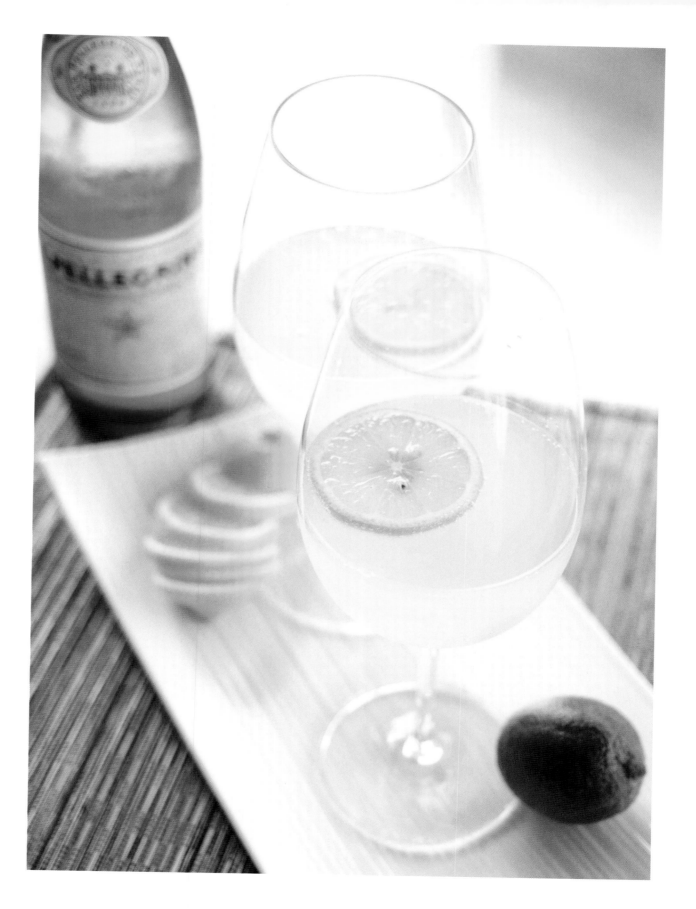

NAKED GIMLET

KETO

Ice

1 (12-ounce) can sparkling water or seltzer water, preferably lime flavored (see Note)

¼ cup olive juice (from the jar of olives below)

Juice of 1 lime

6 pimento-stuffed green olives, for garnish

Special Equipment:

Cocktail sticks (optional)

Fill a large martini shaker or mason jar with ice. Add the sparkling water, olive juice, and lime juice, then cover and shake well. Strain into 2 martini glasses. Spear the olives with cocktail sticks, if desired, and garnish each cocktail with 3 olives. Serve immediately.

Note: *If using a lime-flavored sparkling or seltzer water, look for a clean, naturally flavored water with no added sugars. I use LaCroix brand sparkling water.*

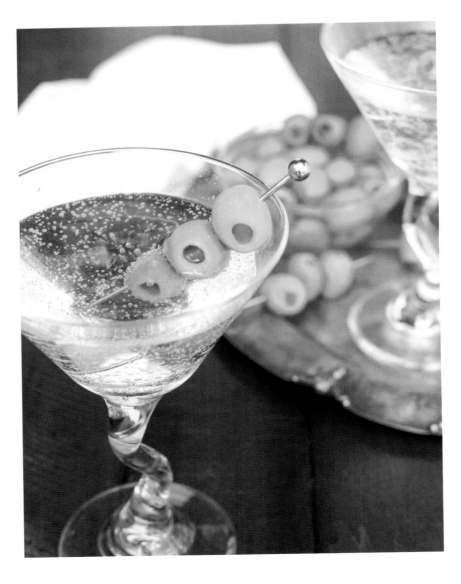

nutritional info (per serving)				
calories	fat	protein	carbs	fiber
22	2g	0.3g	3g	1g

VIRGIN STRAWBERRY MARGARITA

prep time: **4 minutes** *yield:* **4 servings**

For the Rims (optional):

Medium-coarse sea salt (see Note)

Lime wedge

2 cups strong brewed hibiscus tea, chilled

¼ cup Swerve confectioners'-style sweetener or equivalent amount of liquid or powdered sweetener (see page 29)

¼ cup lime juice

2 teaspoons strawberry extract

Ice, for serving

4 lime wedges, for garnish

Note: *A sea salt about the size of kosher salt works well here.*

1. To coat the rims of the glasses, if desired, fill a saucer with about ⅛ inch of medium-coarse sea salt. Run a lime wedge around the rims of 4 tumblers. Take one of the glasses and roll the edge of the dampened rim in the salt until the entire rim is coated. Repeat with the other 3 glasses.

2. Place the tea, sweetener, lime juice, and extract in a blender and blend until smooth. To serve, carefully fill the salt-rimmed tumblers with ice. Pour the margarita mixture into the glasses and garnish with lime wedges.

3. Store in a pitcher in the refrigerator for up to 5 days. Stir well before serving.

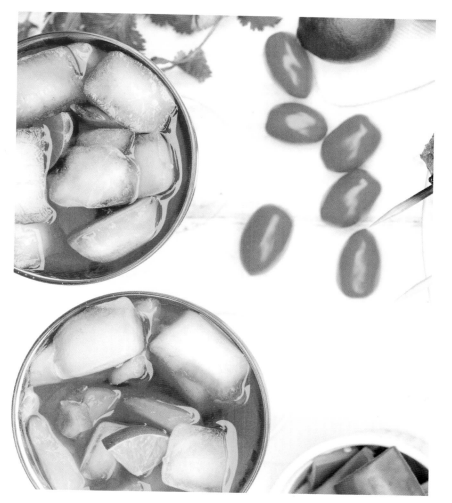

nutritional info (per serving)				
calories	fat	protein	carbs	fiber
4	0g	0g	1g	0.1g

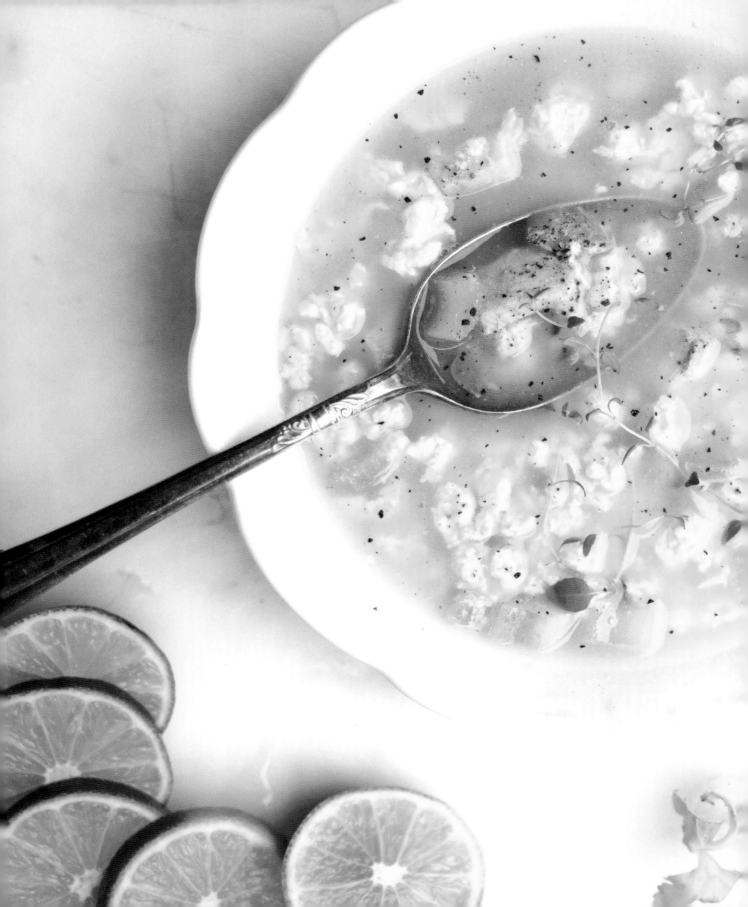

Chapter 4:
Soups and Stews

SUPER FAST BONE BROTH

This time-saving recipe uses a pressure cooker, which enables you to make rich, nutritious bone broth in a fraction of the time. If you don't have a pressure cooker, you can make bone broth in a slow cooker (see the variation below).

When making bone broth, adding an acid such as vinegar helps extract more minerals from the bones. The extracted minerals then become the alkalizing agents to neutralize the acidity of the vinegar. I use organic coconut vinegar, which exceeds all other vinegars in terms of amino acid, vitamin, and mineral content. It is also a fructooligosaccharaide (FOS), a type of prebiotic that promotes digestive health. Don't worry, it doesn't taste like coconut!

prep time: 12 minutes *cook time:* 35 minutes *yield:* 4 quarts (1 cup per serving)

3½ pounds beef, chicken, ham, or fish bones

2 stalks celery, chopped

1 medium onion, chopped

7 cloves garlic, whacked with the side of a knife and peeled

2 bay leaves

2 teaspoons fine sea salt

¼ cup coconut vinegar

Cold filtered water

¼ cup fresh herb leaves, or 1 teaspoon dried herb leaves of choice (optional)

Special Equipment:

Pressure cooker

1. Place the bones, celery, onion, garlic, bay leaves, salt, and vinegar in a pressure cooker, then add enough cold filtered water to cover everything. Add the herbs, if using.

2. Seal the lid on the pressure cooker and cook on low pressure for 30 minutes. Cooking on low allows more gelatin and minerals to be extracted from the bones. Slowly release the pressure.

3. Pour the broth through a strainer and discard the solids.

4. Store in the refrigerator for up to 5 days or freeze for up to several months.

Note: *When chilled, the broth will become gelatinous. To use in a recipe or for drinking, scoop the meaty gelatin into a microwave-safe mug or glass measuring cup and heat in the microwave until it becomes a nice, thick liquid again.*

Busy Family Tip: *I make a huge batch of broth and store it in freezer-safe mason jars in the freezer for easy additions to recipes.*

Variation: *Slow Cooker Bone Broth. Place all of the ingredients in a 6-quart slow cooker. Cover and cook on low for 48 hours. Pour the broth through a strainer and discard the solids.*

nutritional info (per serving)				
calories	fat	protein	carbs	fiber
21	1g	2g	1g	0.2g

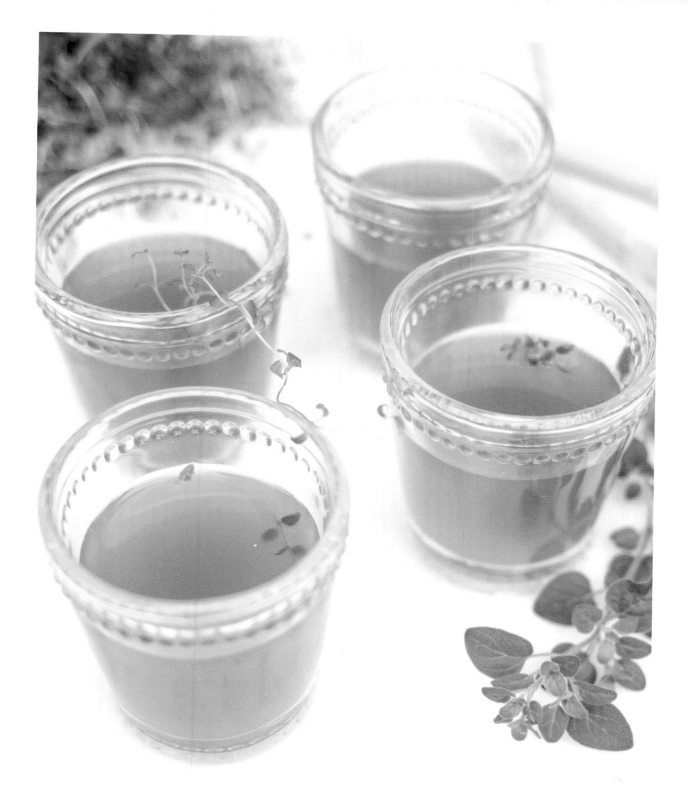

CHINESE BEEF AND BROCCOLI SOUP

prep time: **10 minutes, plus at least 1 hour to marinate beef**
cook time: **18 minutes** *yield:* **8 servings**

2 pounds cubed beef stew meat

1 tablespoon wheat-free tamari, or ¼ cup coconut aminos

2 tablespoons plus 2 teaspoons coconut oil, divided

1 cup diced onions

5 cloves garlic, minced

1 tablespoon peeled and grated fresh ginger (optional)

¼ teaspoon fine sea salt

½ teaspoon ground black pepper

6 cups broccoli florets, cut into bite-sized pieces

6 cups beef bone broth, homemade (page 106) or store-bought

2 tablespoons fish sauce

2 tablespoons Swerve confectioners'-style sweetener or equivalent amount of liquid or powdered sweetener (see page 29)

Scallions, sliced diagonally, for garnish

1. If any of the stew meat pieces are larger than about 1 inch, cut them down to size. Place the meat in a medium-sized bowl. Add the tamari and toss to coat. Place in the refrigerator to marinate for at least 1 hour or overnight.

2. Heat 1 tablespoon of coconut oil in a large pot or Dutch oven over medium-high heat. When the oil is rippling hot, add half of the beef. Spread the beef across the pot and cook, without stirring, for 1 minute. Stir or toss with tongs, spread the beef across the pot again, and cook for 1 minute more. Be careful not to overcook the meat; it should be just barely cooked through and still very tender. Transfer the meat to a dish with a lid.

3. Drain any excess liquid from the pot. Repeat Step 2 with another tablespoon of coconut oil and the remaining meat. Add the second batch of cooked meat and any juices from the pot to the dish and cover tightly with the lid.

4. Add the remaining 2 teaspoons of coconut oil and the onions, garlic, and ginger, if using, to the hot pot. Toss to coat the onions with the oil, sprinkle with the salt and pepper, and cook for about 5 minutes, stirring occasionally, until the onions are tender. Add the broccoli and beef broth and bring to a simmer. Stir in the fish sauce and sweetener and taste; add more salt or sweetener, if desired. Simmer for 4 minutes or until the broccoli is soft.

5. Remove from the heat and stir in the cooked meat and any juices. Ladle the soup into bowls, garnish with sliced scallions, and serve.

6. Store in an airtight container in the refrigerator for up to 3 days. To reheat, place the soup in a saucepan over medium heat for a few minutes, until warmed through.

nutritional info (per serving)				
calories	fat	protein	carbs	fiber
426	28g	35g	9g	4g

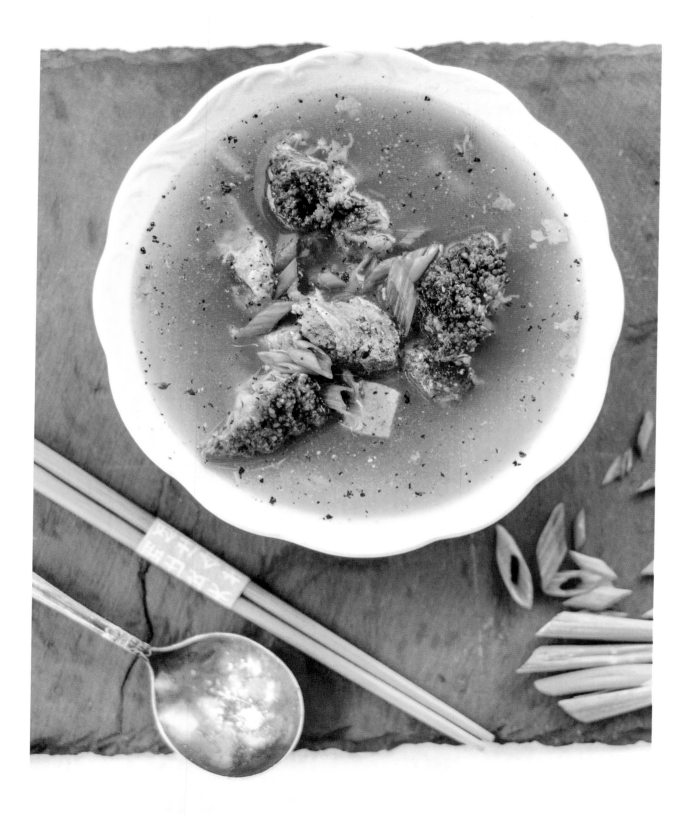

COCONUT GINGER CHICKEN SOUP

prep time: **10 minutes**   *cook time:* **50 minutes**   *yield:* **8 servings**

Ginger Paste:

¼ cup peeled and grated fresh ginger

3 cloves garlic, chopped

4 stalks lemongrass, hard outer layers removed and top third discarded, then chopped

3 shallots, chopped

1 teaspoon ground white pepper

4 cups full-fat coconut milk

4 boneless, skinless chicken breast halves (about 2 pounds), chopped into bite-sized pieces

Grated zest of 2 limes

3 tablespoons fish sauce

5 serrano chile peppers, minced (seeded for less heat)

½ teaspoon fine sea salt

For Garnish:

Chopped fresh chives

Chopped fresh cilantro leaves

Lime wedges

1. Make the ginger paste: Place the ginger and garlic in a food processor or mortar and pulse or pound (using the pestle) into a paste. Add the lemongrass, shallots, and white pepper and pulverize. Set aside.

2. In a medium-sized saucepan, bring the coconut milk to a gentle simmer over medium heat. Do not overheat or it will curdle. Add the ginger paste and stir well, then add the chicken and bring to a boil. Add the lime zest, fish sauce, chiles, and salt. Cover and simmer over medium-low heat for about 45 minutes, until the chicken is fully cooked.

3. Ladle the soup into bowls, then garnish with chives, cilantro, and lime wedges and serve.

4. Store in an airtight container in the refrigerator for up to 3 days. To reheat, place the soup in a saucepan over medium heat for a few minutes, until warmed through.

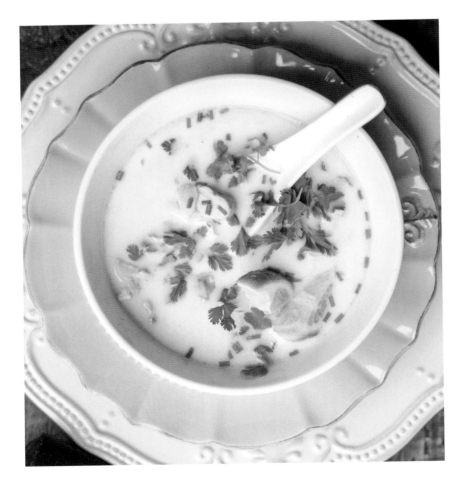

nutritional info (per serving)				
calories	fat	protein	carbs	fiber
441	27g	39g	7g	1g

MEXICAN LIME CHICKEN SOUP

prep time: **5 minutes**   cook time: **20 minutes**   yield: **6 servings**

6 cups chicken bone broth, homemade (page 106) or store-bought

2¼ cups chopped fresh cilantro, divided

4 scallions, chopped

2 tablespoons dried chives

3 cloves garlic, smashed to a paste

1 teaspoon ground cumin

1¼ pounds boneless, skinless chicken thighs, cut into 1-inch chunks (or leftover cooked turkey or chicken)

Fine sea salt and ground black pepper

2 tablespoons lime juice

Lime wedges, for garnish (optional)

1. Place the broth, 2 cups of the cilantro, scallions, chives, garlic, and cumin in a blender and blend until well combined.

2. Pour the broth mixture into a large pot. Add the chicken and bring to a boil, then reduce the heat to low and simmer until the chicken is cooked through, about 20 minutes. If using precooked chicken, reduce the simmering time to about 5 minutes.

3. Season to taste with salt and pepper. Stir in the remaining ¼ cup of cilantro and the lime juice. Ladle the soup into bowls and serve with lime wedges.

4. Store in an airtight container in the refrigerator for up to 3 days. To reheat, place the soup in a saucepan over medium heat for a few minutes, until warmed through.

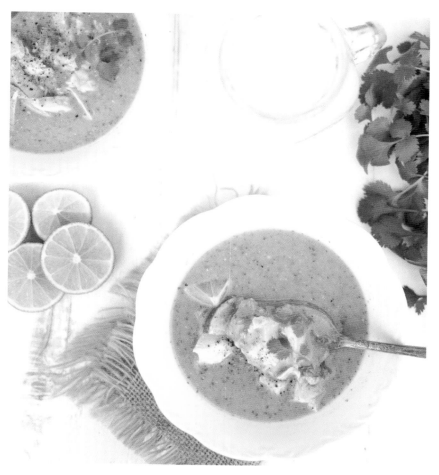

nutritional info (per serving)				
calories	fat	protein	carbs	fiber
207	13g	21g	3g	1g

CALDO DE COSTILLA
(Colombian Beef Rib Broth)

This soup is traditionally made with potatoes, but I swapped in cauliflower, a tasty ketogenic vegetable that absorbs the lovely flavor of the broth.

prep time: **10 minutes**   *cook time:* **8 hours 20 minutes**   *yield:* **6 servings**

1 pound beef short ribs

1 small tomato, diced, or ½ cup jarred diced tomatoes

1 teaspoon ground cumin

¼ teaspoon ground achiote (see Note) or paprika

Fine sea salt and ground black pepper

½ cup sliced scallions

¼ cup diced onions

2 cloves garlic, peeled

3 cups cauliflower florets, cut into ½-inch chunks

¼ cup chopped fresh cilantro

For Garnish:

Fresh cilantro leaves

Lime wedges

Diced avocado

1. Place the short ribs, tomato, cumin, achiote, 2 teaspoons of salt, 1 teaspoon of pepper, and 4½ cups of water in a 6-quart slow cooker.

2. Place the scallions, onions, and garlic in a blender with ½ cup of water and blend until smooth. Add the puree to the slow cooker. Turn the short ribs in the mixture to coat. Cover and cook on low for 8 hours, until the meat is falling off the bones.

3. Shred the meat with 2 forks and discard the bones.

4. Add the cauliflower and cilantro to the slow cooker and season with a couple pinches each of salt and pepper. Cover and cook on low for 10 to 20 more minutes, until the cauliflower is tender.

5. Ladle the soup into bowls and garnish with cilantro, lime wedges, and diced avocado before serving.

6. Store in an airtight container in the refrigerator for up to 3 days. To reheat, place the soup in a saucepan over medium heat for a few minutes, until warmed through.

Note: *Achiote is a traditional Mexican spice that you can find at specialty food stores or online.*

nutritional info (per serving)				
calories	fat	protein	carbs	fiber
377	32g	17g	5g	1g

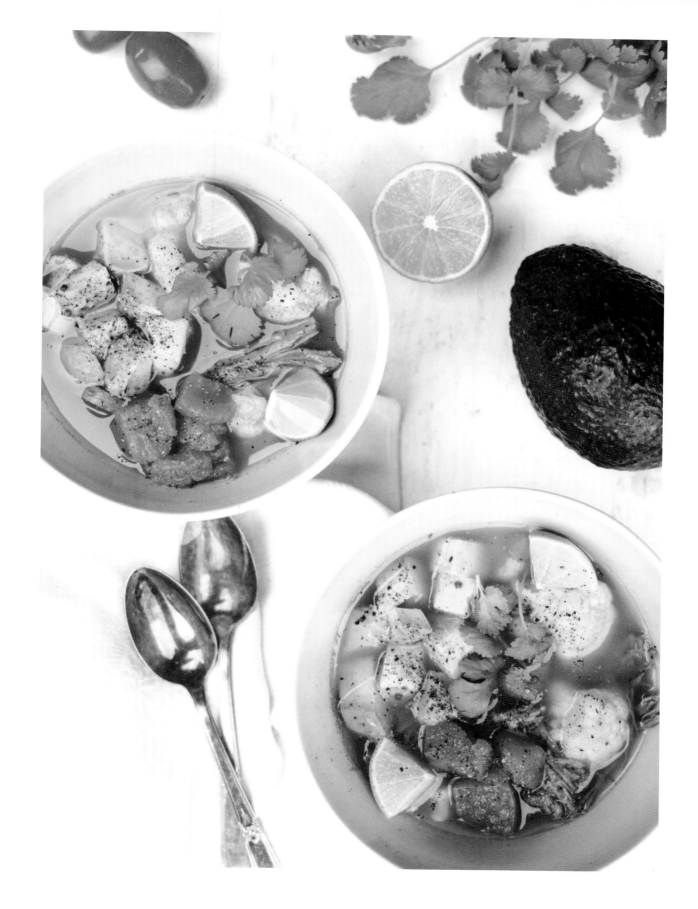

TEXAS BBQ BRISKET SOUP

prep time: **10 minutes**   *cook time:* **40 minutes**   *yield:* **8 servings**

¼ cup coconut oil or avocado oil

1½ cups diced onions

1 green bell pepper, diced

6 cloves garlic, smashed to a paste

1½ pounds brisket, cut into 2-inch chunks

Fine sea salt and ground black pepper

1 medium zucchini, diced

2 tomatoes, chopped

6 cups beef bone broth, homemade (page 106) or store-bought

¾ cup tomato sauce

3 tablespoons Swerve confectioners'-style sweetener or equivalent amount of liquid or powdered sweetener (see page 29)

3 tablespoons smoked paprika

2 teaspoons chili powder

1 teaspoon liquid smoke

For Garnish:

Fresh cilantro

Lime wedges

1. Heat the oil in a Dutch oven or soup pot over medium-high heat. Add the onions and bell pepper and sauté until the onions are soft and starting to caramelize, about 8 minutes. Add the garlic and sauté for another minute.

2. Season the brisket on all sides with salt and pepper. Add to the hot pot with the onions and garlic and sauté until browned on all sides.

3. Add the zucchini, tomatoes, broth, tomato sauce, sweetener, paprika, chili powder, 2 teaspoons of salt, 2 teaspoons of pepper, and liquid smoke. Simmer over medium heat for 20 to 30 minutes, until the brisket is tender. Shred the meat using 2 forks, then ladle the soup into bowls. Garnish with cilantro and lime wedges and serve.

4. Store in an airtight container in the refrigerator for up to 3 days. To reheat, place the soup in a saucepan over medium heat for a few minutes, until warmed through.

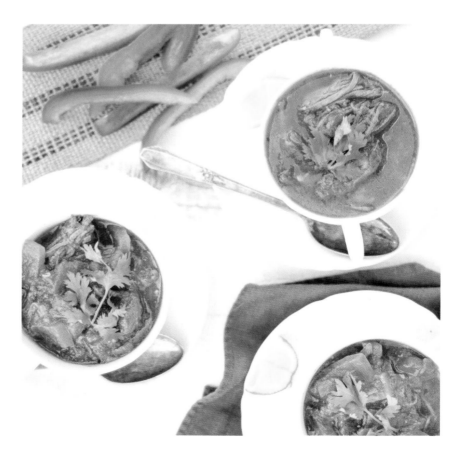

nutritional info (per serving)				
calories	fat	protein	carbs	fiber
399	30g	23g	9g	3g

PIZZA SOUP

prep time: **6 minutes**   *cook time:* **about 30 minutes**   *yield:* **4 servings**

1 tablespoon avocado oil, coconut oil, or lard

2 cups sliced mushrooms

¼ cup diced onions

¼ cup diced red bell peppers

2 cloves garlic, minced

4 ounces Italian sausage, cut into ¼-inch pieces

4 ounces uncured pepperoni, cut into quarters

1 (25-ounce) jar pizza sauce or marinara sauce (see Note)

1 (14½-ounce) can fire-roasted tomatoes

1 (3-ounce) can sliced black olives (optional)

1 tablespoon dried ground oregano

½ teaspoon fine sea salt

Fresh oregano or basil leaves, for garnish

Note: *When buying pizza sauce or marinara sauce, make sure to check the ingredients. Purchase a sauce with no added sugar or oil.*

1. Heat the oil in a deep cast-iron skillet or pot over medium heat. Add the mushrooms and onions and sauté until the mushrooms are golden brown and the onions are soft, about 5 minutes. Add the bell peppers and garlic and sauté for another 2 minutes.

2. Add the sausage and sauté until cooked through, about 3 minutes. Add the pepperoni, pizza sauce, tomatoes, olives (if using), oregano, and salt. Cook for another 15 minutes. Taste and adjust the seasoning to your liking.

3. Ladle the soup into bowls. Garnish with oregano or basil leaves and serve.

4. Store in an airtight container in the refrigerator for up to 3 days. To reheat, place the soup in a saucepan over medium heat for a few minutes, until warmed through.

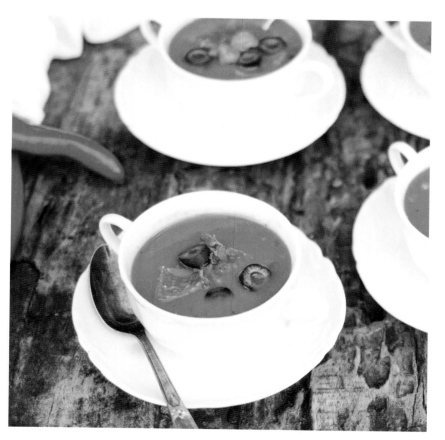

nutritional info (per serving)				
calories	fat	protein	carbs	fiber
430	35g	15g	17g	5g

CILANTRO LIME MEATBALL SOUP

Meatballs:

2 pounds ground beef

1 cup finely chopped mushrooms

¼ cup chopped onions

2 cloves garlic, minced

1 pickled jalapeño pepper, seeded and finely chopped

1 teaspoon fine sea salt

½ teaspoon ground cumin

1 large egg

1 tablespoon lard or coconut oil

¼ cup chopped onions

2 cloves garlic, minced

5 cups beef bone broth, homemade (page 106) or store-bought

1 medium tomato, diced

¼ cup chopped fresh cilantro leaves

2 tablespoons lime juice

Lime wedges, for garnish

1. Preheat the oven to 350°F.

2. Make the meatballs: Put the ground beef, mushrooms, onions, garlic, jalapeño, salt, cumin, and egg in a bowl. Work everything together with your hands.

3. Shape the meat mixture into 1-inch balls and place on a rimmed baking sheet. Bake for 15 minutes or until cooked through.

4. Meanwhile, heat the lard in a large saucepan over medium-high heat. Add the onions and sauté for 3 minutes or until soft. Add the garlic and sauté for 1 minute more. Add the broth, tomato, and cilantro, bring to a boil, and boil for 4 minutes. Reduce the heat and simmer until the meatballs are done baking.

5. Just before serving, stir in the lime juice and add the meatballs. Taste and add more salt, if desired. Ladle the soup into bowls and serve with lime wedges.

6. The soup is best served fresh, but leftovers can be stored in an airtight container in the refrigerator for up to 5 days or frozen in a freezer-safe container for up to a month. To reheat, place the soup in a saucepan over medium heat for a few minutes, until warmed through.

nutritional info (per serving)				
calories	fat	protein	carbs	fiber
309	23g	21g	3g	1g

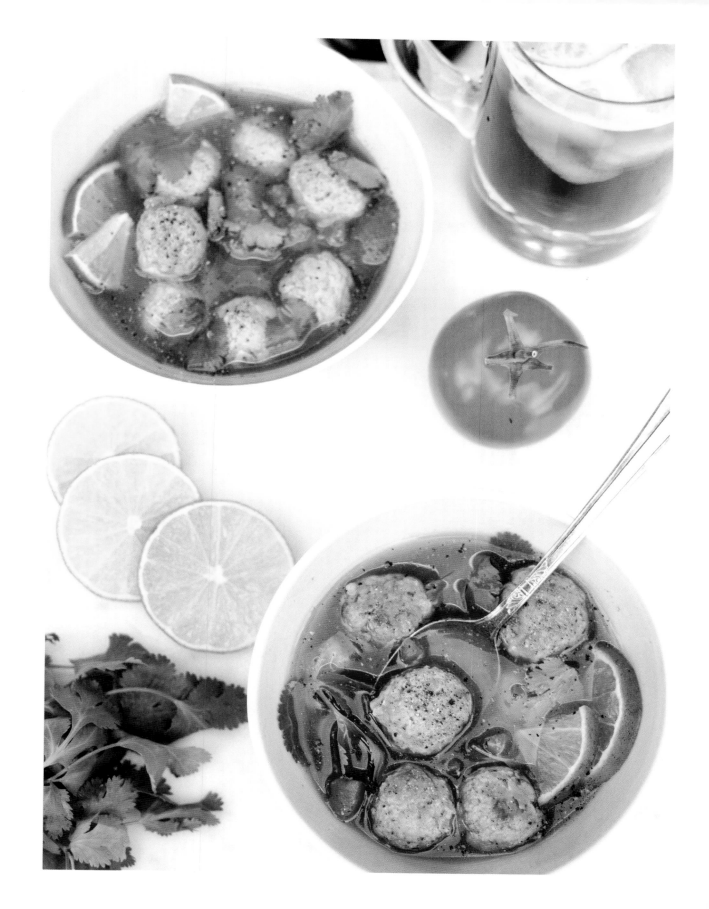

CHILLED TOMATO AND HAM SOUP

¾ pound plum tomatoes, quartered

1 clove garlic, whacked with the side of a large knife and peeled

¼ cup avocado oil, MCT oil, or extra-virgin olive oil, plus more for serving

1 tablespoon coconut vinegar, plus more for serving

Fine sea salt and ground black pepper

2 hard-boiled eggs (see page 81), peeled (omit for egg-free)

4 thin slices prosciutto (about 1 ounce), sliced into strips about ¼ inch wide

Fresh herbs of choice, for garnish (optional)

1. Place the tomatoes, garlic, oil, and vinegar in a blender or food processor and pulse until smooth. Season with salt and pepper and refrigerate for about 15 minutes, until cold.

2. Press the eggs through a sieve or colander with tiny holes.

3. Ladle the chilled soup into bowls and drizzle a little vinegar and oil on top. Serve the soup topped with the sieved hard-boiled eggs and strips of ham. Garnish with fresh herbs, if desired.

4. Store in an airtight container in the refrigerator for up to 3 days. To reheat, place the soup in a saucepan over medium heat for a few minutes, until warmed through.

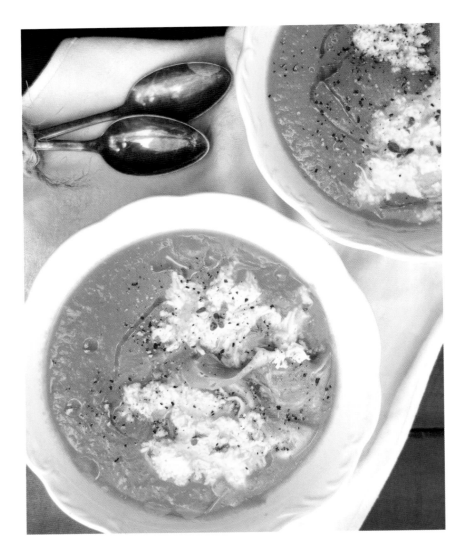

nutritional info (per serving)				
calories	fat	protein	carbs	fiber
406	36g	15g	8g	2g

TURKEY AND "ORZO" SOUP

prep time: **5 minutes**   *cook time:* **10 minutes**   *yield:* **6 servings**

1 tablespoon coconut oil

2 tablespoons finely diced onions

2 cups coarsely chopped cauliflower florets

6 cups chicken bone broth, homemade (page 106) or store-bought

1½ cups diced roasted turkey or chicken

Fine sea salt (optional)

3 tablespoons chopped fresh dill, plus extra for garnish

Freshly ground black pepper, for garnish

1. Melt the coconut oil in a Dutch oven or stockpot over medium-high heat. Add the onions and sauté for 4 minutes or until translucent. Add the cauliflower and sauté for another 3 minutes. Add the broth, turkey, and dill and simmer for 3 minutes or until heated through. Taste and add salt, if needed.

2. Ladle the soup into bowls and garnish with a sprig of dill and some freshly ground pepper before serving.

3. Store in an airtight container in the refrigerator for up to 3 days. To reheat, place the soup in a saucepan over medium heat for a few minutes, until warmed through.

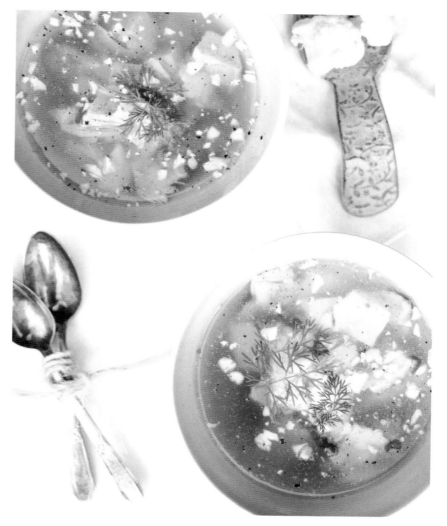

nutritional info (per serving)				
calories	fat	protein	carbs	fiber
179	10g	18g	4g	2g

MANHATTAN CLAM CHOWDER

prep time: **8 minutes** *cook time:* **20 minutes** *yield:* **4 servings**

4 strips bacon, diced

¼ cup diced onions

2 cloves garlic, minced

1 stalk celery, diced

1 green bell pepper, diced

1 small zucchini, diced

½ teaspoon dried thyme leaves

1 teaspoon fine sea salt

½ teaspoon ground black pepper

1 large tomato, diced, with juices, or 1½ cups jarred diced tomatoes with juices

2 tablespoons tomato paste

4 cups chicken bone broth, homemade (page 106) or store-bought

1 (8-ounce) bottle clam juice

2 bay leaves

2 (10-ounce) cans baby clams with liquid

For Garnish:

Avocado oil or extra-virgin olive oil

Chopped fresh parsley, oregano, or other herb of choice

1. Sauté the bacon in a stockpot or Dutch oven over medium-high heat until crisp, about 4 minutes.

2. Add the onions and garlic to the pot and sauté for 2 minutes, then add the celery, bell pepper, zucchini, and thyme. Season the veggies with the salt and pepper and sauté for 4 more minutes.

3. Add the tomato, tomato paste, broth, clam juice, and bay leaves. Bring to a boil, then lower the heat and simmer for 10 minutes.

4. Just before serving, add the clams and cook just until the clams are warmed through. Taste and add more seasoning, if desired. Ladle the soup into bowls and garnish with a drizzle of oil and parsley leaves.

5. Store in an airtight container in the refrigerator for up to 3 days. To reheat, place the soup in a saucepan over medium heat for a few minutes, until warmed through.

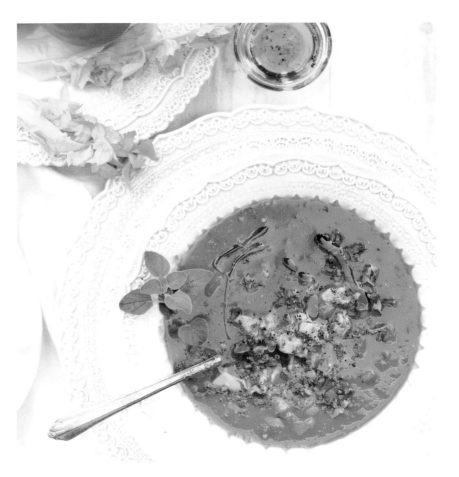

nutritional info (per serving)				
calories	fat	protein	carbs	fiber
306	14g	32g	13g	3g

STEAK FAJITA SOUP

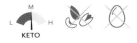

prep time: **5 minutes**   *cook time:* **4 or 7 hours**   *yield:* **4 servings**

6 cups beef or chicken bone broth, homemade (page 106) or store-bought

½ cup diced onions (about 1 medium)

1 green bell pepper, thinly sliced

1 cup sugar-free salsa

¼ cup diced jalapeño pepper

2½ teaspoons fine sea salt

2 teaspoons chili powder

1 teaspoon paprika

1 teaspoon ground cumin

½ teaspoon ground black pepper

1 pound boneless beef roast, cut into 2-inch pieces

2 limes, halved

For Garnish (optional):

Chopped fresh cilantro

Sliced avocado

Lime wedges

1. Place the broth, onions, bell pepper, salsa, jalapeño, salt, and spices in a 4-quart slow cooker. Place the beef on top.

2. Cover and cook on low for 7 hours or on high for 4 hours, until the beef is tender. Shred the meat with 2 forks. Squeeze the lime juice into the slow cooker. Taste and add more salt, if desired. Stir well. Ladle the soup into bowls and garnish with cilantro, sliced avocado, and lime wedges, if desired.

3. Store in an airtight container in the refrigerator for up to 5 days. To reheat, place the soup in a saucepan over medium heat for a few minutes, until warmed through.

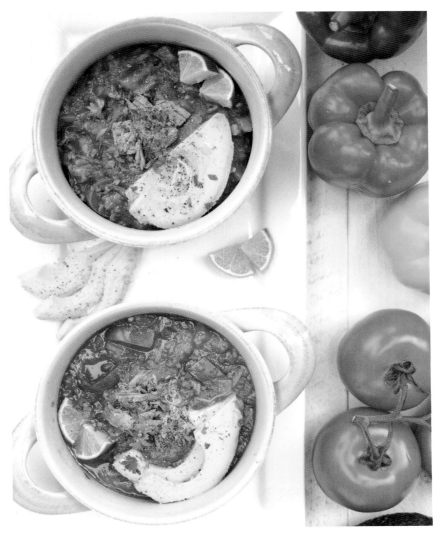

nutritional info (per serving)				
calories	fat	protein	carbs	fiber
486	32g	37g	11g	2g

SMOKY SPICY CHICKEN STEW

prep time: **7 minutes**   *cook time:* **16 minutes**   *yield:* **12 servings**

1 tablespoon lard or coconut oil

2 pounds ground chicken

2 boneless, skinless chicken thighs, cut into ½-inch dice

1 cup chopped onions

3 tablespoons minced garlic

2 tablespoons smoked paprika

1 tablespoon ground cumin

1 tablespoon dried oregano leaves

2 teaspoons fine sea salt

1 teaspoon cayenne pepper

1 (28-ounce) can diced tomatoes, with juices

2 cups chicken bone broth, homemade (page 106) or store-bought

1 (12-ounce) can lime-flavored sparkling water or seltzer water (see Note)

1 ounce unsweetened baking chocolate, finely chopped

¼ cup lime juice

¼ cup chopped fresh cilantro

For Garnish (optional):

Chopped fresh cilantro

Lime wedges or slices

Crushed red pepper

1. Combine the lard, ground chicken, diced chicken thighs, and onions in a large soup pot over medium-high heat. Cook until the onions are soft and the chicken is cooked through, about 6 minutes.

2. Add the garlic, paprika, cumin, oregano, salt, and cayenne to the pot and sauté for another minute, while stirring. Add the tomatoes with juices, broth, sparkling water, and chocolate. Simmer gently for 10 minutes to allow the flavors to develop.

3. Just before serving, stir in the lime juice and cilantro. Garnish with additional cilantro, lime wedges or slices, and some crushed red pepper, if desired.

4. Store in an airtight container in the refrigerator for up to 3 days. To reheat, place the stew in a saucepan over medium heat for 5 minutes or until warmed through.

Note: *When choosing a lime-flavored sparkling or seltzer water, look for a clean, naturally flavored water with no added sugars. I use LaCroix brand lime-flavored sparkling water.*

nutritional info (per serving)				
calories	fat	protein	carbs	fiber
278	16g	26g	6g	2g

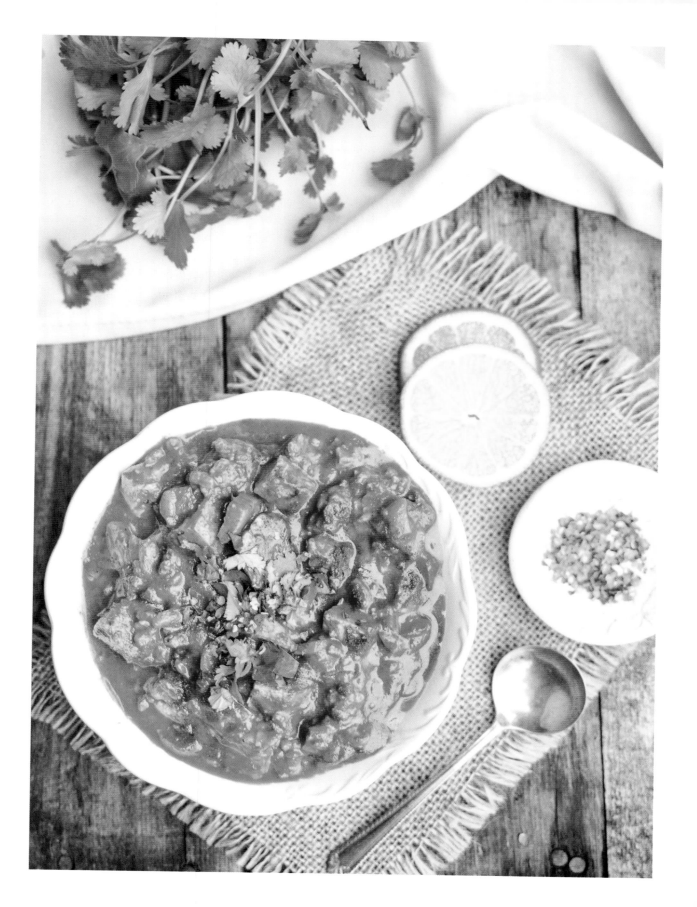

TUSCAN SAUSAGE AND "RICE" STEW

prep time: **5 minutes** *cook time:* **25 minutes** *yield:* **4 servings**

2 tablespoons coconut oil or lard, divided

1 cup diced onions

1 pound bulk Italian sausage

3 cloves garlic, minced

2 teaspoons Italian seasoning

6 large eggs

4 cups chicken bone broth, homemade (page 106) or store-bought, divided

½ teaspoon fine sea salt

½ teaspoon ground black pepper

1 cup diced fire-roasted tomatoes

½ cup fresh basil leaves

For Garnish (optional):

Crushed red pepper

Fresh oregano leaves

1. Heat 1 tablespoon of coconut oil in a stockpot over medium-high heat. Add the onions and sauté until translucent, about 3 minutes. Add the sausage, garlic, and Italian seasoning and sauté, stirring often to break up the meat, until the sausage is cooked through, about 4 minutes. Remove the sausage mixture from the pot and set aside.

2. Add the remaining tablespoon of coconut oil to the pot and heat over medium heat. In a bowl, whisk together the eggs, ¼ cup of the broth, salt, and pepper. Add the beaten egg mixture to the pot and use a whisk to cook the eggs into a ricelike consistency, scraping the bottom of the pot to deglaze, about 3 minutes.

3. Add the reserved sausage mixture, the rest of the broth, and the tomatoes to the pot. Simmer over medium heat for 6 to 8 minutes to develop the flavors.

4. Just before serving, add the basil leaves and cook for 2 minutes or until the basil is just wilted. Taste and add more salt, if desired. Garnish with crushed red pepper and fresh oregano leaves, if desired.

5. Store in an airtight container in the refrigerator for up to 4 days or freeze in a freezer-safe container for up to a month. To reheat, place the stew in a saucepan over medium heat for 5 minutes or until warmed through.

nutritional info (per serving)				
calories	fat	protein	carbs	fiber
583	45g	33g	8g	1g

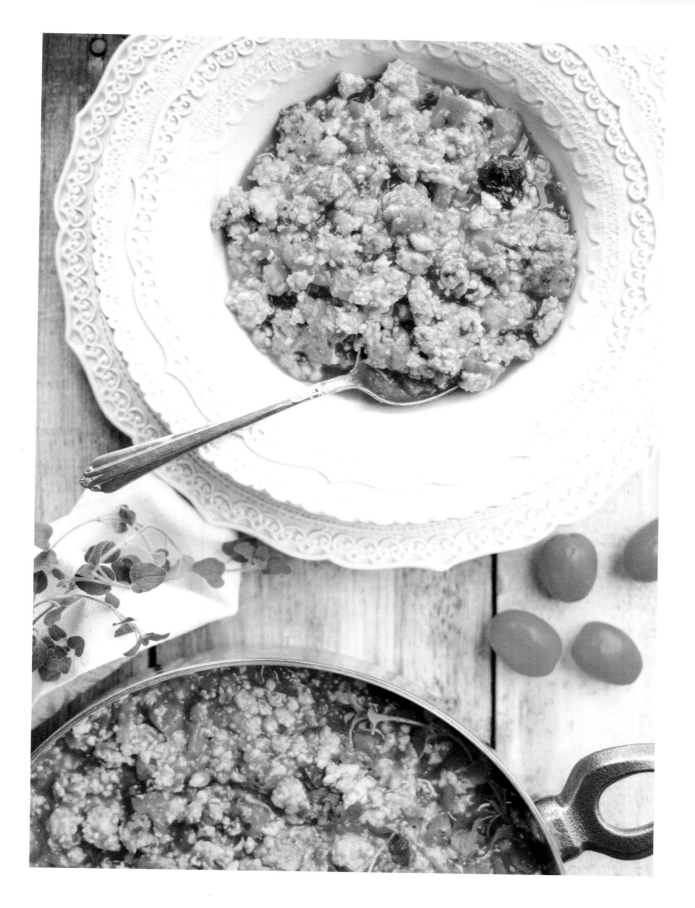

FRENCH ONION MEATBALL SOUP

Meatballs:

1 tablespoon avocado oil or lard

¼ cup chopped onions

1 clove garlic, minced

1 teaspoon fine sea salt

2 pounds ground beef

2 tablespoons beef bone broth, homemade (page 106) or store-bought

1 teaspoon dried thyme leaves

1 large egg

Soup:

3 tablespoons avocado oil or lard

2 cups thinly sliced onions

4 cups beef bone broth, homemade (page 106) or store-bought

1 teaspoon dried thyme leaves

Fine sea salt

For Garnish:

Fresh thyme leaves

Freshly ground black pepper

1. Preheat the oven to 425°F.

2. Make the meatballs: Heat the oil in a skillet over medium heat. Add the onions and garlic and season with the salt; sauté until the onions are translucent, about 5 minutes. Transfer the onion mixture to a small bowl and set aside to cool.

3. Combine the ground beef, broth, thyme, and egg in a large bowl. When the onion mixture is no longer hot to the touch, add it to the bowl with the meat mixture and work everything together with your hands.

4. Shape the meat mixture into 1¼-inch balls and place on a rimmed baking sheet. Bake for 15 minutes or until cooked through.

5. Meanwhile, make the soup: Heat the oil in a Dutch oven over medium-high heat. Add the sliced onions and sauté for 5 minutes, stirring often, until golden brown. Add the broth and thyme and boil for 10 minutes or until the onions are very soft. Taste and add salt, if desired. Ladle the onion broth into bowls and add the meatballs. Garnish with fresh thyme and freshly ground pepper.

6. Store in an airtight container in the refrigerator for up to 5 days or freeze in an freezer-safe container for up to a month. To reheat, place the soup in a saucepan over medium heat for a few minutes, until warmed through.

Note: Adding a little water or other liquid to the meatball mixture helps bind the fat to the meat when cooking, which creates a moist cooked meatball. Here I've used a couple tablespoons of broth to add both moisture and flavor. Baking the meatballs in a very hot oven results in meatballs that are crispy on the outside and tender inside.

nutritional info (per serving)				
calories	fat	protein	carbs	fiber
385	31g	22g	5g	1g

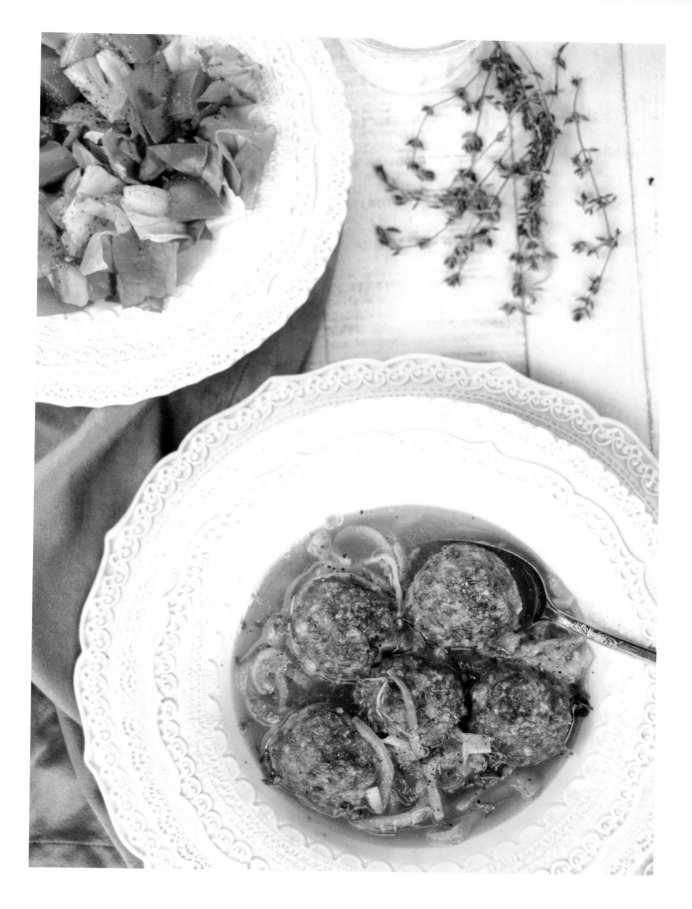

HAM AND FAUXTATO SOUP

prep time: **5 minutes**   *cook time:* **15 minutes**   *yield:* **8 servings**

3½ cups chopped cauliflower florets

⅓ cup diced celery

⅓ cup finely chopped onions

¾ cup diced cooked ham

3¼ cups chicken bone broth, homemade (page 106) or store-bought

½ teaspoon sea salt

1 teaspoon ground black pepper

5 tablespoons Kite Hill brand cream cheese style spread

1. Combine the cauliflower, celery, onions, ham, broth, salt, and pepper in a stockpot. Bring to a boil, then cover and cook over medium heat until the cauliflower is tender, 10 to 15 minutes.

2. Remove from the heat and scoop about half of the hot soup into a blender or food processor. Add the cream cheese spread and pulse until very smooth. Return the puree to the pot and stir to combine. Taste and add more salt and pepper, if desired. Ladle the soup into bowls and serve immediately.

3. Store in an airtight container in the refrigerator for up to 4 days or freeze in a freezer-safe container for up to a month. To reheat, place the soup in a saucepan over medium heat for 4 minutes or until warmed through.

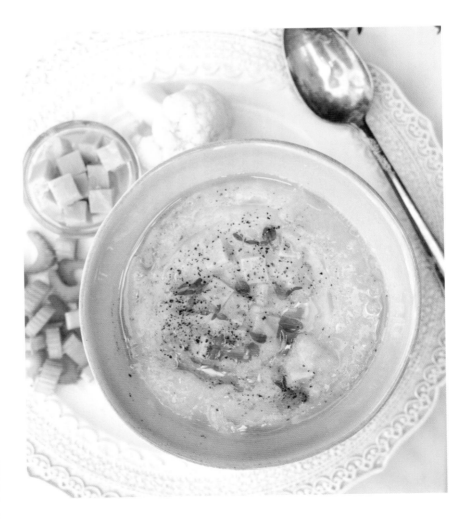

nutritional info (per serving)				
calories	fat	protein	carbs	fiber
118	8g	7g	4g	2g

SLOW COOKER THAI SOUP

prep time: 10 minutes   *cook time:* 6 hours   *yield:* 4 servings

1½ pounds boneless, skinless chicken thighs, cut into bite-sized chunks

4 cups mushrooms, sliced

½ cup sliced red bell peppers

4 scallions, white and green parts, sliced

3 cups chicken bone broth, homemade (page 106) or store-bought

1 (13½-ounce) can full-fat coconut milk

2 tablespoons Swerve confectioners'-style sweetener or equivalent amount of liquid or powdered sweetener (see page 29)

2 tablespoons red curry paste

1 teaspoon dried lemongrass

1 tablespoon peeled and grated fresh ginger

3 tablespoons lime juice

For Garnish:

⅓ cup chopped fresh cilantro

Lime wedges

Sliced scallions

Extra-virgin olive oil or avocado oil

1. Grease a 6-quart slow cooker. Place the chicken, mushrooms, bell peppers, scallions, broth, coconut milk, sweetener, curry paste, lemongrass, and ginger in the slow cooker. Cover and cook on low for 6 hours or until the chicken is very tender.

2. Stir in the lime juice, then ladle the soup into bowls. Garnish with cilantro, lime wedges, scallions, and a drizzle of oil before serving.

3. Store in an airtight container in the refrigerator for up to 4 days or freeze in a freezer-safe container for up to a month. To reheat, place the soup in a saucepan over medium heat for 4 minutes or until warmed through.

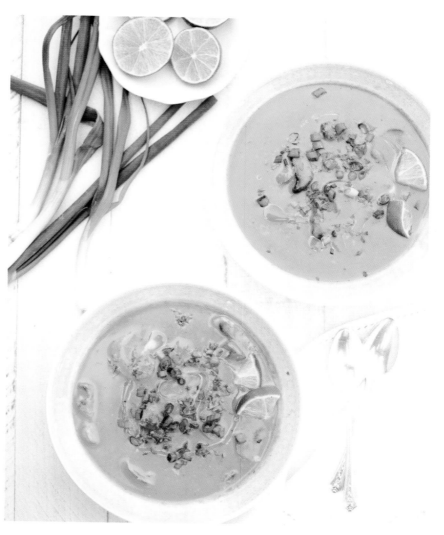

nutritional info (per serving)				
calories	fat	protein	carbs	fiber
466	32g	37g	7g	2g

CHICKEN AND "RICE" SOUP

prep time: **5 minutes**   *cook time:* **20 minutes**   *yield:* **8 servings**

6 large eggs, beaten

8 cups chicken bone broth, homemade (page 106) or store-bought, divided

½ teaspoon fine sea salt

½ teaspoon ground black pepper

2 tablespoons lard or coconut oil

1 cup diced onions

1 cup diced celery

4 boneless, skinless chicken thighs, cut into ½-inch chunks

2 sprigs fresh thyme, or 1 teaspoon dried thyme leaves

1 bay leaf

2 tablespoons lime juice

For Garnish (optional):

Fresh thyme sprigs

Extra-virgin olive oil

1. In a medium-sized bowl, combine the eggs, ¼ cup of the broth, salt, and pepper.

2. Heat the lard in a stockpot over medium-high heat. Add the onions and sauté for 3 minutes or until soft. Add the celery and cook for another 2 minutes. Add the egg mixture and use a whisk to deglaze the bottom of the pot as the eggs cook, about 3 minutes. Whisk continuously to create small pieces that resemble rice.

3. Add the remaining broth, chicken, thyme, and bay leaf to the pot. Boil for 10 minutes or until the chicken is cooked through and no longer pink. Discard the bay leaf and stir in the lime juice. Taste and adjust the seasoning to your liking.

4. Ladle the soup into bowls. Garnish with thyme leaves and a drizzle of olive oil, if desired.

5. Store in an airtight container in the refrigerator for up to 3 days. To reheat, place the soup in a saucepan over medium heat for 4 minutes or until warmed through.

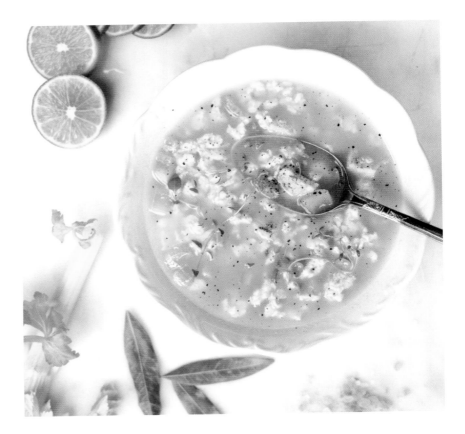

nutritional info (per serving)				
calories	fat	protein	carbs	fiber
223	14g	20g	4g	1g

ITALIAN "ORZO" SOUP

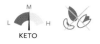

prep time: **5 minutes**   *cook time:* **18 minutes**   *yield:* **4 servings**

2 tablespoons coconut oil or lard

1 cup diced onions

1 cup diced celery

3 cloves garlic, minced

2 teaspoons Italian seasoning

8 large eggs

4 cups chicken bone broth, homemade (page 106) or store-bought, divided

½ teaspoon fine sea salt

½ teaspoon ground black pepper

1 cup chunky marinara sauce or diced fire-roasted tomatoes

1 cup fresh basil leaves

Crushed red pepper or freshly ground black pepper, for garnish

Note: *To make this soup vegetarian, simply swap out the chicken broth for vegetable broth.*

1. Heat the coconut oil in a stockpot over medium-high heat. Add the onions and celery and sauté until the onions are translucent, about 3 minutes. Add the garlic and Italian seasoning and sauté for another minute.

2. In a bowl, whisk the eggs with ¼ cup of the broth and the salt and pepper. Pour the whisked egg mixture into the pot and use a whisk to cook the eggs into a ricelike consistency, scraping the bottom of the pot to deglaze, about 3 minutes.

3. Add the remaining 3¾ cups of the broth and the marinara sauce. Simmer over medium heat for 6 to 8 minutes to develop the flavors.

4. Just before serving, add the basil leaves and cook for 2 minutes or until the basil is just getting soft. Taste and add more salt, if desired. Ladle the soup into bowls. Garnish with crushed red pepper or freshly ground black pepper and serve.

5. Store in an airtight container in the refrigerator for up to 4 days. To reheat, place the soup in a saucepan over medium heat for 4 minutes or until warmed through.

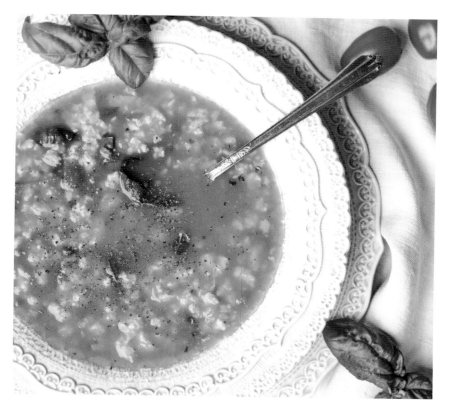

nutritional info (per serving)				
calories	fat	protein	carbs	fiber
341	26g	17g	9g	2g

THAI RED CURRY SHRIMP SOUP

prep time: **5 minutes**   *cook time:* **25 to 45 minutes**   *yield:* **4 servings**

1 tablespoon avocado oil or coconut oil

1 pound medium shrimp, peeled and deveined

Fine sea salt and ground black pepper

3 shallots, finely diced

1½ cups chicken bone broth, homemade (page 106) or store-bought

1 (13½-ounce) can full-fat coconut milk

1½ tablespoons red curry paste

¼ cup fresh cilantro leaves

¼ cup scallion pieces (about ½ inch long)

Juice of 1 lime

For Garnish:

Sliced scallions

Fresh cilantro leaves

Lime wedges

1. Heat the oil in a large cast-iron skillet over medium heat. Season the shrimp with salt and pepper and sauté for 2 minutes or until cooked through. Remove from the pan and set aside.

2. Add the shallots and sauté until tender, about 2 minutes. Reduce the heat to low. Whisk in the broth, coconut milk, and curry paste. Simmer, uncovered, stirring often, for 10 minutes or until the broth has reduced a bit. The longer you simmer, the thicker your sauce will be.

3. Stir in the cilantro, scallions, and lime juice. Return the shrimp to the pan and stir to coat in the sauce. Immediately remove the pan from the heat and ladle the soup into bowls. Garnish with sliced scallions, cilantro leaves, and lime wedges.

4. Store in an airtight container in the refrigerator for up to 4 days. To reheat, place the soup in a saucepan over medium heat for 4 minutes or until warmed through.

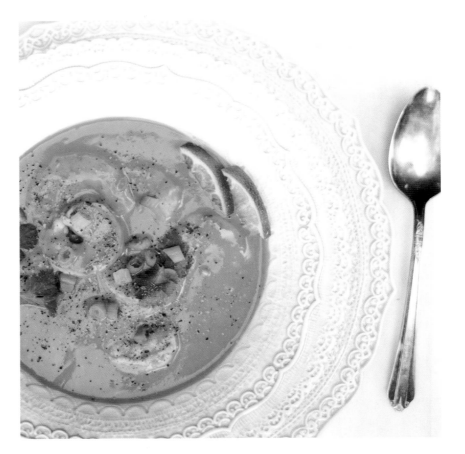

nutritional info (per serving)				
calories	fat	protein	carbs	fiber
362	23g	32g	6g	1g

SALMON SOUP

This is one amazingly flavorful soup. If you like salmon, you will love it! However, if the flavor of salmon is too intense for you, feel free to use a mild white fish, such as cod, instead.

prep time: **10 minutes** *cook time:* **20 minutes** *yield:* **4 servings**

1 tablespoon avocado oil or coconut oil

¼ cup thinly sliced red onions

2 tablespoons minced garlic

1 pound skinned salmon fillets, cut into 1-inch chunks

1 large tomato, seeded and coarsely chopped

1 tablespoon fish sauce (optional, for umami flavor)

¼ teaspoon fine sea salt

4 cups fish or chicken bone broth, homemade (page 106) or store-bought

3 tablespoons chopped fresh dill

For Garnish:

Sprigs of fresh dill

Capers

Sliced fresh chives (optional)

Freshly ground black pepper

1. Heat the oil in a saucepan over medium heat. Add the onions and cook for 4 minutes or until soft, stirring occasionally. Add the garlic and sauté for another minute or until fragrant.

2. Add the salmon, tomato, fish sauce (if using), salt, and broth. Bring to a boil over high heat, then reduce the heat to low and simmer gently for 12 minutes or until the salmon is cooked through. Serve immediately, garnished with sprigs of fresh dill, capers, chives (if using), and freshly ground pepper.

3. Store in an airtight container in the refrigerator for up to 3 days. To reheat, place in a saucepan over medium heat for 5 minutes or until warmed through.

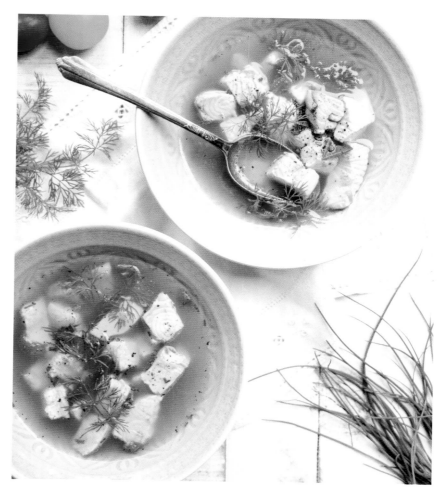

nutritional info (per serving)				
calories	fat	protein	carbs	fiber
259	14g	27g	4g	1g

CREAMY SMOKED SALMON SOUP

Looking for a soup with the creamy mouthfeel that you would get from dairy? Look no further! This creamy soup will leave your body satisfied.

prep time: 10 minutes   *cook time:* 20 minutes   *yield:* 4 servings

1 tablespoon avocado oil or coconut oil

¼ cup diced red onions

1 teaspoon minced garlic

¼ cup chopped fresh dill, or 2 teaspoons dried dill weed

4 cups chicken bone broth, homemade (page 106) or store-bought

Fine sea salt and ground black pepper

2 large eggs

2 tablespoons lemon juice

12 ounces smoked salmon

For Garnish:

2 tablespoons finely diced red onions

2 tablespoons capers

Sprigs of fresh dill

¼ cup extra-virgin olive oil or MCT oil, for drizzling (optional)

1. Heat the avocado oil in a saucepan over medium heat. Add the onions and sauté for 3 minutes or until soft. Add the garlic and dill and sauté for another minute or until fragrant. Add the broth and bring to a boil. Remove from the heat. Season with a pinch each of salt and pepper.

2. In a medium-sized bowl, whisk the eggs and lemon juice. While whisking, very slowly pour in ½ cup of the hot broth (if you add the hot broth too quickly, the eggs will curdle). Slowly pour another cup of the hot broth into the egg mixture while continuing to whisk.

3. Pour the egg and broth mixture into the pot while stirring. Reduce the heat and gently simmer for 10 minutes, stirring constantly. The soup will thicken slightly as it cooks.

4. Ladle the soup into bowls, then top each bowl with one-quarter of the smoked salmon. Garnish with the red onions, capers, and dill sprigs. Drizzle 1 tablespoon of olive oil over each bowl, if desired.

5. This soup is best served fresh because the eggs can curdle when reheating, but leftovers can be stored in an airtight container in the refrigerator for up to 2 days. To reheat, place the soup in a saucepan over medium-low heat until warmed, stirring constantly to prevent the eggs from curdling.

nutritional info (per serving)				
calories	fat	protein	carbs	fiber
365	29g	23g	4g	1g

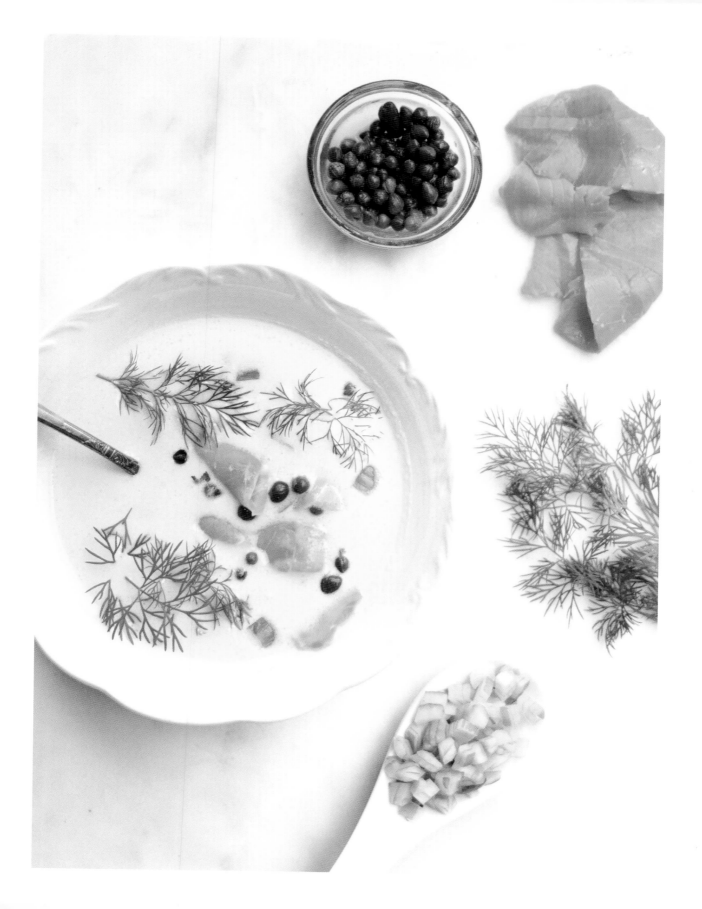

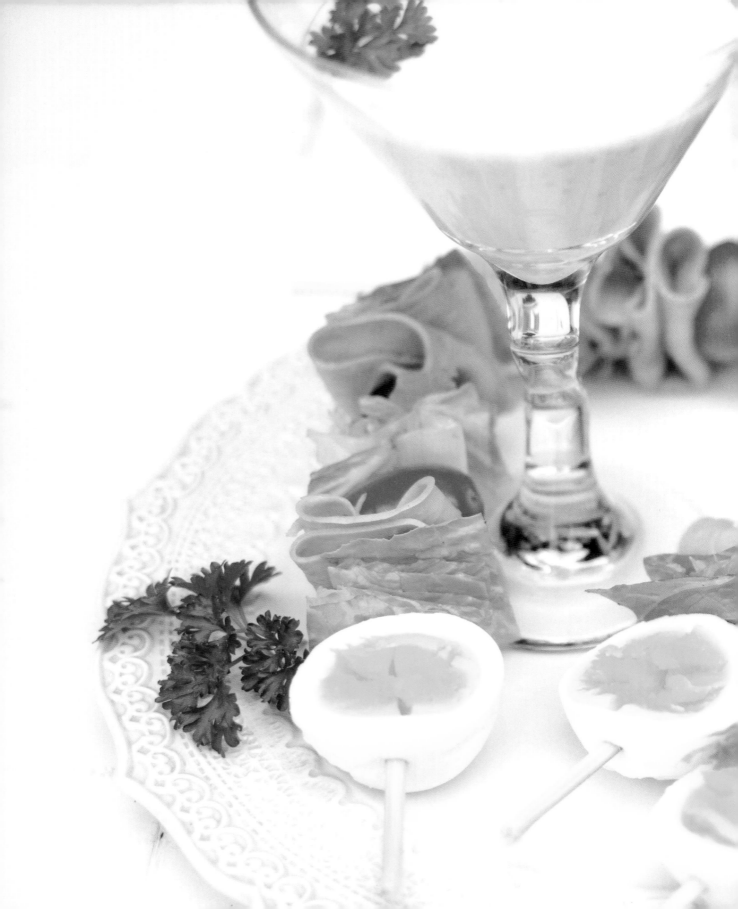

Chapter 5:
Salads and Sides

ASPARAGUS COBB SALAD
with Ranch Dressing

prep time: **8 minutes** (not including time to cook eggs) *cook time:* **10 to 20 minutes**
yield: **4 servings**

1 pound asparagus, ends trimmed

2 tablespoons melted lard, tallow, or coconut oil

½ teaspoon fine sea salt

¼ teaspoon ground black pepper

5 cloves garlic, minced

2 tablespoons chopped fresh chives, plus extra for garnish

1 cup diced ham

2 hard-boiled eggs (see page 81), peeled and chopped (omit for egg-free)

¼ cup dairy-free ranch dressing, homemade (page 45) or store-bought

1. Preheat the oven to 400°F.

2. Place the asparagus on a rimmed baking sheet. Drizzle with the melted lard and season with the salt and pepper. Turn the asparagus in the fat to coat evenly, then spread the spears out in a single layer. Top with the garlic and chives.

3. Roast the asparagus until slightly charred on the ends, 10 minutes for thin spears or 20 minutes for medium to thick spears.

4. Transfer the asparagus to a platter and top with the ham, eggs, and dressing. Garnish with additional chives.

5. This salad is best served fresh; however, you can store the salad and dressing in separate airtight containers in the refrigerator for up to 4 days.

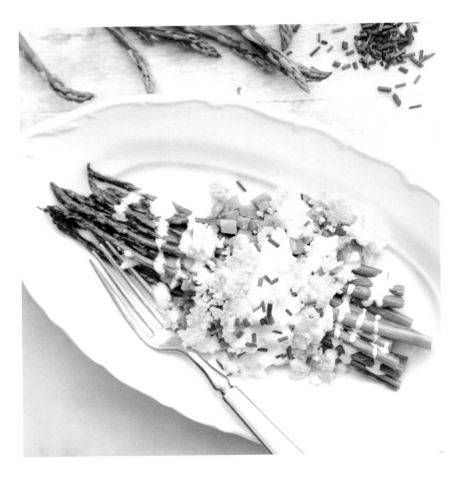

nutritional info (per serving)				
calories	fat	protein	carbs	fiber
336	26g	19g	6g	2g

BLT GRILLED ROMAINE

prep time: 5 minutes   *cook time:* 5 minutes   *yield:* 2 servings

1 medium head romaine lettuce

2 tablespoons avocado oil or extra-virgin olive oil

¼ cup dairy-free ranch dressing, homemade (page 45) or store-bought

2 tablespoons chopped tomatoes

2 tablespoons chopped scallions or chives

2 strips bacon, cooked and chopped

Lemon slices, for garnish (optional)

1. Preheat a grill to medium-high heat. Rinse the lettuce and pat completely dry.

2. Cut the head of lettuce in half lengthwise, keeping the core end intact. Brush the lettuce with the oil and grill for 4 to 5 minutes, turning occasionally, until the leaves are slightly charred.

3. Place each wedge on a plate and drizzle with the dressing. Top with the tomatoes and scallions. Garnish with the bacon and lemon slices, if desired.

4. Store the salad and dressing in separate airtight containers in the refrigerator for up to 3 days.

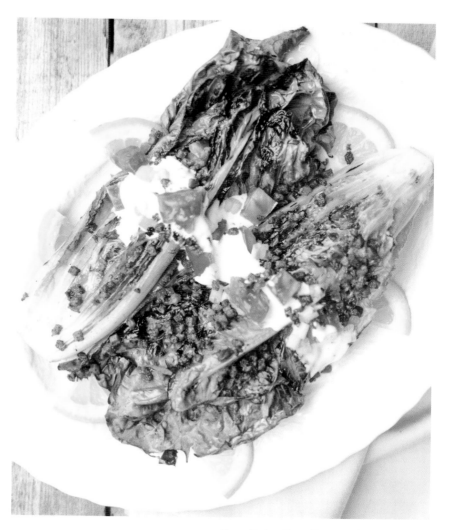

nutritional info (per serving)				
calories	fat	protein	carbs	fiber
240	25g	1g	3g	1g

CRAB LOUIE SALAD

KETO · OPTION

Once I ordered a crab Louie salad at a somewhat upscale restaurant in Hawaii, assuming that I would be getting real crab. Nope! It was imitation crab . . . yuck! This version uses canned crabmeat, which is real crab.

prep time: **6 minutes (not including time to cook eggs)** *cook time:* **3 minutes**
yield: **4 servings**

4 strips bacon, diced

1 head romaine lettuce, chopped

8 ounces canned crabmeat

4 hard-boiled eggs (see page 81), peeled and quartered (omit for egg-free)

1 tomato, diced

¼ cup diced red onions

½ cup sliced black olives

¾ cup Crab Louie Dressing (page 44), for serving

Freshly ground black pepper, for garnish

1. Fry the bacon in a skillet over medium heat, stirring often, until slightly crisp, about 3 minutes. Remove from the skillet and set aside on a paper towel–lined plate to drain and cool.

2. Make a bed of romaine lettuce on a platter. Top with a row each of egg quarters, tomatoes, onions, cooked bacon, crabmeat, and olives. Drizzle with the dressing and garnish with freshly ground pepper.

3. Store the salad and dressing in separate airtight containers in the refrigerator for up to 4 days.

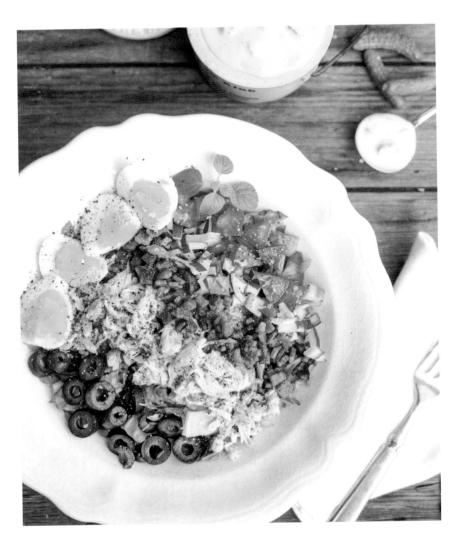

nutritional info (per serving)				
calories	fat	protein	carbs	fiber
402	31g	22g	6g	1g

SALAD KABOBS

I love to make food fun. One way I get my boys to enjoy salads is to put them on sticks and let them dip the goodness into a tasty dressing!

You can use shaved ham for this recipe if that's what you have on hand, but I usually use a large piece of ham and cut it into 1-inch chunks.

prep time: **7 minutes** *(not including time to cook eggs)* *yield:* **4 servings**

½ head iceberg lettuce, cut into 1-inch squares

8 hard-boiled eggs (see page 81), peeled and halved

1 pound sliced or cubed ham

1 cup pitted black olives

1 cup cherry tomatoes

½ cup dairy-free ranch dressing, homemade (page 45) or store-bought, for serving

Special Equipment:

8 skewers, about 8 inches long

1. Thread a few squares of lettuce onto a skewer. Add a slice of ham folded twice to form a square or cube, an olive, a few more squares of lettuce, a tomato, another cube of ham, a few more squares of lettuce, and an egg half.

2. Place the kabob on a platter and repeat with the remaining ingredients and skewers. Serve with a bowl of dressing for dipping.

3. These kabobs are best served fresh; however, you can store the kabobs and dressing in separate airtight containers in the refrigerator for up to 2 days.

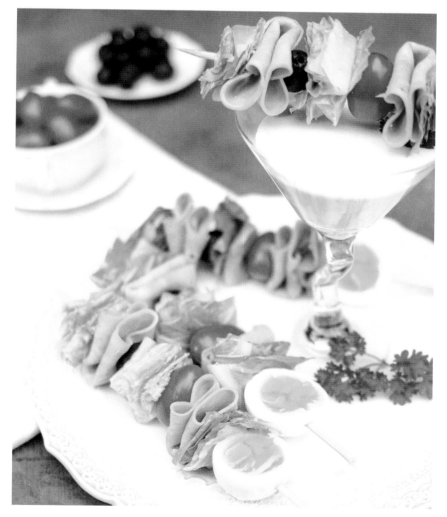

nutritional info (per serving)				
calories	fat	protein	carbs	fiber
561	44g	37g	5g	1g

CHEF'S SALAD

Dressing:

½ cup Baconnaise (page 34) or mayonnaise, homemade (page 34) or store-bought

½ cup tomato sauce

¼ cup diced dill pickles

2 tablespoons Swerve confectioners'-style sweetener or equivalent amount of liquid or powdered sweetener (see page 29)

Salad:

1 head romaine lettuce, chopped

½ pound thinly sliced roast beef

1 small avocado, pitted and sliced

4 hard-boiled (see page 81) or soft-boiled eggs , peeled and sliced

¼ small red onion, thinly sliced

Cherry tomatoes, halved, for garnish (optional)

Baby dill pickles, for garnish (optional)

Freshly ground black pepper, for garnish

I always keep hard-boiled eggs in my fridge, but to make this salad even easier, you can pick up precooked hard-boiled eggs from the grocery store!

prep time: 5 minutes (not including time to cook eggs) *yield:* 4 servings

1. Make the dressing: Place the baconnaise, tomato sauce, pickles, and sweetener in a bowl and stir to combine. Taste and adjust for seasoning, adding salt or more sweetener, if desired.

2. Arrange the chopped romaine on a platter. Top the lettuce with the roast beef slices, avocado slices, sliced hard-boiled eggs, and onion slices. Garnish with freshly ground pepper, cherry tomatoes, and baby dill pickles, if desired. Pour the dressing over the salad or serve on the side.

3. Store the salad and dressing in separate airtight containers in the refrigerator for up to 3 days.

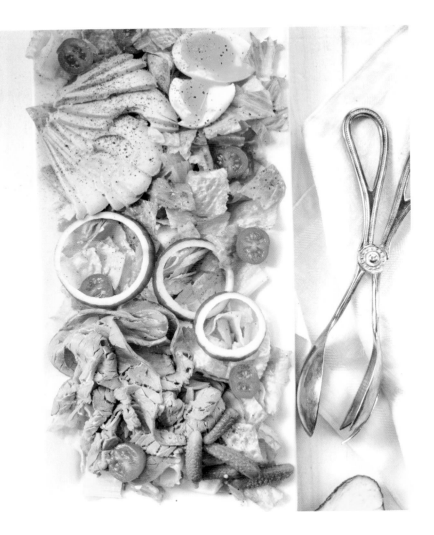

nutritional info (per serving)				
calories	fat	protein	carbs	fiber
373	31g	19g	5g	2g

GRILLED AVOCADO

prep time: **4 minutes**   *cook time:* **3 minutes**   *yield:* **4 servings**

2 ripe avocados

2 tablespoons lime or lemon juice

1 tablespoon MCT oil, avocado oil, or melted coconut oil

Fine sea salt and ground black pepper

Chopped fresh parsley, basil, or cilantro, for garnish

Sugar-free salsa, for serving (optional)

1. Preheat a grill to high heat.

2. Cut the avocados in half and remove the pits with a spoon. Drizzle with the lime juice and brush with the oil. Season well with salt and pepper.

3. Place the avocados cut side down on the grill and grill for 3 minutes or until they have softened and have grill marks. Garnish with fresh herbs and serve with salsa on the side, if desired.

4. Store in an airtight container in the refrigerator for up to 3 days. To reheat, place the avocados on a baking sheet in a preheated 350°F oven for a few minutes, until warmed through.

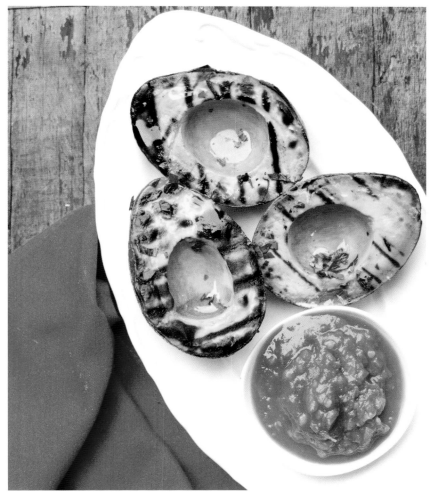

nutritional info (per serving)				
calories	fat	protein	carbs	fiber
183	17g	2g	9g	6g

KETO BRIOCHE

KETO

This very low-carb bread is not only simple to make, but also very versatile. You can bake the bread and freeze it for easy additions to future meals or use it to make sandwiches. You can even make it into Avocado Toast (page 306) or garlic toast to serve alongside my Italian Beef Tips (page 230).

prep time: 5 minutes (not including time to cook eggs) *cook time:* 1 to 40 minutes, depending on cooking method *yield:* 4 servings

3 hard-boiled eggs (see page 81), peeled

3 large eggs

2 tablespoons unflavored egg white powder

1 teaspoon baking powder

½ teaspoon fine sea salt

Optional Flavorings:

1 teaspoon garlic powder

1 teaspoon onion powder

1. If baking the brioche, preheat the oven to 350°F. Grease a standard-size 12-well muffin pan, an 8 by 4-inch loaf pan, or four 4-ounce ramekins.

2. Place all of the ingredients (including the optional flavorings, if using) in a blender and puree until smooth.

3. Pour the batter into the prepared muffin pan, filling each well about two-thirds full, or into the loaf pan, or into the ramekins, filling them about two-thirds full. Bake until a toothpick inserted in the middle comes out clean, about 12 minutes for muffins, 35 to 40 minutes for a loaf, or 13 to 17 minutes in ramekins.

4. To cook in the microwave, grease four 4-ounce microwave-safe ramekins and fill them about two-thirds full with the batter. Microwave on high for 1 minute or until a toothpick inserted in the middle of a brioche comes out clean.

5. Let cool slightly before removing the brioche from the pan or ramekins. To serve the loaf, cut it into 12 slices; to serve brioche prepared in ramekins, cut each into 3 round slices.

6. Store in an airtight container in the refrigerator for up to 4 days or in the freezer for up to a month.

nutritional info (per serving)				
calories	fat	protein	carbs	fiber
114	7g	12g	1g	0.1g

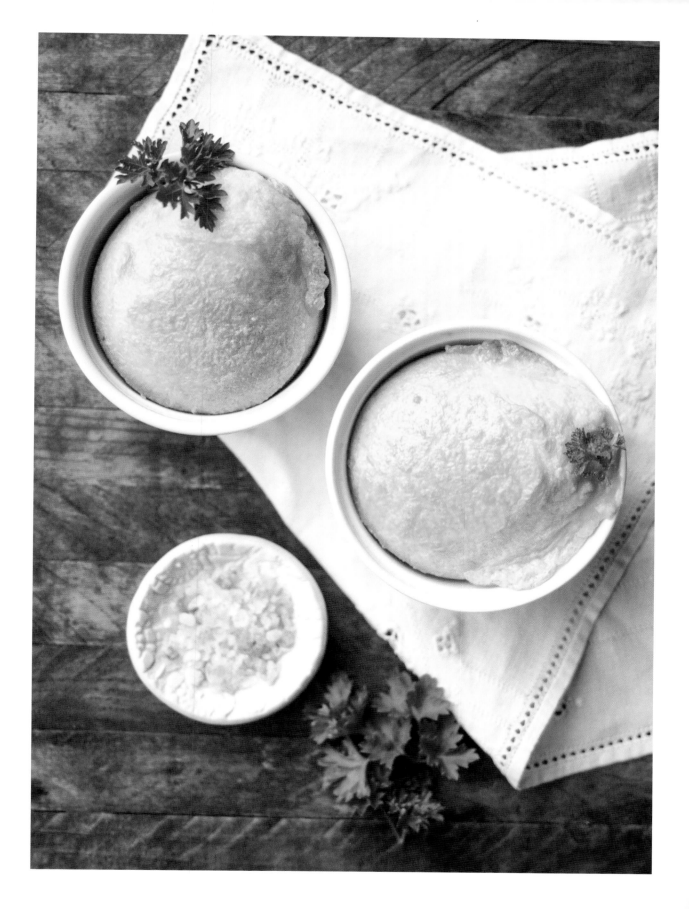

BRIOCHE CROUTONS

prep time: 5 minutes (not including time to make brioche)   cook time: 10 minutes
yield: 12 servings

1 batch Keto Brioche (page 144)

5 strips bacon, diced (see Note)

1 clove garlic, smashed to a paste

1. Preheat the oven to 350°F. Cut the brioche into 1-inch cubes and place in a large bowl. Set aside.

2. Place the bacon in a large cast-iron skillet over medium heat. Cook, stirring occasionally, until the bacon is just starting to brown but isn't crisp. Remove from the heat. Add the garlic to the pan and stir well.

3. Pour the bacon and drippings into the bowl with the brioche and toss to coat the cubes well. Place on a rimmed baking sheet and bake for 7 minutes or until the cubes are crisp and browned and the bacon has crisped. Serve over soups or salads.

4. Store in an airtight container in the refrigerator for up to 5 days or in the freezer for up to a month.

Note: *If you prefer to make these croutons without the bacon, drizzle 5 tablespoons of avocado oil or melted coconut oil over the cubed brioche and sprinkle with 1½ teaspoons of salt. Toss to coat the cubes and bake as described above. Store in an airtight container in the refrigerator for up to 4 days or in the freezer for up to a month.*

nutritional info (per serving)				
calories	fat	protein	carbs	fiber
68	5g	6g	0.4g	0g

KETO "RICE"

This amazing side tastes great with Sweet 'n' Sour Pork Meatballs (page 250), Kung Pao Meatballs (page 222), or Paella (page 184), as well as any recipe you prefer served over "rice."

prep time: **3 minutes**   *cook time:* **11 minutes**   *yield:* **4 servings**

8 large eggs

½ cup full-fat coconut milk

2 tablespoons beef bone broth, homemade (page 106) or store-bought

1 teaspoon fine sea salt

½ teaspoon ground black pepper

Chopped fresh herbs, such as cilantro, rosemary, or thyme, for garnish (optional; see Note)

1. Place the eggs, coconut milk, broth, salt, and pepper in a bowl and whisk until well combined.

2. Pour the egg mixture into a medium-sized saucepan and cook over medium heat until the mixture thickens and small curds form, continuously scraping the bottom of the pan and stirring to keep larger curds from forming. (A whisk works well for this task.) This will take about 5 minutes.

3. Place the "rice" on a platter. If extra liquid is released, soak it up with a paper towel before serving. Garnish with herbs, if desired.

4. Store in an airtight container in the refrigerator for up to 4 days. To reheat, place the rice in a lightly greased skillet over medium heat and sauté, stirring often, for 3 minutes or until warmed through.

Note: *Feel free to use your favorite herb for garnish. For the best flavor, keep in mind the flavors of the main dish that the rice will be accompanying when choosing an herb.*

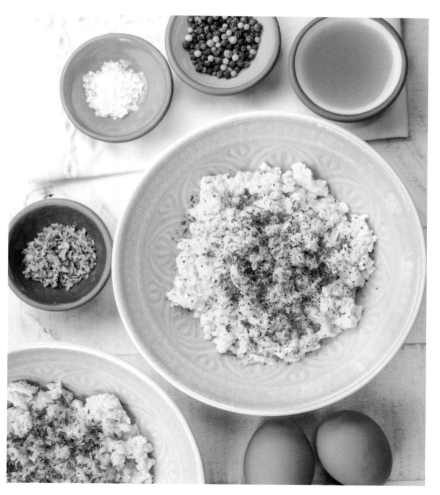

nutritional info (per serving)				
calories	fat	protein	carbs	fiber
194	14g	13g	1g	0.1g

KETO FRIED "RICE"

8 large eggs

⅓ cup full-fat coconut milk

1 tablespoon plus 1 teaspoon beef bone broth, homemade (page 106) or store-bought

¼ teaspoon wheat-free tamari, or 2 teaspoons coconut aminos

½ teaspoon fine sea salt

Pinch of ground black pepper

2 strips bacon, diced

3 tablespoons diced onions

½ teaspoon minced garlic

Sliced scallions, for garnish

1. Place the eggs, coconut milk, broth, tamari, salt, and pepper in a bowl and whisk until well combined.

2. In a large saucepan, cook the diced bacon over medium heat until crisp, about 2 minutes. Using a slotted spoon, remove the bacon, leaving the drippings in the pan. Add the onions and garlic and sauté until the onions are translucent, about 2 minutes.

3. Pour the egg mixture into the pan and cook until the mixture thickens and small curds form, continuously scraping the bottom of the pan and stirring to keep large curds from forming. (A whisk works well for this task.) This will take about 7 minutes.

4. Stir in the reserved bacon. Place the "rice" on a platter. Garnish with scallions.

5. Store in an airtight container in the refrigerator for up to 4 days or freeze for up to a month. To reheat, place the rice in a skillet over medium-high heat and sauté for 3 minutes or until warmed through.

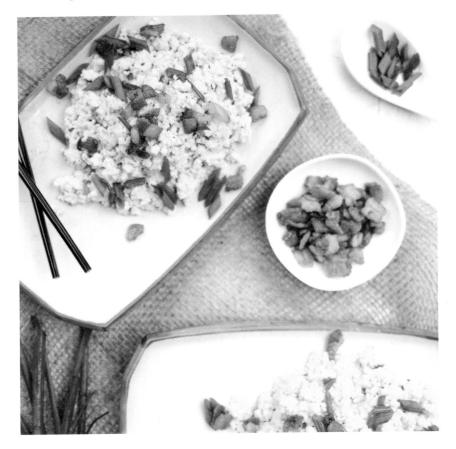

nutritional info (per serving)				
calories	fat	protein	carbs	fiber
217	16g	15g	2g	0.2g

CAULIFLOWER RICE

prep time: 5 minutes   *cook time:* 5 minutes   *yield:* 4 servings (½ cup per serving)

2 cups small cauliflower florets, about 1 inch in size

2 tablespoons coconut oil

Fine sea salt

1. Place the cauliflower florets in a food processor. Pulse until you have small pieces of "rice."

2. Heat the oil in a large skillet over medium-low heat. When hot, add the riced cauliflower and cook for 4 minutes, stirring occasionally, or until the cauliflower is soft but not mushy. Season with salt to taste.

3. Store in an airtight container in the refrigerator for up to 3 days. To reheat, place the cauliflower rice in a lightly greased sauté pan over medium heat, stirring, for 2 minutes or until warmed through.

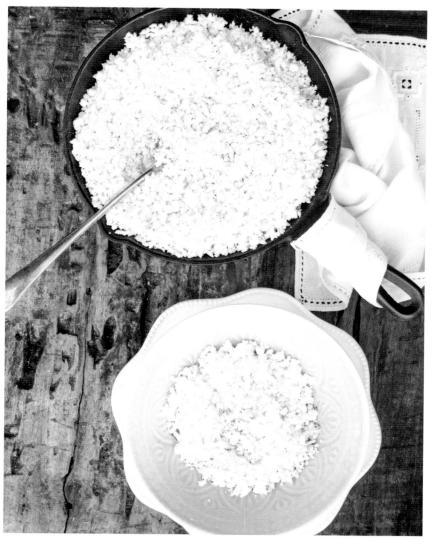

nutritional info (per serving)				
calories	fat	protein	carbs	fiber
70	7g	1g	2g	1g

KETO TORTILLAS

These tortillas taste great with Chicken Tinga (page 162), Chicken Shawarma (page 158), or South of the Border Steak (page 200), or whenever you want a tortilla-like bread to scoop up all the good flavors on your plate.

prep time: **8 minutes**   *cook time:* **4 minutes per tortilla**
yield: **8 tortillas (2 per serving)**

3 large eggs, separated (see Note)

2 tablespoons unflavored egg white or beef protein powder

1 teaspoon onion powder (optional)

Coconut oil or lard, for frying

1. Place the egg whites in a clean, dry bowl and whip with a hand mixer, or whip in a stand mixer, until they are very stiff. Slowly add the protein powder and onion powder, if using.

2. Place the egg yolks in a small bowl and beat with a fork, then gently stir the yolks into the egg white mixture.

3. Heat 2 tablespoons of oil in an 8-inch skillet over medium-high heat. Scoop ¼ cup of the dough into the skillet and flatten with a spoon to form a 5-inch circle that is about ¼ inch thick. Fry the tortilla until firm and golden brown on both sides, about 2 minutes per side.

4. Remove the tortilla from the skillet and set on paper towels to drain the excess oil. Then transfer the tortilla to a platter and cover to keep warm until ready to serve. Repeat with the remaining dough, adding more oil to the skillet between tortillas as needed.

5. Store in an airtight container in the refrigerator for up to a week or in the freezer for up to a month. To reheat, place one tortilla at a time in a skillet over medium-high heat and warm each side for about 30 seconds.

Note: *Make sure there are no spots of yolk in the egg whites or this recipe won't work.*

nutritional info (per serving)				
calories	fat	protein	carbs	fiber
68	4g	7g	0.3g	0g

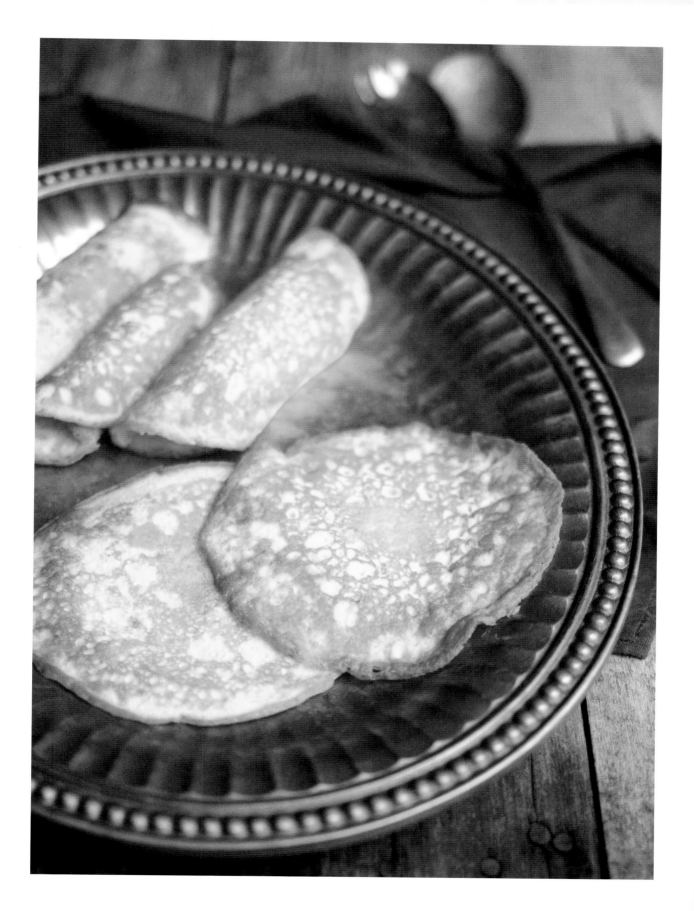

CABBAGE PASTA

KETO

¼ cup coconut oil

4 cups very thinly sliced green cabbage (about 1 small head)

I prefer cabbage pasta over zoodles. One reason is that cabbage pasta does not get soggy when sauced. It also can be stored with the sauce—not only will it hold up well, but it also grabs onto flavors and tastes even better as leftovers!

prep time: **10 minutes** *cook time:* **15 minutes** *yield:* **4 servings (¾ cup per serving)**

Melt the oil in a large sauté pan over medium heat. Add the cabbage and sauté until very tender, about 15 minutes, stirring often to prevent it from burning. Store in an airtight container in the refrigerator for up to 5 days.

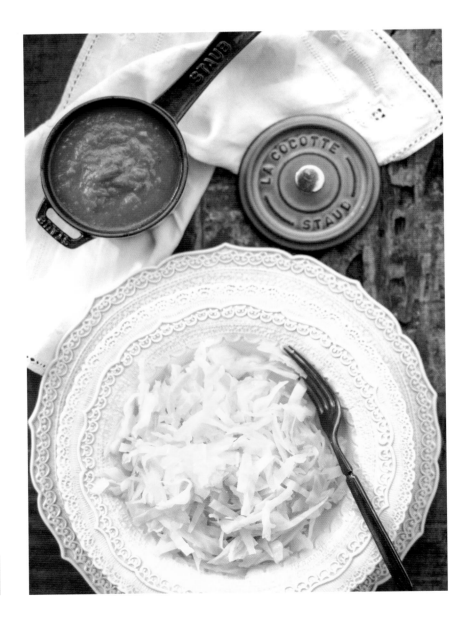

nutritional info (per serving)				
calories	fat	protein	carbs	fiber
117	11g	1g	4g	2g

CHOW CHOW

Chow chow is a popular condiment that tastes great over hot dogs and brats. It's readily available at most grocery stores, but most store brands are sweetened with sugar. If you want your chow chow to taste like these sweetened versions, add the sweetener; however, if you want it to have more of a tang without the added sweetness, feel free to omit the sweetener.

prep time: **10 minutes**   *cook time:* **10 minutes**   *yield:* **10 servings**

¼ cup Swerve confectioners'-style sweetener or equivalent amount of liquid or powdered sweetener (see page 29) (optional)

1 tablespoon fine sea salt

1 teaspoon dry mustard

1 teaspoon mustard seeds

½ teaspoon crushed red pepper

¼ teaspoon celery seeds

¼ teaspoon ginger powder

¼ teaspoon turmeric powder

½ cup coconut vinegar or apple cider vinegar

2 cups diced green bell peppers

2 cups diced red bell peppers

1 cup diced firm green tomatoes

1 cup diced white onions

1 cup diced cabbage

1. In a large non-reactive skillet, bring 3 tablespoons of water along with the sweetener, salt, and spices to a simmer. Add the vinegar and bring to a boil, then add the vegetables.

2. Stir to coat the vegetables, then reduce the heat to medium and continue to cook, stirring occasionally, until the vegetables are tender, 5 to 10 minutes.

3. Transfer to glass jars and, once cool, seal and refrigerate.

4. Store in the refrigerator for up to 3 weeks or in the freezer for up to a month.

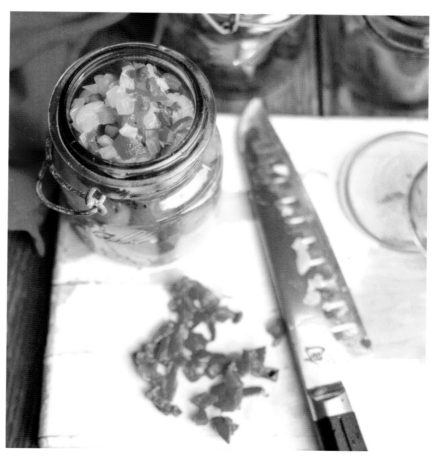

nutritional info (per serving)				
calories	fat	protein	carbs	fiber
30	0.2g	1g	6g	2g

BACON-WRAPPED PORTOBELLO FRIES

prep time: **7 minutes**   *cook time:* **15 minutes**   *yield:* **2 servings**

6 strips thin-cut bacon, cut in half lengthwise

2 large portobello mushrooms, sliced into ¼-inch-thick fries

Chopped fresh parsley or cilantro, for garnish

¼ cup Creamy Lime Sauce (page 38) or dairy-free ranch dressing, homemade (page 45) or store-bought, for serving

1. Preheat the oven to 400°F.

2. Wrap a strip of bacon around each mushroom "fry." Secure the ends with toothpicks. Place the bacon-wrapped fries on a rimmed baking sheet. Bake for 15 minutes or until the bacon is crispy. Place on a platter. Garnish with parsley and serve with the dipping sauce.

3. Store in an airtight container in the refrigerator for up to 3 days. To reheat, place the fries on a rimmed baking sheet in a preheated 400°F oven for a few minutes, until warmed through.

Note: *To make this dish egg-free, omit the dipping sauces or make them with Egg-Free Mayo (page 35).*

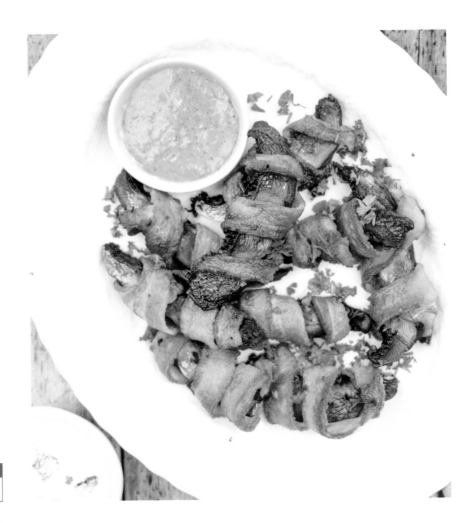

nutritional info (per serving)				
calories	fat	protein	carbs	fiber
230	18g	15g	3g	1g

ASIAN COLESLAW

prep time: **10 minutes** *yield:* **4 servings**

1 tablespoon wheat-free tamari, or ¼ cup coconut aminos

2 tablespoons avocado oil or extra-virgin olive oil

2 tablespoons Swerve confectioners'-style sweetener or equivalent amount of liquid or powdered sweetener (see page 29), or more to taste

2 tablespoons lime juice, or more to taste

½ tablespoon peeled and grated fresh ginger

4 drops orange oil, or 1 teaspoon orange extract (optional)

2 cups shredded red or green cabbage

¼ cup chopped scallions

½ teaspoon fine sea salt

For Garnish:

1 tablespoon toasted sesame seeds

1 tablespoon sliced scallions

1. Place the tamari, oil, sweetener, lime juice, ginger, and orange oil, if using, in a medium-sized bowl. Stir well to combine. Add the cabbage and scallions and toss to coat well.

2. Season with the salt. Taste and adjust seasoning to your liking, adding more salt, sweetener, or lime juice. Garnish with the toasted sesame seeds and sliced scallions before serving.

3. Store in an airtight container in the refrigerator for up to 5 days.

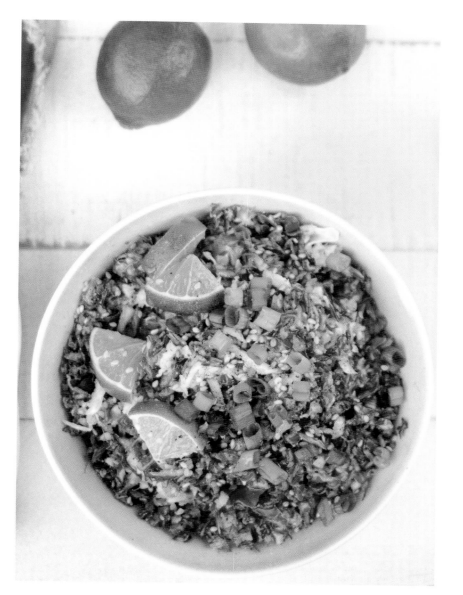

nutritional info (per serving)				
calories	fat	protein	carbs	fiber
100	9g	2g	5g	2g

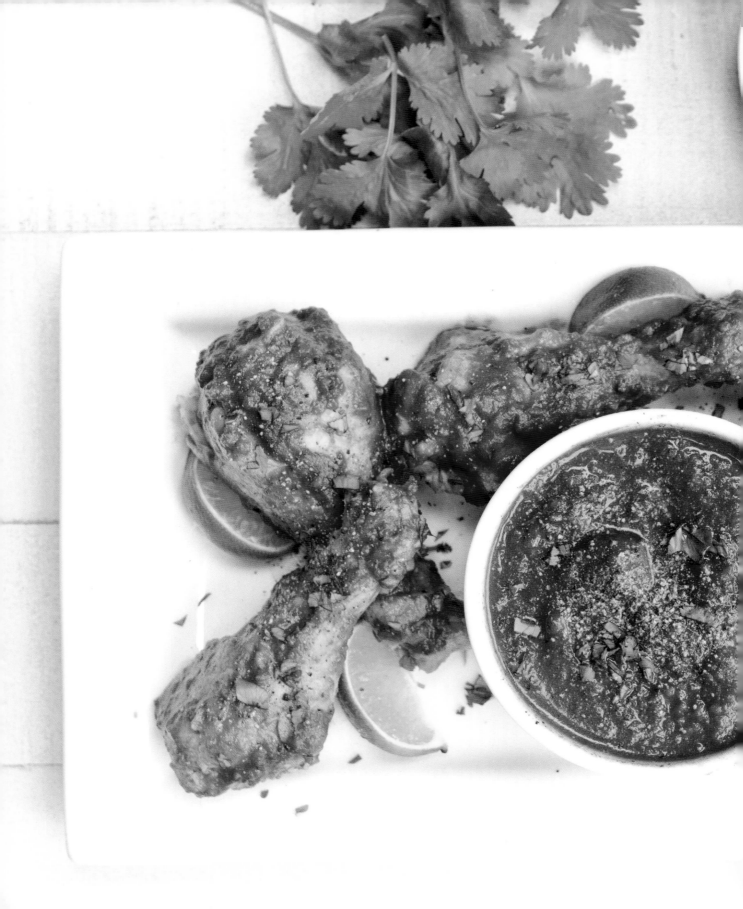

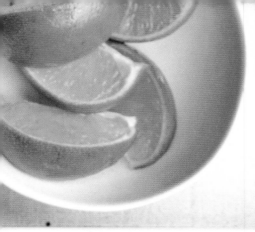
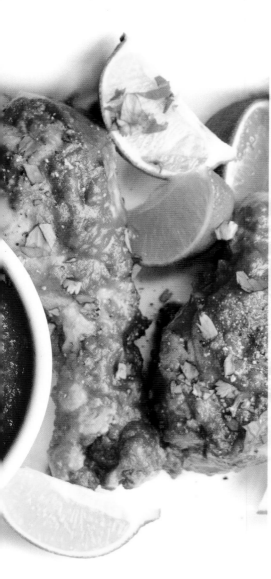

Chapter 6:
Poultry

CHICKEN SHAWARMA

L M H
KETO   OPTION

This tasty chicken dish tastes great served with Cauliflower Rice (page 149) or Keto Tortillas (page 150).

prep time: 10 minutes, plus 1 hour to marinate (not including time to make tortillas)
cook time: 30 minutes *yield:* 4 servings

Marinade:

¼ cup avocado oil or extra-virgin olive oil

Juice of 2 lemons

3 cloves garlic, smashed to a paste

½ teaspoon fine sea salt

1 teaspoon ground cumin

1 teaspoon paprika

½ teaspoon ground black pepper

½ teaspoon turmeric powder

⅛ teaspoon ground cinnamon

⅛ teaspoon crushed red pepper

1 pound boneless, skinless chicken thighs

¼ cup sliced red onions

1 batch Keto Tortillas (page 150), for serving (omit for egg-free)

Topping Suggestions:

Cucumber slices

Lemon slices

Chopped fresh parsley

Handful of Greek olives

Diced red onions

Handful of grape tomatoes

Greek Vinaigrette (page 46), for drizzling

1. Make the marinade: Combine the oil, lemon juice, garlic, salt, and spices in a baking dish. Place the chicken thighs and onions in the dish and turn to coat well. Cover and refrigerate for 1 hour or overnight.

2. Preheat the oven to 425°F. Grease a rimmed baking sheet.

3. Remove the chicken and onions from the marinade and place on the prepared baking sheet. Bake for 30 minutes or until the chicken is no longer pink in the center.

4. When the chicken is done, remove the pan from the oven and transfer the chicken to a cutting board to rest for a few minutes. Slice the chicken into thin strips. Serve the chicken and onions with tortillas along with the toppings of your choice.

5. Store in an airtight container in the refrigerator for up to 3 days. To reheat, place the chicken on a rimmed baking sheet in a preheated 350°F oven for 5 minutes or until warmed through.

nutritional info (per serving)				
calories	fat	protein	carbs	fiber
358	26g	28g	5g	1g

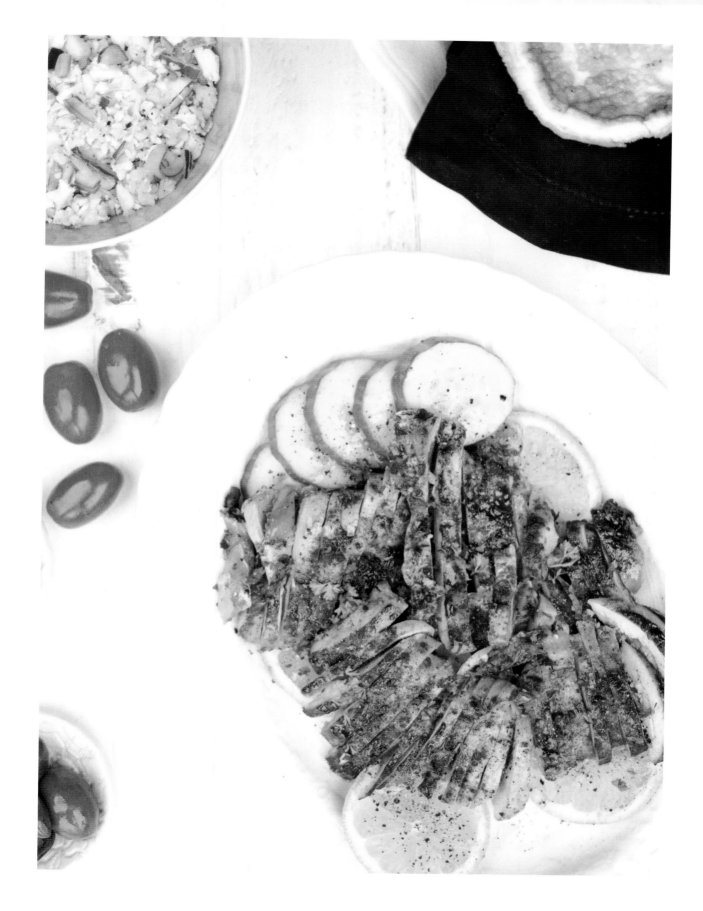

BLT CHICKEN KABOBS

prep time: 8 minutes, plus time to marinate chicken   cook time: 15 minutes

yield: 4 servings (2 kabobs per serving)

Marinade:

½ cup MCT oil or extra-virgin olive oil

Juice of 1 lime

3 cloves garlic, chopped

1 teaspoon fine sea salt

1 teaspoon ground black pepper

1 tablespoon chopped fresh tarragon or parsley

1 teaspoon chopped fresh oregano

Kabobs:

2 whole boneless, skinless chicken breasts (about 2 pounds), or 4 boneless, skinless thighs, cut into 1 by ½-inch pieces

16 grape tomatoes

8 strips thin-cut bacon

Boston lettuce leaves, for serving (optional)

Suggested Dipping Sauces:

Comeback Sauce (page 37)

Cilantro Lime Dressing (page 39)

Dairy-free ranch dressing, homemade (page 45) or store-bought

Special Equipment:

8 wood skewers, soaked in water for 15 minutes

1. In a large bowl, combine the ingredients for the marinade. Add the chicken pieces and toss to coat. Cover and refrigerate for at least 6 hours or overnight.

2. Preheat a grill to high heat.

3. Take a grape tomato and place it on a skewer, about 2 inches from the bottom of the skewer. Next, take a strip of bacon and thread one end onto the skewer. Take a piece of the marinated chicken and place it on the skewer, next to the bacon. Drape the bacon over the chicken, then add another piece of chicken.

4. Repeat Step 3 three more times, weaving the strip of bacon between pieces of chicken. End with another grape tomato. Repeat with the remaining skewers and ingredients.

5. Lightly brush the hot grill grate with oil. Place the kabobs on the grill and cook for about 15 minutes, turning once halfway through cooking, until the bacon is slightly crispy and the juices of the chicken run clear when a piece of chicken is pierced.

6. Remove from the grill and allow to rest for 5 minutes.

7. Remove the kabobs from the skewers and wrap in lettuce leaves, if desired. Serve with the dipping sauces.

8. Store in an airtight container in the refrigerator for up to 4 days. The leftover kabobs taste great chilled.

Busy Family Tip: *To save time, prepare and refrigerate the dipping sauces you want to serve with the kabobs the night before.*

nutritional info (per serving)				
calories	fat	protein	carbs	fiber
295	18g	30g	3g	1g

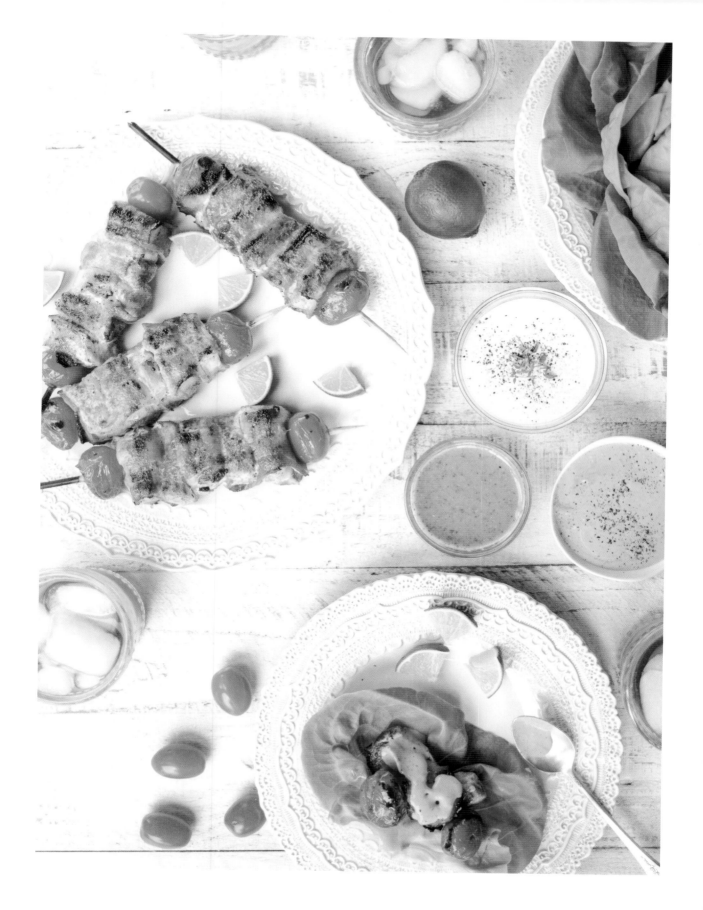

CHICKEN TINGA
with Keto Tortillas

prep time: **10 minutes** *cook time:* **40 minutes** *yield:* **4 servings**

Chicken:

1 pound bone-in, skin-on chicken thighs

¼ cup chopped onions

1 tablespoon minced garlic

1 tablespoon fine sea salt

½ tablespoon ground black pepper

4 ounces Mexican-style fresh (raw) chorizo, removed from casings

½ large white onion, chopped

1 clove garlic, minced

3 cups chopped tomatoes

1 cup husked and chopped tomatillos

2 tablespoons pureed chipotle

1½ teaspoons fine sea salt

1 teaspoon ground black pepper

½ teaspoon dried oregano leaves

1 sprig fresh marjoram

1 sprig fresh thyme

½ cup chicken bone broth, homemade (page 106) or store-bought

1 batch Keto Tortillas (page 150) (omit for egg-free), or 8 large lettuce leaves, for serving

1. Place the chicken, onions, garlic, salt, and pepper in a deep saucepan with 5 cups of water. Bring to a boil over high heat, then reduce the heat to medium and simmer for 20 minutes.

2. Remove the chicken to a cutting board. Using 2 forks, remove the chicken from the bones and shred it; discard the bones and set the shredded chicken aside.

3. Crumble the chorizo into a large cast-iron skillet. Place the skillet over medium heat, add the onion and garlic, and cook, stirring often, until the sausage is cooked through, about 5 minutes. Add the shredded chicken, tomatoes, tomatillos, chipotle, salt, pepper, and herbs. Continue cooking for 5 minutes, then add the chicken broth and cook for 5 more minutes. Remove the marjoram and thyme sprigs. Serve with tortillas or lettuce leaves.

4. Store in an airtight container in the refrigerator for up to 3 days. To reheat, place the chicken in a saucepan over medium heat for a few minutes, until warmed to your liking.

nutritional info (per serving)				
calories	fat	protein	carbs	fiber
506	33g	41g	10g	2g

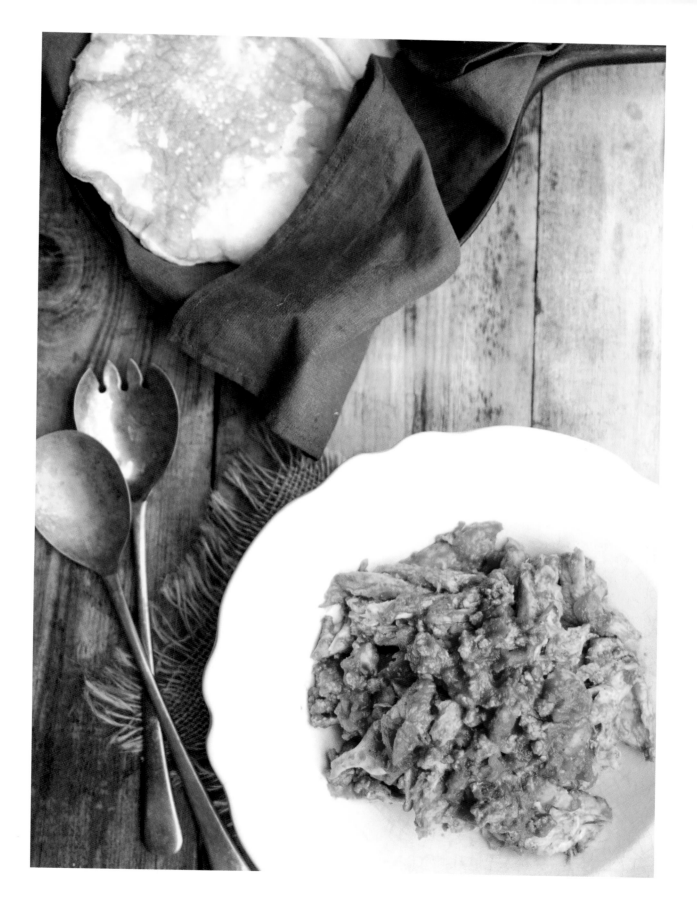

GUACAMOLE LOVERS' STUFFED CHICKEN

To make this dish even easier to prepare, ask your butcher to pound out the chicken to a ¼-inch thickness! I do so all the time to save myself time and effort in the kitchen.

prep time: **10 minutes**   *cook time:* **17 minutes**   *yield:* **4 servings**

Guacamole:

1 avocado, peeled and pitted

1½ tablespoons lime juice, or more to taste

1 small plum tomato, diced

¼ cup finely diced onions

1 small clove garlic, smashed to a paste

1½ tablespoons chopped fresh cilantro leaves

¼ scant teaspoon fine sea salt

¼ scant teaspoon ground cumin

4 boneless, skinless chicken breast halves (about 2 pounds), pounded to ¼ inch thick

8 strips thin-cut bacon

For Serving:

Lime wedges

Grape tomatoes

1 batch Pico de Gallo (page 85) (optional)

1. Preheat the oven to 425°F.

2. Make the guacamole: Place the avocado and lime juice in a large bowl and mash until it reaches your desired consistency. Add the tomato, onions, garlic, cilantro, salt, and cumin and stir until well combined. Taste and add more lime juice, if desired. Place in a large resealable plastic bag, squeeze out all the air, and seal shut. (*Note:* If making the guacamole ahead of time, it will keep in the refrigerator for up to 3 days when stored this way.)

3. Place a chicken breast on a cutting board. Take a sharp knife and, holding it parallel to the chicken, make a 1-inch-wide incision at the top of the breast. Carefully cut into the breast to form a large pocket, leaving a ½-inch border along the sides and bottom. Repeat with the other 3 chicken breasts.

4. Cut a ¾-inch hole in one corner of the plastic bag with the guacamole, then squirt the guacamole into the pockets in the chicken breasts, dividing the guacamole evenly among them.

5. Wrap 2 strips of bacon around each chicken breast and secure the ends with toothpicks. Place the bacon-wrapped chicken on a rimmed baking sheet. Bake until the bacon is crisp and the chicken is cooked through, about 17 minutes. Serve with lime wedges, tomatoes, and pico de gallo, if desired.

6. Store in an airtight container in the refrigerator for up to 3 days. To reheat, place the chicken on a rimmed baking sheet in a preheated 400°F oven for 5 minutes or until warmed through.

nutritional info (per serving)				
calories	fat	protein	carbs	fiber
469	28g	45g	8g	4g

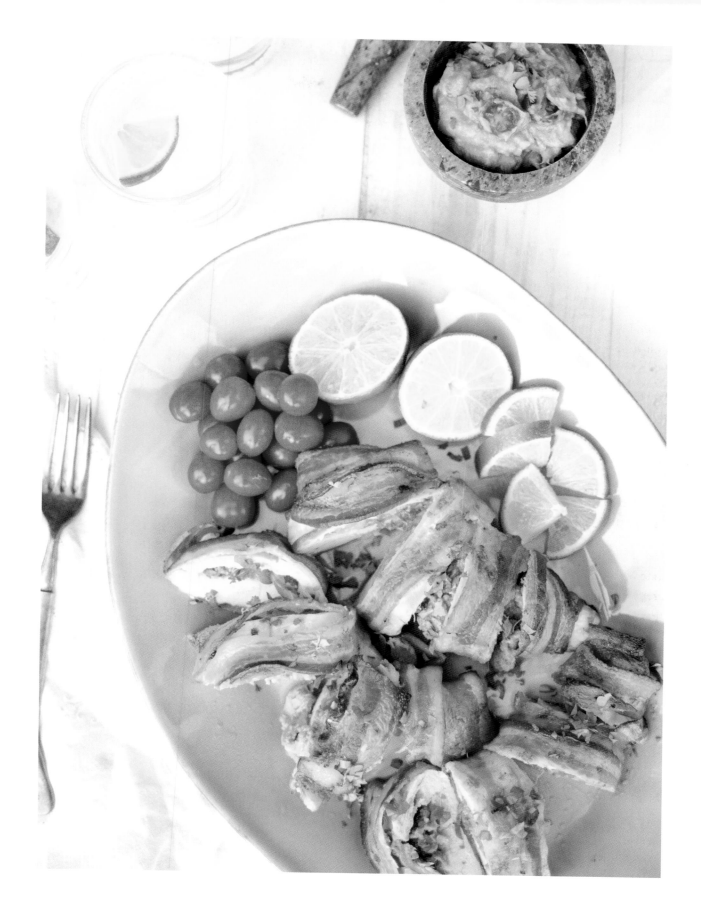

CHICKEN AND ASPARAGUS CURRY

prep time: **5 minutes**   *cook time:* **15 minutes**   *yield:* **4 servings**

1 tablespoon coconut oil

½ cup chopped onions

1 cinnamon stick

2 teaspoons ground fenugreek

2 teaspoons dry mustard

1 teaspoon ground cumin

2 boneless, skinless chicken thighs, cut into ½-inch pieces

Fine sea salt and ground black pepper

1 pound asparagus, trimmed and cut into 2-inch pieces

1 (13½-ounce) can full-fat coconut milk

¼ cup chicken bone broth, homemade (page 106) or store-bought

2 teaspoons Swerve confectioners'-style sweetener or equivalent amount of liquid or powdered sweetener (see page 29)

½ teaspoon turmeric powder

1 tablespoon red curry paste

Juice of 1 lime

Fresh cilantro leaves, for garnish

Lime wedges, for serving

1. Heat the oil in a cast-iron skillet over medium-high heat. Add the onions, cinnamon stick, fenugreek, dry mustard, and cumin and cook for 4 minutes or until the onions are soft.

2. Meanwhile, pat the chicken dry and season well on all sides with salt and pepper. Place in the skillet and cook for 5 minutes on each side, until the chicken is golden brown and no longer pink inside.

3. Add the asparagus, coconut milk, broth, sweetener, turmeric, curry paste, and lime juice. Stir well to combine. Bring to a simmer, then continue to simmer for 5 minutes or until the asparagus is cooked to your liking. Remove from the heat. Garnish with cilantro and serve with lime wedges.

4. Store in an airtight container in the refrigerator for up to 3 days. To reheat, place the curry in a saucepan over medium heat for a few minutes, until warmed to your liking.

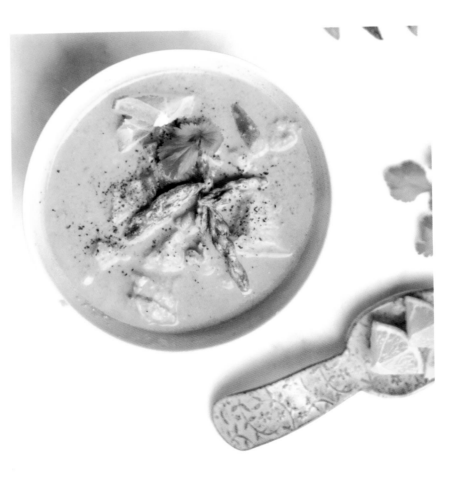

nutritional info (per serving)				
calories	fat	protein	carbs	fiber
313	24g	15g	9g	3g

CURRY BRAISED CHICKEN LEGS

prep time: **10 minutes**   cook time: **45 minutes**   yield: **8 servings**

¼ cup avocado oil or coconut oil

¼ cup diced onions

1 tablespoon peeled and grated fresh ginger

1 tablespoon minced garlic

1 cup sliced button mushrooms

8 chicken legs

1 teaspoon fine sea salt

1 cup chicken bone broth, homemade (page 106) or store-bought

½ cup full-fat coconut milk

2 tablespoons red curry paste

2 tablespoons lime juice

Sliced scallions, for garnish

Lime wedges, for serving

1. Heat the oil in a large cast-iron skillet over medium-high heat. Add the onions and cook for 2 minutes or until soft. Add the ginger and garlic and cook for another minute. Add the mushrooms and sauté until golden brown, about 2 minutes.

2. Season the chicken on all sides with the salt. Place the chicken in the skillet and sear on all sides for about 2 minutes per side, until golden brown. Add the broth, coconut milk, and curry paste and whisk to combine. Cover and cook for 30 to 40 minutes, until the chicken is cooked through and fork-tender; during cooking, lift the lid occasionally and stir to deglaze the bottom of the pan.

3. Stir in the lime juice. Taste and add more salt, if desired. Garnish with scallions and serve with lime wedges.

4. Store in an airtight container in the refrigerator for up to 3 days or in the freezer for up to a month. To reheat, place the chicken in a skillet over medium heat, cover, and cook until warmed through, about 5 minutes.

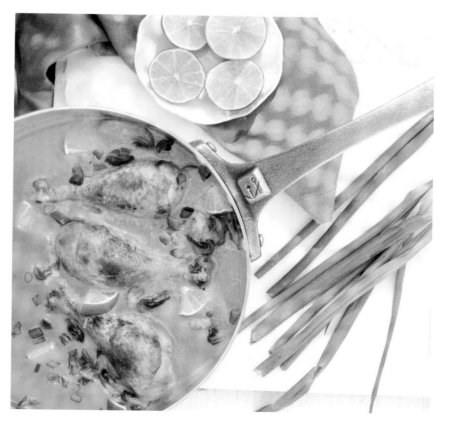

nutritional info (per serving)				
calories	fat	protein	carbs	fiber
363	25g	30g	2g	0.5g

GRILLED JERK CHICKEN THIGHS

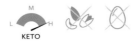

prep. time: **5 minutes, plus time to marinate**   *cook time:* **18 minutes**
yield: **6 servings**

Jerk Marinade:

6 scallions, chopped

1 onion, chopped

1 jalapeño pepper, seeded and minced

¾ cup wheat-free tamari

½ cup coconut vinegar or apple cider vinegar

¼ cup avocado oil or MCT oil

2 tablespoons Swerve confectioners'-style sweetener or equivalent amount of liquid or powdered sweetener (see page 29)

1 tablespoon chopped fresh thyme

½ teaspoon ground allspice

½ teaspoon ground cloves

½ teaspoon ground nutmeg

1½ pounds bone-in, skin-on chicken thighs

1. Place the ingredients for the marinade in a food processor or blender. Pulse until smooth, about 15 seconds.

2. Place the chicken in a medium-sized bowl and coat with the marinade. Refrigerate for 4 to 6 hours, or overnight.

3. Preheat a grill to high heat. Lightly oil the grill grate. Grill the marinated chicken for 2 minutes, then lower the heat to medium and grill for 6 to 8 minutes on each side, until the juices run clear.

4. Store in an airtight container in the refrigerator for up to 3 days. To reheat, place the chicken on a rimmed baking sheet in a preheated 400°F oven for a few minutes or until warmed through.

Note: Jerk chicken tastes great with a side of red cabbage dressed with Creamy Lime Sauce (page 38).

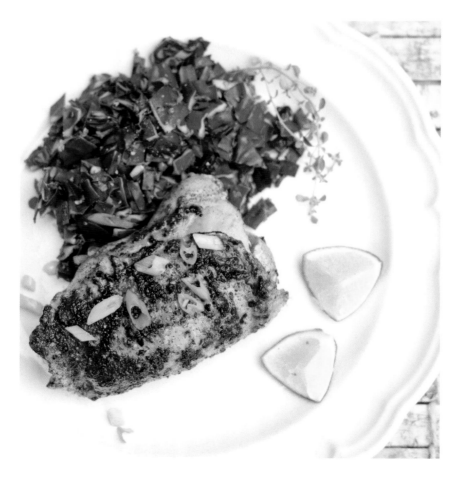

nutritional info (per serving)				
calories	fat	protein	carbs	fiber
408	27g	33g	7g	2g

EASY ASIAN CHICKEN LEGS

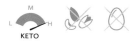

prep time: 5 minutes   cook time: 35 minutes   yield: 4 servings

½ cup chicken bone broth, homemade (page 106) or store-bought

⅓ cup Swerve confectioners'-style sweetener or equivalent amount of liquid or powdered sweetener (see page 29)

⅓ cup wheat-free tamari

¼ cup tomato sauce

1 tablespoon coconut vinegar or apple cider vinegar

¾ teaspoon crushed red pepper

¼ teaspoon peeled and grated fresh ginger

1 clove garlic, smashed to a paste

5 drops orange oil (optional)

1 pound bone-in, skin-on chicken legs or thighs

For Garnish:

1 lime, quartered

1 tablespoon toasted sesame seeds

4 scallions, sliced

Fresh cilantro leaves

1. Preheat the oven to 400°F.

2. Place the broth, sweetener, tamari, tomato sauce, vinegar, crushed red pepper, ginger, garlic, and orange oil, if using, in a small bowl. Stir well, then pour half of the sauce into another bowl and set aside for serving.

3. Place the chicken in an 8-inch square baking dish and baste with the other half of the sauce. Cover and bake for 25 minutes. Uncover and bake for another 10 minutes or until the chicken is cooked through and no longer pink inside.

4. Serve the chicken with the reserved sauce. Garnish with lime quarters, toasted sesame seeds, sliced scallions, and cilantro leaves.

5. Store in an airtight container in the refrigerator for up to 4 days or in the freezer for up to a month. To reheat, place the chicken in a preheated 375°F oven for 10 minutes or until warmed to your liking.

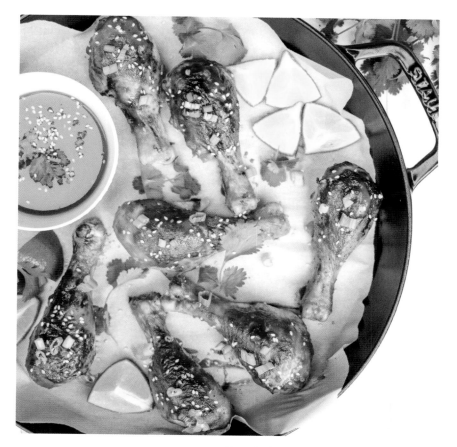

nutritional info (per serving)				
calories	fat	protein	carbs	fiber
322	16g	33g	6g	2g

CHICKEN AND MUSHROOM KABOBS

prep time: **10 minutes, plus time to marinate chicken**   *cook time:* **12 minutes**
yield: **2 servings**

Marinade:

½ cup MCT oil, avocado oil, or extra-virgin olive oil

3 tablespoons lime juice

1 tablespoon chopped fresh tarragon or parsley

1 teaspoon chopped fresh oregano

1 teaspoon fine sea salt

1 teaspoon ground black pepper

3 cloves garlic, minced

2 boneless, skinless chicken thighs, cut into ½-inch pieces

6 large button mushrooms, cut into quarters

Dipping Sauce:

¼ cup mayonnaise, homemade (page 34 or 35) or store-bought

1 tablespoon lime juice

1 tablespoon sliced fresh chives, or 2 teaspoons dried chives

Fine sea salt and ground black pepper

Special Equipment:

6 wood skewers, soaked in water for 15 minutes

1. Place the ingredients for the marinade in a large bowl and stir to combine. Add the chicken and stir well to coat. Cover and refrigerate for at least 3 hours or overnight.

2. Preheat a grill to high heat. Thread a piece of marinated chicken onto a skewer, followed by a mushroom quarter. Repeat 3 more times to fill the skewer. Then repeat with the remaining skewers, chicken, and mushrooms. Discard the marinade.

3. Lightly brush the hot grill grate with oil, then place the kabobs on the grill and cook for 6 minutes. Flip and grill for another 6 minutes or until the chicken is cooked through.

4. Meanwhile, prepare the dipping sauce: Place the mayonnaise, lime juice, and chives in a small food processor or blender and blend until smooth. Season to taste with salt and pepper.

5. Place the kabobs on a platter and serve with a bowl of the dipping sauce on the side.

6. Store leftover kabobs and sauce in separate airtight containers in the refrigerator for up to 4 days; the kabobs can be frozen for up to a month. Reheat the kabobs in a lightly greased skillet for 2 minutes per side or until warmed to your liking.

nutritional info (per serving)				
calories	fat	protein	carbs	fiber
436	36g	24g	6g	1g

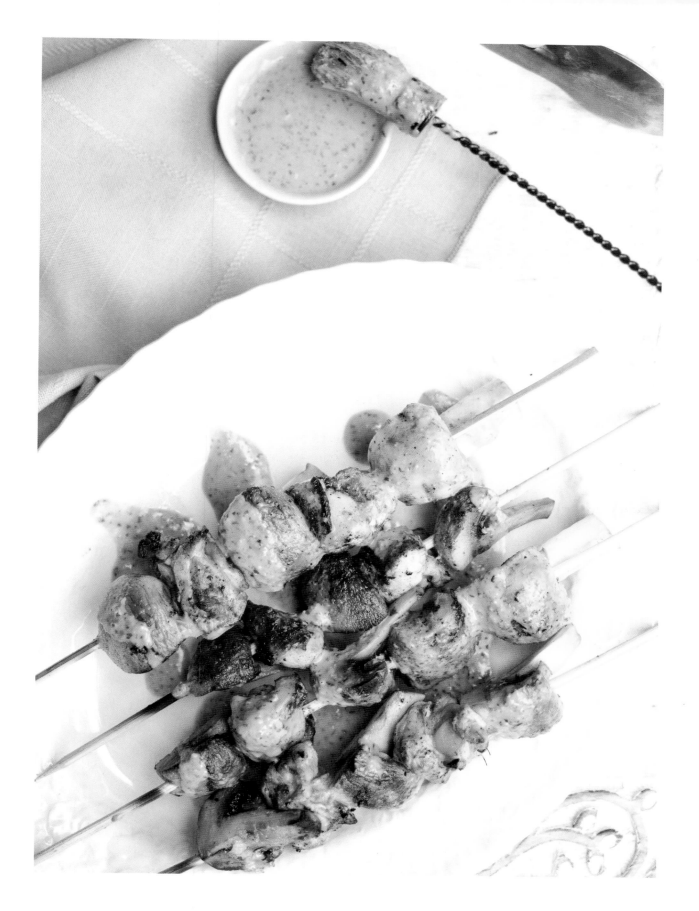

CHICKEN
with Sausage and Greens

KETO

2 tablespoons avocado oil or lard, divided

4 bone-in, skin-on chicken thighs

2 teaspoons fine sea salt, divided

¼ cup diced onions

1 pound Italian sausage, removed from casings

2 cloves garlic, minced

1 cup chopped radicchio

1 cup chopped kale

¼ cup broccoli slaw (see Note)

To make this recipe even faster, you can sauté the sausage while the chicken is cooking; however, you will have more pans to clean at the end. I like making it in one pan to save time on cleanup.

prep time: **5 minutes** *cook time:* **20 minutes** *yield:* **4 servings**

1. Heat 1 tablespoon of the oil in a large heavy skillet over medium-high heat. Season the chicken on all sides with 1 teaspoon of the salt. When the oil is hot, place the chicken in the pan, skin side down. Place a heavy cast-iron skillet (or a brick covered in parchment paper) on top of the chicken to crisp up the skin. Cook for 6 minutes.

2. Remove the top skillet or brick, flip the chicken over, and cook for another 5 minutes or until the chicken is cooked through and no longer pink inside. Remove the chicken from the skillet and set aside on a warm plate.

3. In the same skillet, heat the remaining tablespoon of oil over medium-high heat. Add the onions and sauté for 2 minutes, then add the sausage and garlic. Sauté while crumbling until the sausage is cooked through, about 5 minutes. Season with the remaining teaspoon of salt.

4. Add the radicchio, kale, and broccoli slaw and sauté until wilted, about 2 minutes. Season with salt to taste. Place the chicken on top of the vegetables in the pan and serve.

5. Store extras in an airtight container in the refrigerator for up to 3 days. To reheat, fry in a greased cast-iron skillet for 5 minutes or until warmed through. Leftover chicken can be served cold over salad greens.

Note: *Packaged broccoli slaw is available in the produce section of most grocery stores.*

nutritional info (per serving)				
calories	fat	protein	carbs	fiber
539	41g	36g	4g	1g

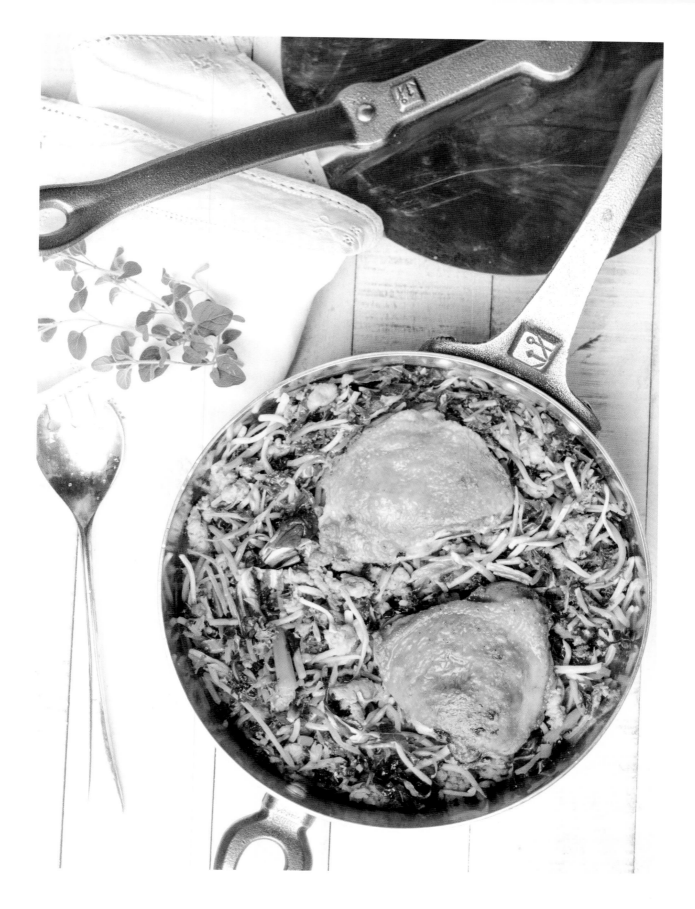

TENDER COCONUT CHICKEN

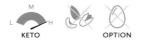

prep time: 5 minutes, plus time to marinate (optional)
cook time: 35 minutes   *yield:* 4 servings

2 tablespoons peeled and grated fresh ginger

1½ mounded tablespoons minced garlic

2 tablespoons lime juice

1 teaspoon fine sea salt, divided

½ teaspoon fish sauce (optional, for umami flavor)

4 tablespoons chicken bone broth, homemade (page 106) or store-bought, divided

8 bone-in, skin-on chicken thighs

1 tomato, seeded and chopped

3 cups lightly packed cilantro leaves and stems

3 tablespoons coconut oil

1 cup full-fat coconut milk

1 batch Keto "Rice" (page 147), for serving (optional; omit for egg-free)

1. Place the ginger, garlic, lime juice, ¼ teaspoon of the salt, fish sauce (if using), and 2 tablespoons of the broth in a blender and pulse until smooth.

2. Place the chicken in a bowl and rub the ginger mixture all over the chicken. For the best flavor, cover the bowl and refrigerate for up to 24 hours.

3. In same blender jar, combine the tomato, cilantro, remaining ¾ teaspoon of salt, and remaining 2 tablespoons of broth. Puree until smooth.

4. Heat the oil in a large cast-iron skillet over high heat. Place the chicken in the skillet and cook, turning occasionally, until lightly browned on all sides, about 10 minutes. Pour the cilantro mixture over the chicken. Cook, stirring often, until the sauce thickens and the oil separates, about 10 minutes.

5. Pour the coconut milk into the pan and bring to a boil, then continue to boil for 5 minutes, stirring occasionally. Reduce the heat to low and simmer until the chicken is tender and no longer pink inside, about 10 minutes.

6. Serve over rice, if desired.

7. Store in an airtight container in the refrigerator for up to 3 days or in the freezer for up to a month. To reheat, place the chicken in a skillet over medium heat, cover, and cook until warmed through, about 5 minutes.

nutritional info (per serving)				
calories	fat	protein	carbs	fiber
515	40g	32g	4g	1g

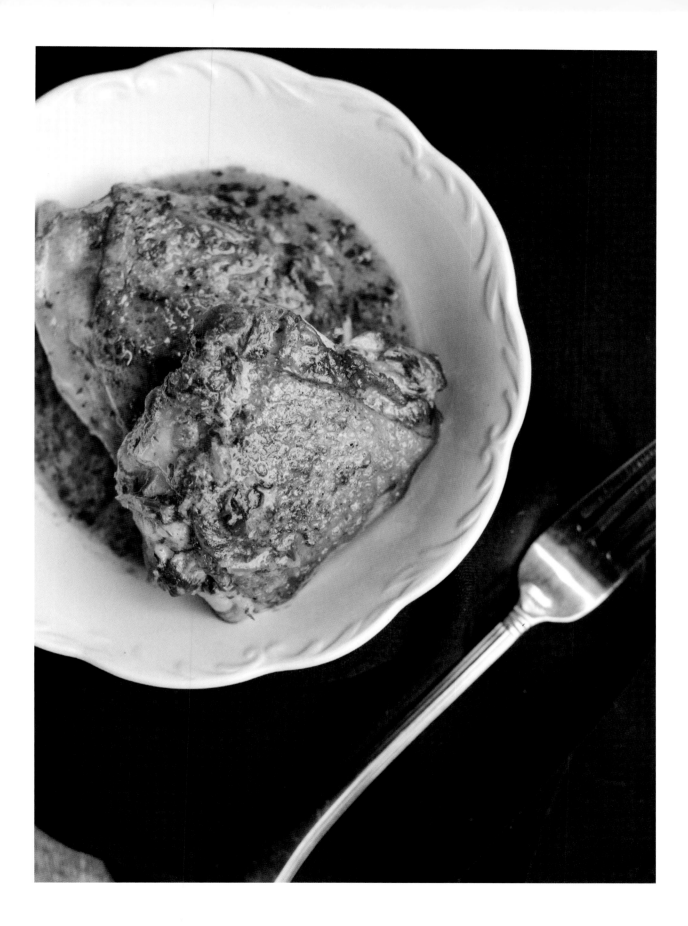

LEMON PEPPER CHICKEN TENDERS

prep time: **7 minutes** *cook time:* **20 minutes** *yield:* **4 servings**

¼ cup avocado oil or melted coconut oil

1 tablespoon minced garlic

2 lemons, divided

4 boneless, skinless chicken breast halves (about 2 pounds), cut into 1-inch-wide strips

2 tablespoons lemon pepper seasoning

2 teaspoons fine sea salt

1 teaspoon black peppercorns, for garnish

Chopped fresh parsley or oregano, for garnish

1. Preheat the oven to 400°F.

2. Make the lemon sauce: Place the oil and garlic in a small bowl. Grate the zest of one of the lemons and add 2 teaspoons of the zest to the bowl. Juice the zested lemon and add the juice to the bowl. Stir well.

3. Cut the second lemon into thin slices. Arrange the slices on a rimmed baking sheet or a 13 by 9-inch baking dish.

4. Season all sides of the chicken strips with the lemon pepper seasoning and salt. Place on top of the lemon slices and drizzle with the lemon sauce.

5. Bake for 18 to 20 minutes, until the chicken is no longer pink inside. Serve garnished with peppercorns and fresh parsley.

6. Store in an airtight container in the refrigerator for up to 3 days or in the freezer for up to a month. To reheat, place the chicken on a rimmed baking sheet in a preheated 375°F oven for 5 minutes or until warmed through.

nutritional info (per serving)				
calories	fat	protein	carbs	fiber
432	25g	44g	5g	2g

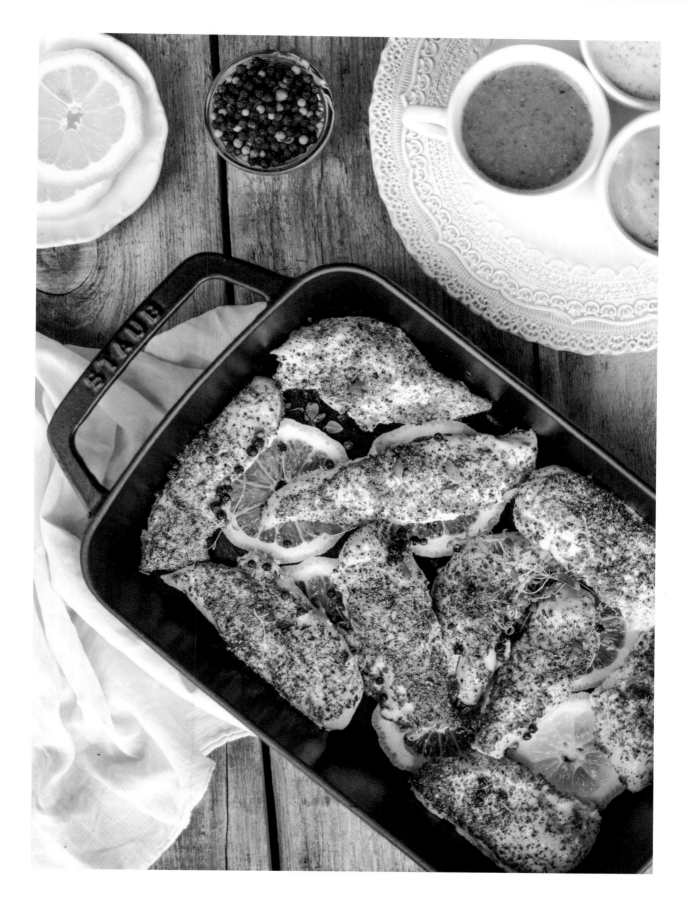

BUNDT PAN CHICKEN

KETO

prep time: **7 minutes**   *cook time:* **45 minutes**   *yield:* **8 servings**

2 medium zucchini, sliced ½ inch thick (about 2½ cups)

½ small onion, cut into 1-inch pieces

1 tablespoon plus 1 teaspoon minced garlic

4 teaspoons fine sea salt, divided

2 teaspoons ground black pepper, divided

4 tablespoons avocado oil or melted lard, duck fat, or bacon fat, divided

3 sprigs fresh thyme, divided

1 (3-pound) whole chicken (see Note)

1. Place all of the oven racks in the lower portion of the oven. (The chicken stands tall and needs a lot of space above it.) Preheat the oven to 425°F.

2. Place the zucchini, onion, and garlic in a medium-sized bowl. Season with 3 teaspoons of the salt and 1½ teaspoons of the pepper. Drizzle with 1 tablespoon of the oil and toss to coat well. Place in the Bundt pan. Top with a thyme sprig.

3. Place a piece of aluminum foil over the hole of the Bundt pan, then place parchment paper over the foil so the food doesn't touch the foil while roasting.

4. Pat the chicken dry and use your hands to rub the remaining 3 tablespoons of oil all over the outside. Season the inside and outside of the chicken well with the remaining teaspoon of salt and remaining ½ teaspoon of pepper. Place the remaining 2 sprigs of thyme inside the cavity.

5. Place the chicken in the middle of the Bundt pan with the neck facing up. Roast in the oven for 45 minutes or until the chicken is cooked through and the juices run clear. Serve with the roasted veggies.

6. Store in an airtight container in the refrigerator for up to 3 days or in the freezer for up to a month. To reheat, place on a rimmed baking sheet in a preheated 375°F oven for 8 minutes or until warmed through.

Note: If you use a chicken larger than 3 pounds, it will take much longer to roast, and this will cause the vegetables to be overcooked. You can give the bird a head start and roast it alone for 15 to 20 minutes, then add the zucchini, onion, and garlic to the pan and continue to roast for 45 minutes, or until the chicken is cooked through.

nutritional info (per serving)				
calories	fat	protein	carbs	fiber
445	33g	33g	4g	1g

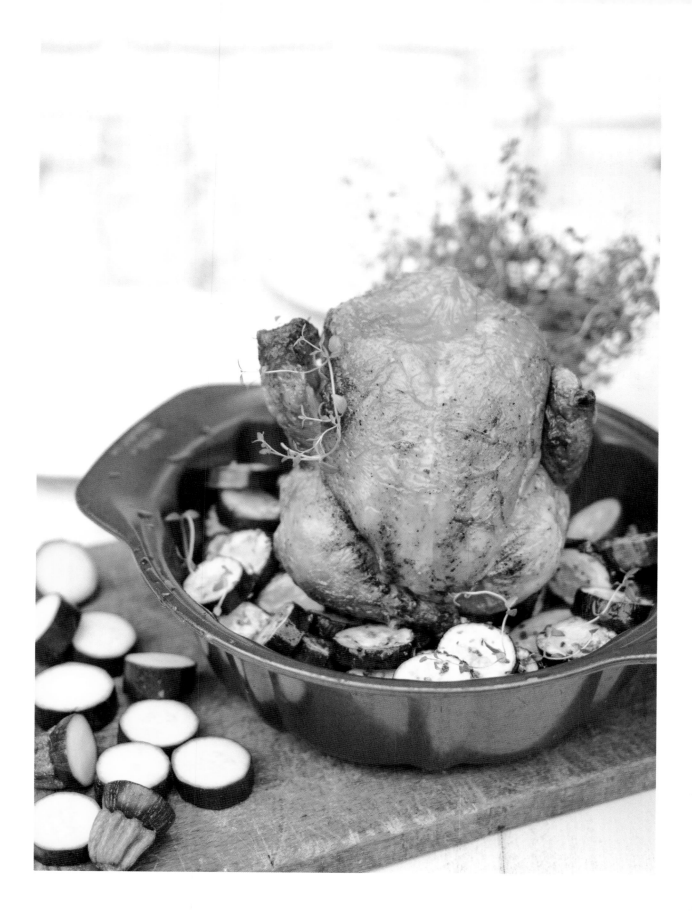

SHEET PAN BBQ CHICKEN BREASTS
with Bacon-Wrapped Avocado Fries

prep time: **8 minutes** *cook time:* **25 minutes** *yield:* **8 servings**

4 boneless, skinless chicken breast halves (about 2 pounds), sliced into 1½ by 4-inch strips

½ cup Simple BBQ Sauce (page 43)

3 firm and barely ripe avocados

1 (1-pound) package thin-cut bacon (about 20 strips)

1. Preheat the oven to 425°F. Line a rimmed baking sheet with parchment paper.

2. Baste the chicken strips with the BBQ sauce.

3. Peel and pit the avocados, then slice into thick french fry shapes. Wrap each slice with a strip of bacon and secure with a toothpick.

4. Place the chicken and bacon-wrapped avocado slices on the lined baking sheet. Bake for 20 to 25 minutes, until the avocados are tender and the juice of the chicken runs clear when the center of the thickest part is cut and the internal temperature is at least 165°F.

5. Store in an airtight container in the refrigerator for up to 3 days or in the freezer for up to a month. To reheat, place the chicken and fries on a baking sheet in a preheated 375°F oven for 5 minutes or until warmed through.

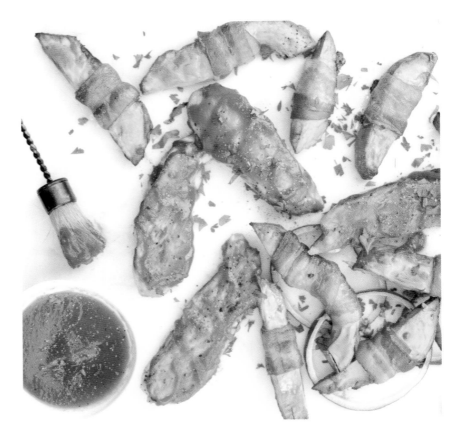

nutritional info (per serving)				
calories	fat	protein	carbs	fiber
464	40g	23g	7g	5g

BACON-WRAPPED CHICKEN FINGERS

prep time: **5 minutes**   *cook time:* **14 minutes**   *yield:* **4 servings**

4 boneless, skinless chicken breast halves (about 2 pounds)

8 strips thin-cut bacon

1 tablespoon coconut oil or avocado oil

½ cup Simple BBQ Sauce (page 43), for serving

1. Preheat the oven to 400°F.

2. Cut each chicken breast crosswise into four 1-inch-thick strips. Cut the bacon down the middle to make 16 long, narrow strips. Starting at one end of each chicken strip, wrap a strip of bacon around while spiraling so the bacon slightly overlaps at the edges and covers the whole strip. Use toothpicks to secure the ends of the bacon.

3. Heat the oil in a large cast-iron skillet over medium-high heat. Sear the bacon-wrapped strips in the hot oil for 2 minutes per side. Using a hand mitt, transfer the skillet to the oven and bake for 10 minutes or until the bacon is crisp and the chicken is cooked through and no longer pink. Serve the chicken fingers with the BBQ sauce.

4. Store in an airtight container in the refrigerator for up to 4 days. To reheat, place the chicken on a rimmed baking sheet in a preheated 375°F oven for 5 minutes or until warmed through.

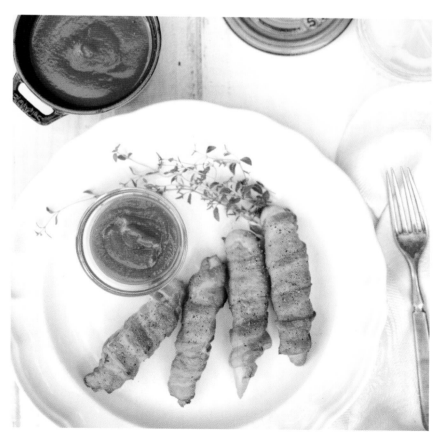

nutritional info (per serving)				
calories	fat	protein	carbs	fiber
451	27g	51g	0g	0g

SIMPLE SESAME CHICKEN

prep time: **10 minutes**   *cook time:* **25 minutes**   *yield:* **4 servings**

2 tablespoons avocado oil or coconut oil

1 pound boneless, skinless chicken thighs, cut into bite-sized pieces

Fine sea salt

½ cup chicken bone broth, homemade (page 106) or store-bought

⅓ cup Swerve confectioners'-style sweetener or equivalent amount of liquid or powdered sweetener (see page 29)

2 tablespoons wheat-free tamari, or ½ cup coconut aminos

2 tablespoons toasted (dark) sesame oil

2 tablespoons tomato sauce

1 tablespoon lime juice

¼ teaspoon peeled and grated fresh ginger

1 clove garlic, smashed to a paste

1 batch Keto Fried "Rice" (page 147), for serving (optional)

For Garnish:

Sesame seeds

Sliced scallions

Lime wedges

1. Heat the oil in a large wok or cast-iron skillet over medium-high heat. Pat the chicken pieces dry with a paper towel and season well on all sides with salt.

2. Fry the chicken in the hot oil until light golden brown on all sides, about 4 minutes. Remove the chicken from the wok and set aside.

3. Add the remaining ingredients to the wok and boil over medium heat until reduced and thickened, about 10 minutes.

4. Return the chicken to the wok and bring to a hard boil. Reduce the heat to medium and simmer for 10 minutes, until the chicken is cooked through and no longer pink inside.

5. Garnish with sesame seeds, sliced scallions, and lime wedges. Serve over fried "rice," if desired.

6. Store in an airtight container in the refrigerator for up to 3 days. To reheat, place the chicken in a greased skillet over medium heat for 5 minutes or until warmed to your liking.

nutritional info (per serving)				
calories	fat	protein	carbs	fiber
301	22g	24g	3g	0.1g

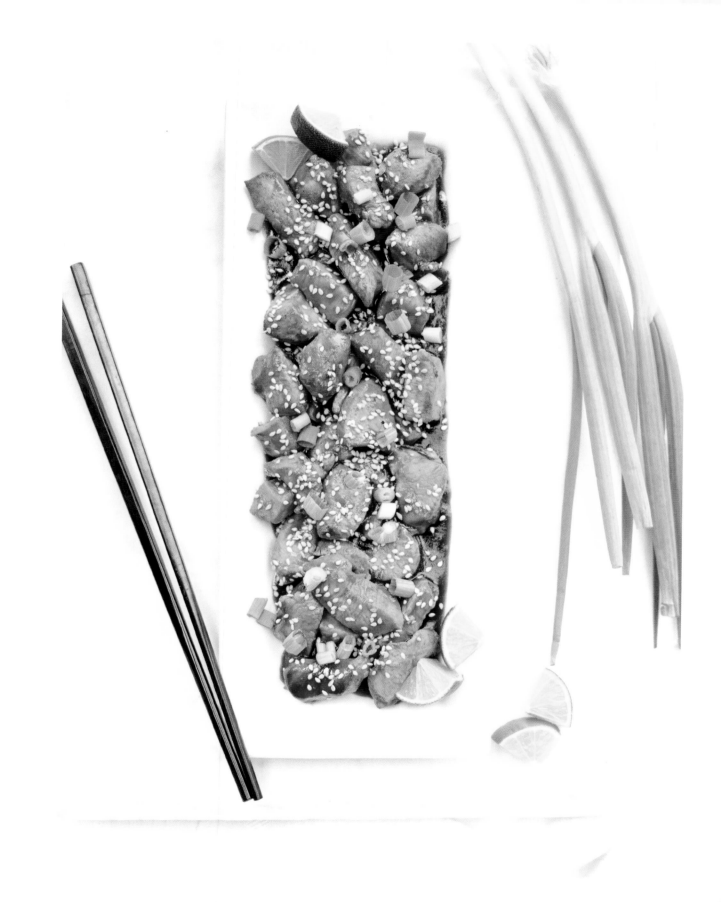

PAELLA

People often complain to me that they don't have time to cook. Well, using things like cauliflower rice reduces the time significantly. Traditional rice takes a long time to cook; cauliflower rice takes only 3 minutes. I rice the cauliflower the night before, so all I have to do is stir-fry it until soft. You can even buy packaged cauliflower rice at the grocery store to cut down on prep time even more.

prep time: **8 minutes, plus time to marinate**   *cook time:* **10 minutes**
yield: **8 servings**

Marinade:

2 tablespoons MCT oil or extra-virgin olive oil

1 tablespoon paprika

2 teaspoons dried oregano leaves

½ teaspoon fine sea salt

2 pounds boneless, skinless chicken thighs, cut into 2-inch pieces

"Rice":

1 head cauliflower, cored and cut into large pieces

2 tablespoons coconut oil

3 cloves garlic, crushed

1 teaspoon crushed red pepper

1 pinch of saffron threads

1 bay leaf

½ bunch fresh parsley, chopped

Grated zest of 2 lemons

2 tablespoons coconut oil

½ cup chopped onions

1 red bell pepper, coarsely chopped

½ pound Mexican-style fresh (raw) chorizo, removed from casings and crumbled

½ pound shrimp, peeled and deveined

½ pound precooked mussels, thawed if frozen (optional)

1. In a medium-sized bowl, mix together the ingredients for the marinade. Stir in the chicken pieces to coat. Cover and refrigerate for 1 hour or up to 24 hours.

2. Make the rice: Pulse the cauliflower in a food processor until broken down into rice-sized pieces. Set aside.

3. Heat 2 tablespoons of coconut oil in a large skillet or paella pan over medium heat. Stir in the garlic, crushed red pepper, saffron threads, bay leaf, parsley, lemon zest, and riced cauliflower. Cook, stirring often, for 3 to 5 minutes, until the cauliflower rice is done to your liking.

4. Meanwhile, heat another 2 tablespoons of coconut oil in a separate skillet over medium heat. Add the marinated chicken and onions and cook for 5 minutes. Stir in the bell pepper and sausage and cook until the chicken and sausage are cooked through, about 5 minutes.

5. Add the shrimp and cook, turning often, until both sides are pink. Add the mussels, if using, and cook just until the mussels are heated, about 1 minute. Spread the cauliflower rice mixture onto a serving platter. Top with the meat and seafood mixture and serve.

6. Store in an airtight container in the refrigerator for up to 3 days. To reheat, place the paella in a greased skillet over medium heat for 5 minutes or until warmed through.

Note: *To make this dish even lower in carbs (but not egg-free), skip Steps 2 and 3 and replace the cauliflower rice with my Keto "Rice" (page 147).*

Busy Family Tip: *You can make the cauliflower rice up to 2 days ahead and store it in the refrigerator for easy lunch/dinner options.*

nutritional info (per serving)				
calories	fat	protein	carbs	fiber
433	28g	36g	9g	2g

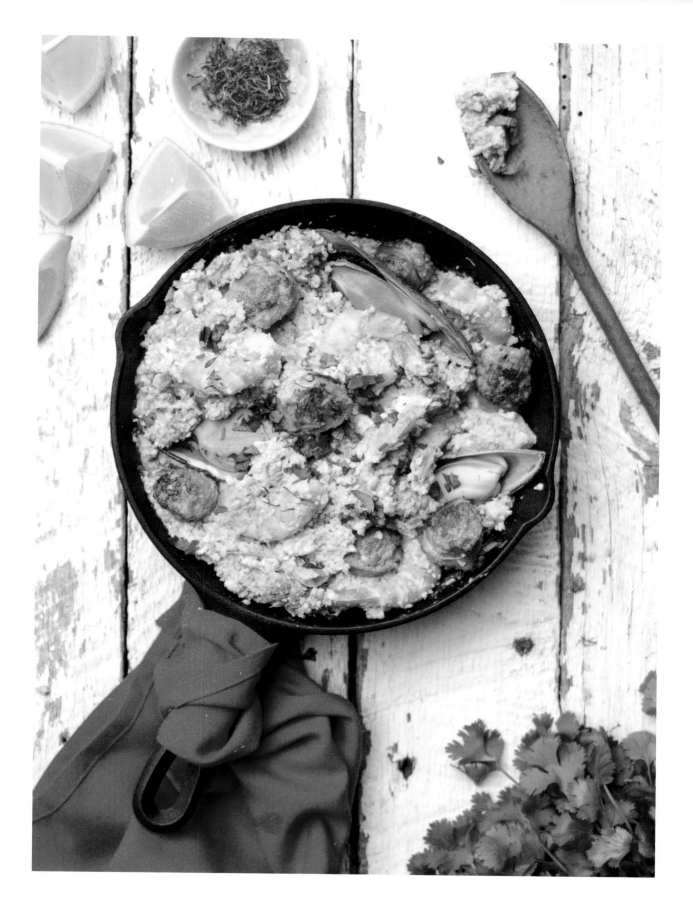

GREEK CHICKEN THIGHS

KETO

prep time: 10 minutes (not including time to make vinaigrette)
cook time: 20 minutes   yield: 4 servings

4 bone-in, skin-on chicken thighs

1 teaspoon fine sea salt

1 teaspoon ground black pepper

1 batch Greek Vinaigrette (page 46; see Note)

2 cups Greek olives, pitted

¼ cup diced red onions

1 medium cucumber, diced

1 medium tomato, diced

4 sprigs fresh oregano

1. Place an oven rack in the upper third of the oven and preheat the broiler to high. Line a rimmed baking sheet with aluminum foil.

2. Place the chicken thighs on the prepared baking sheet and season on all sides with the salt and pepper. Broil, skin side up, for 5 minutes. Flip the chicken and continue to broil skin side down for 10 minutes.

3. Remove the chicken from the oven. Turn it skin side up again. Brush each thigh with a tablespoon of the vinaigrette. Place under the broiler for 5 more minutes or until the chicken is golden brown and no longer pink inside.

4. Meanwhile, toss the olives, onions, cucumber, tomato, and oregano with 3 tablespoons of the vinaigrette, or dress only the amount of salad you plan to eat right away. Serve the chicken thighs with the salad.

5. Store the chicken and salad in separate airtight containers in the refrigerator for up to 3 days; the chicken can be frozen for up to a month. To reheat, place the chicken on a rimmed baking sheet in a preheated 375°F oven for 8 minutes or until warmed through.

Note: A full batch of Greek Vinaigrette is more than you will need for this recipe, but it will keep for up to 2 weeks in the refrigerator and is wonderful to have on hand for easy salads. You can also use the leftovers to make Lamb Chops with Gyro Salad (page 228).

nutritional info (per serving)				
calories	fat	protein	carbs	fiber
647	60g	21g	10g	6g

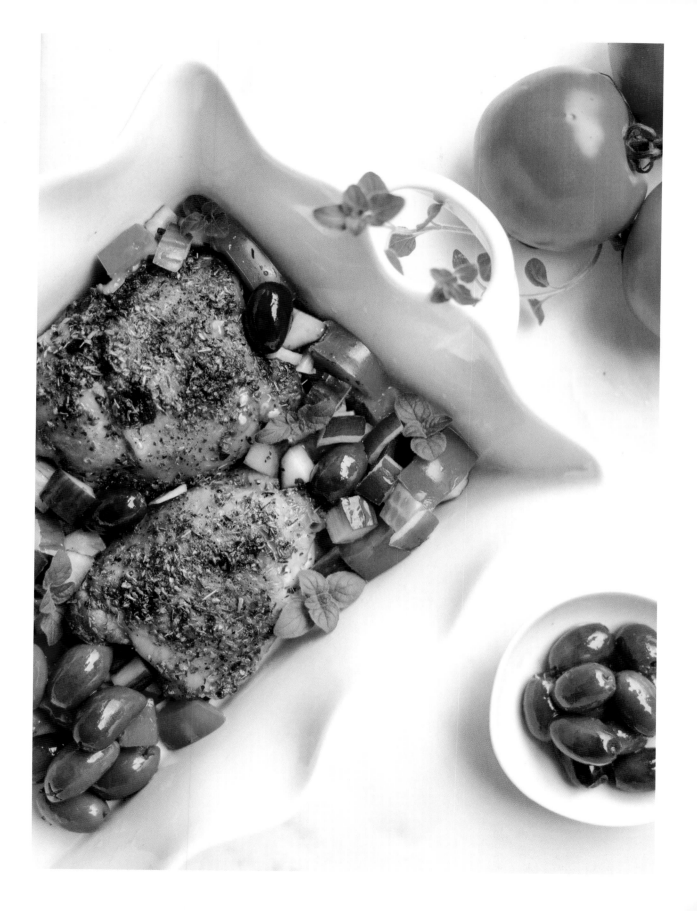

TENDER CHICKEN LIVERS

KETO · OPTION

1 pound chicken livers

1 teaspoon fine sea salt

1 tablespoon avocado oil

1 teaspoon lemon juice

2 cloves garlic, smashed to a paste

1 tablespoon chopped fresh parsley

¼ cup Comeback Sauce (page 37), dairy-free ranch dressing, homemade (page 45) or store-bought, and/or Cilantro Lime Dressing (page 39), for serving

When I purchased the chicken livers for this recipe at the store, the cashier asked if I was going fishing. I responded no and asked why. He said that most people buy chicken livers to fish with. I just giggled to myself.

prep time: 5 minutes   *cook time:* 5 minutes   *yield:* 4 servings

1. Rinse the chicken livers and pat dry. Season on all sides with the salt.

2. Heat a cast-iron skillet over medium-high heat. When hot, add the seasoned chicken livers. Cooking the livers in a dry skillet keeps them very tender. Cook, stirring occasionally, for 3 minutes or until cooked through. (When properly cooked, the livers will be pink in the center.)

3. Add the oil, lemon juice, garlic, and parsley to the skillet and stir well. Serve with the Comeback Sauce or dressing.

4. This dish is best served fresh; however, the livers can be stored in an airtight container in the refrigerator for up to 3 days. They can be served cold over salad greens or reheated in a dry cast-iron skillet over medium heat for 2 minutes or until warmed through.

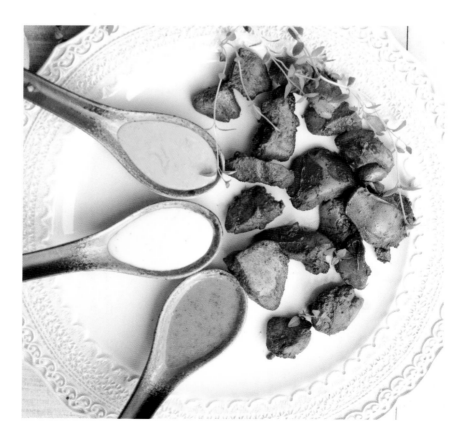

nutritional info (per serving)				
calories	fat	protein	carbs	fiber
170	9g	19g	1g	0g

DIJON CHICKEN

4 bone-in, skin-on chicken legs or thighs

¼ cup chicken bone broth, homemade (page 106) or store-bought

¼ cup Dijon mustard

2 tablespoons avocado oil or melted coconut oil

2 tablespoons chopped fresh chives, or 2 teaspoons dried chives

2 cloves garlic, smashed to a paste

1 teaspoon fine sea salt

1. Preheat the oven to 450°F. Place the chicken on a rimmed baking sheet and set aside.

2. Place the broth, mustard, oil, chives, garlic, and salt in a small bowl and mix well. Use your hands to rub half of the mixture all over the chicken. Reserve the other half for serving.

3. Bake for 22 to 25 minutes, until the chicken is no longer pink inside and the juices run clear. Pour the reserved sauce over the chicken and serve.

4. Store in an airtight container in the refrigerator for up to 3 days. The chicken can be served cold over salad greens or reheated in a greased cast-iron skillet over medium heat for 5 minutes or until warmed through.

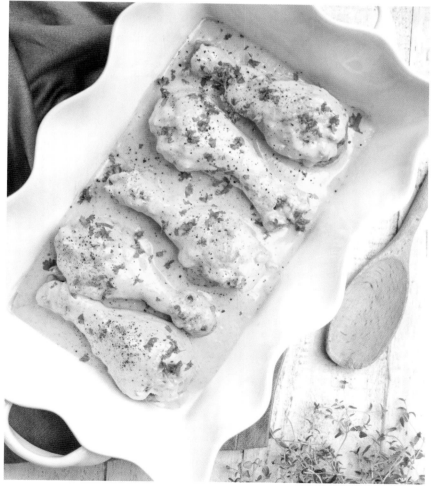

nutritional info (per serving)				
calories	fat	protein	carbs	fiber
335	22g	30g	1g	0.1g

CURRY CHICKEN MEATBALLS

Meatballs:

2 pounds ground chicken

¼ cup diced onions

4 cloves garlic, minced

2 tablespoons peeled and grated fresh ginger

2 tablespoons red curry paste

1½ tablespoons garam masala

1 tablespoon lime juice

2 teaspoons fine sea salt

Sauce:

¼ cup coconut oil

½ cup diced onions

6 cloves garlic, minced

2 tablespoons peeled and grated fresh ginger

3 tablespoons garam masala

2 tablespoons red curry paste

1 tablespoon turmeric powder

1 (14½-ounce) can diced tomatoes

2 teaspoons fine sea salt

1 teaspoon lime juice

For Garnish:

Lime wedges

Chopped fresh cilantro

Scallions, sliced on the diagonal

2 batches Keto "Rice" (page 147), for serving (optional)

1. Preheat the oven to 400°F.

2. Make the meatballs: Place the ingredients for the meatballs in a large bowl. Using your hands, combine until well mixed. Form into 1-inch balls and place on a rimmed baking sheet. Bake for 15 minutes or until cooked through and no longer pink inside.

3. Meanwhile, make the sauce: Heat the coconut oil in a large cast-iron skillet over medium-high heat. Add the onions and sauté for 3 minutes or until soft. Add the garlic and ginger and sauté for another 2 minutes. Add the garam masala, curry paste, and turmeric powder and stir until well mixed. Add the diced tomatoes and salt. Lower the heat to medium and simmer for 10 minutes (or until the meatballs are done baking).

4. Stir the lime juice into the sauce, then add the cooked meatballs and turn to coat in the sauce. Garnish with lime wedges, cilantro, and scallions. Serve with Keto "Rice," if desired.

5. Store in an airtight container in the refrigerator for up to 3 days. To reheat, pan-fry the meatballs in a greased cast-iron skillet over medium heat for 5 minutes or until warmed through.

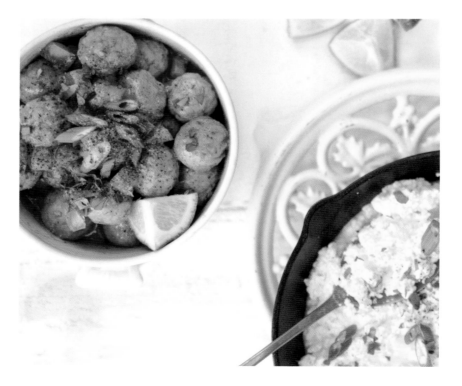

nutritional info (per serving)				
calories	fat	protein	carbs	fiber
367	22g	32g	7g	2g

GRILLED CHICKEN AND AVOCADO

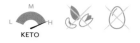

prep time: **8 minutes**   cook time: **30 minutes**   yield: **4 servings**

4 bone-in, skin-on chicken thighs

1 teaspoon fine sea salt

1 teaspoon ground black pepper

1 ripe avocado

2 tablespoons lime or lemon juice

1 teaspoon avocado oil

1 (⅛-inch-thick) slice red onion, separated into rings

2 scallions

1 lime, cut into wedges, for garnish

1. Preheat a grill to high heat.

2. Pat the chicken dry with paper towels and season on both sides with the salt and pepper. Grill the chicken for 10 minutes, then flip and grill for another 10 to 20 minutes, until cooked through and no longer pink inside (the exact cook time will depend on how large the thighs are).

3. Meanwhile, cut the avocado in half and remove the pit with a spoon. Drizzle the halves with the lime juice and brush with the oil. Place the avocado halves cut side down on the grill along with the onion rings and scallions. Grill for 3 minutes.

4. Remove everything from the grill and place on a platter. Season the avocado with salt to taste. Let the chicken rest for 10 minutes before serving. Serve each piece of chicken with one-quarter of the avocado and lime wedges.

5. Store in an airtight container in the refrigerator for up to 3 days. The chicken and avocado can be served cold over salad greens or reheated in a greased cast-iron skillet over medium heat for 5 minutes or until warmed through.

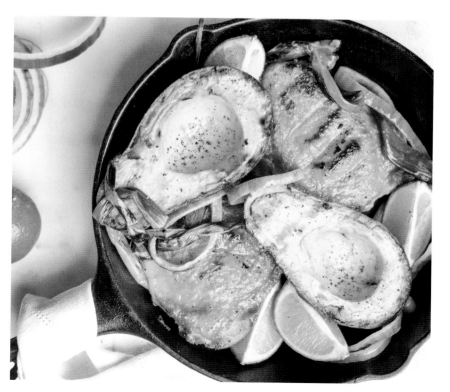

nutritional info (per serving)				
calories	fat	protein	carbs	fiber
248	18g	17g	7g	4g

CHICKEN SATAY
with Dipping Sauce

prep time: **12 minutes, plus 30 minutes to marinate**   *cook time:* **4 minutes**
yield: **4 servings**

Satay Sauce:

1 cup full-fat coconut milk

½ cup crushed pili nuts, macadamia nuts, or sunflower seeds

2 tablespoons creamy almond butter or sunflower seed butter

2 tablespoons lime juice

1 tablespoon fish sauce

1 clove garlic, chopped

½ teaspoon red curry paste

2 tablespoons Swerve confectioners'-style sweetener or equivalent amount of liquid or powdered sweetener (see page 29) (optional)

½ teaspoon paprika

Marinade:

½ cup full-fat coconut milk

2 teaspoons ground coriander

2 teaspoons Swerve confectioners'-style sweetener or equivalent amount of liquid or powdered sweetener (see page 29) (optional)

1 teaspoon curry powder

1 teaspoon fish sauce

½ teaspoon chili oil, or ¼ teaspoon cayenne pepper

Juice of 1 lime

1 pound boneless, skinless chicken thighs or breasts, cut into 3-inch by ¾-inch strips

For Garnish:

Chopped fresh cilantro leaves

Sliced scallions

Chopped pili nuts or macadamia nuts

Special Equipment:

4 wood skewers, soaked in water for 15 minutes

1. Make the sauce: Place the ingredients for the sauce in a blender and puree until very smooth. Transfer to a serving dish, cover, and refrigerate until ready to use. (*Note:* The sauce can be made up to 3 days ahead.)

2. Marinate the chicken: Combine the ingredients for the marinade in a medium-sized bowl. Add the chicken to the bowl with the marinade. Cover the bowl, place in the refrigerator, and marinate for 30 minutes or overnight.

3. Preheat a grill to high heat. Remove the chicken from the marinade, discard the marinade, and thread the chicken onto the skewers.

4. Grill the chicken skewers for 2 minutes per side or until cooked through. Remove from the heat and place on a platter. Garnish with cilantro, scallions, and pili nuts. Sprinkle some chopped pili nuts on top of the sauce and serve alongside the skewers.

5. Store in an airtight container in the refrigerator for up to 3 days. To reheat, place the chicken on a hot grill or under the broiler for 2 minutes or until warmed through.

Note: *The sweetener in this recipe is optional, but if you prefer a traditional-tasting satay, I recommend adding it.*

nutritional info (per serving)				
calories	fat	protein	carbs	fiber
461	39g	26g	6g	2g

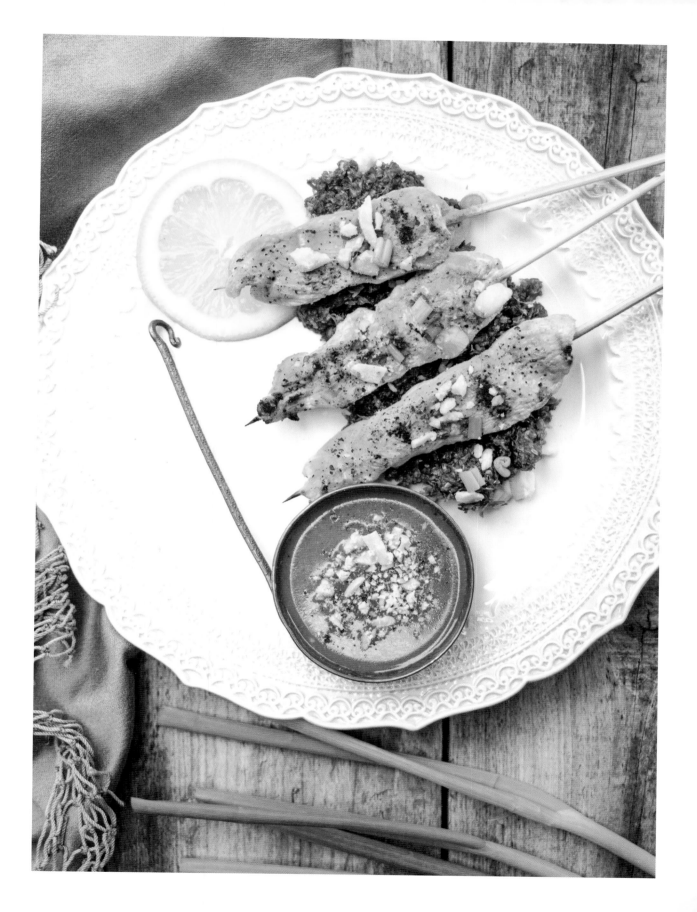

EASY CHICKEN AND ASPARAGUS STIR-FRY

prep time: **5 minutes, plus time to marinate chicken** *cook time:* **8 minutes**
yield: **4 servings**

Marinade:

2¼ teaspoons wheat-free tamari, or 3 tablespoons coconut aminos

1 tablespoon peeled and grated fresh ginger

1 tablespoon fish sauce, or 1 teaspoon fine sea salt

2 cloves garlic, minced

2 tablespoons Swerve confectioners'-style sweetener or equivalent amount of liquid or powdered sweetener (see page 29)

4 boneless, skinless chicken thighs, cut into 1-inch chunks

2 tablespoons avocado oil or coconut oil

1½ pounds thick asparagus, ends trimmed, cut into 1-inch pieces

¼ cup thinly sliced scallions

1 teaspoon peeled and grated fresh ginger

1 teaspoon fine sea salt

¼ cup chicken bone broth, homemade (page 106) or store-bought

1. Place the tamari, ginger, fish sauce, garlic, and sweetener in a medium-sized bowl. Add the chicken pieces and toss to coat. Cover and refrigerate for 15 minutes or overnight.

2. Heat the oil in a large wok or cast-iron skillet over medium-high heat. Add the asparagus, scallions, and ginger and stir-fry for 3 minutes. Season with the salt, then remove from the wok and set aside, leaving the drippings in the pan.

3. Place the wok over medium-high heat, then add the chicken and marinade and stir-fry for 3 minutes or until the chicken is golden and cooked through. Add the reserved asparagus and broth and boil for 2 minutes. Stir well and serve.

4. Store in an airtight container in the refrigerator for up to 3 days. The stir-fry can be served cold over salad greens or reheated in a greased cast-iron skillet for 5 minutes or until warmed through.

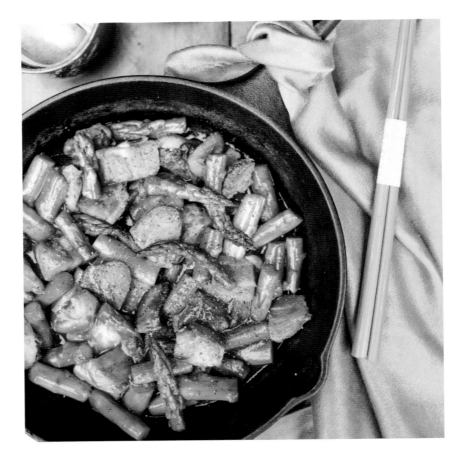

nutritional info (per serving)				
calories	fat	protein	carbs	fiber
274	16g	25g	6g	3g

MOLE CHICKEN LEGS

prep time: **5 minutes** cook time: **6 to 8 hours** yield: **8 servings**

Mole Sauce:

¼ cup finely chopped onions

1 clove garlic, minced

1 tablespoon chopped fresh cilantro

1 cup tomato sauce

1 (4-ounce) can diced green chiles

2 tablespoons MCT oil

1 tablespoon unsweetened cocoa powder

1 teaspoon ground cumin

8 chicken legs (about 4 pounds)

1. Make the sauce: Place the ingredients for the sauce in a 4-quart or larger slow cooker. Stir to combine.

2. Place the chicken legs in the slow cooker. Cover and cook on low for 6 to 8 hours, until the meat is tender and easily pulls away from the bone. Transfer to a serving plate. Serve with the sauce.

3. Store in an airtight container in the refrigerator for up to 4 days. To reheat, place the chicken in a preheated 375°F oven for 5 minutes or until warmed through.

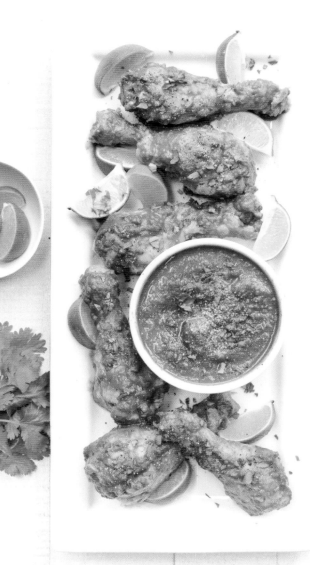

nutritional info (per serving)				
calories	fat	protein	carbs	fiber
310	19g	30g	4g	1g

DEVIL CHICKEN

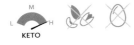

KETO

4 bone-in, skin-on chicken thighs

1 teaspoon fine sea salt

1 teaspoon ground black pepper

½ cup Dijon mustard

1 teaspoon onion powder, or ¼ cup minced onions

4 drops hot sauce, or more to taste

Fresh cilantro leaves, for garnish

I call this dish Devil Chicken because of the spiciness of the Dijon mustard and hot sauce. I am a traditional German girl who is still fairly new to spicy food, and this dish certainly opened up my flavor profile!

prep time: **5 minutes**   *cook time:* **20 minutes**   *yield:* **2 servings**

1. Preheat the oven broiler to high. Line a rimmed baking sheet with aluminum foil.

2. Place the chicken thighs on the prepared baking sheet and season on all sides with the salt and pepper.

3. Broil the chicken skin side up for 5 minutes. Flip and broil skin side down for 10 more minutes.

4. Meanwhile, place the mustard, onion powder, and hot sauce in a small bowl and stir well to combine.

5. Remove the chicken from the oven and turn it skin side up again. Brush each thigh with a tablespoon of the mustard mixture. Place back under the broiler and broil for 5 more minutes or until the chicken is golden brown on the outside and no longer pink inside. Garnish with cilantro leaves and serve with the remaining sauce.

6. Store in an airtight container in the refrigerator for up to 3 days. To reheat, place the chicken in a preheated 375°F oven for 5 minutes or until warmed through.

nutritional info (per serving)				
calories	fat	protein	carbs	fiber
366	19g	31g	1g	0.3g

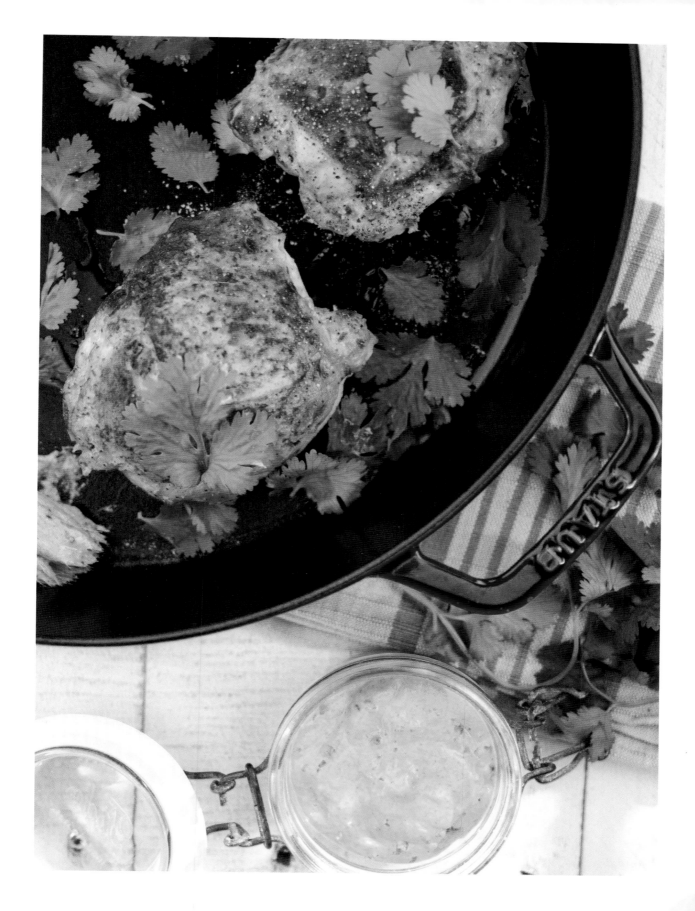

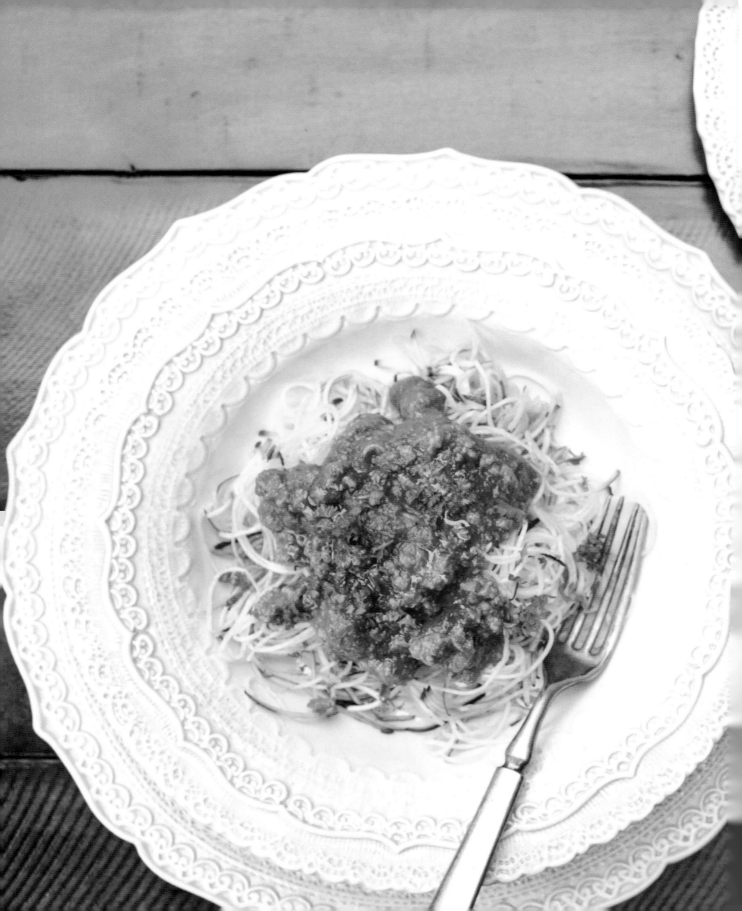

Chapter 7:
Beef and Lamb

SOUTH OF THE BORDER STEAK

Marinade:

⅓ cup avocado oil

¼ cup lime juice

2 tablespoons Swerve confectioners'-style sweetener or equivalent amount of liquid or powdered sweetener (see page 29)

1 tablespoon wheat-free tamari, or ¼ cup coconut aminos

1 tablespoon chili powder

1 tablespoon ground cumin

2 teaspoons fine sea salt

1 teaspoon ground black pepper

4 cloves garlic, minced

6 drops orange oil (optional)

2 pounds flank steak or skirt steak

Serving Suggestions:

Diced avocado

Lime slices or wedges

Sliced radishes

Fresh cilantro leaves

Shredded lettuce

Pico de Gallo (page 85)

1. Place the ingredients for the marinade in a large baking dish and stir to combine. Place the steak in the dish and turn to coat in the marinade. Cover and place in the refrigerator for 3 hours or overnight.

2. Preheat a grill to medium-high heat or set a large cast-iron skillet over medium-high heat. Remove the steak from the marinade. When the grill or pan is hot, sear the steak for 3 minutes, then flip and cook for another 3 minutes.

3. Use a meat thermometer to check that the steak is cooked to your liking: 115°F for rare, 125°F for medium-rare, or 140°F for medium. (I don't recommend cooking this cut of steak beyond medium doneness.) Remove from the grill or skillet and place on a cutting board to rest for 10 minutes before slicing.

4. Meanwhile, set out the avocado, lime, radishes, cilantro, lettuce, and pico de gallo.

5. Using a sharp knife, slice the steak across the grain. Serve with the accompaniments.

6. This steak is best served fresh; however, you can store it in an airtight container in the refrigerator for up to 3 days. To reheat, place the steak in a baking dish in a preheated 350°F oven for 3 minutes or until warmed through.

nutritional info (per serving)				
calories	fat	protein	carbs	fiber
329	23g	25g	6g	4g

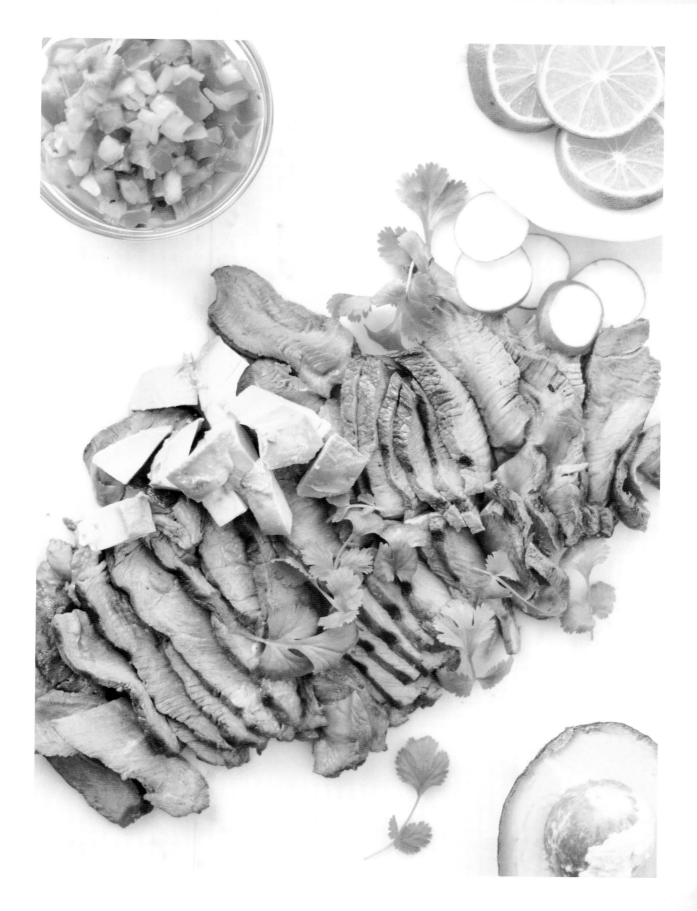

SPANISH SPICED LAMB CHOPS

prep time: **5 minutes**   *cook time:* **6 minutes**   *yield:* **6 servings**

1½ teaspoons paprika

1 teaspoon ground coriander

1 teaspoon ground cumin

½ teaspoon ground allspice

½ teaspoon ground cinnamon

¼ teaspoon cayenne pepper

6 (5-ounce) lamb loin chops

4 tablespoons avocado oil, divided

4 cloves garlic, smashed to a paste

2 tablespoons lime juice

Fine sea salt and ground black pepper (optional)

Fresh thyme, for garnish

1. In a small bowl, combine the spices. Reserve 2 teaspoons of the spice mixture for the pan sauce. Rub the lamb chops with the remaining spice mixture.

2. Heat 2 tablespoons of the avocado oil in a large cast-iron skillet over medium heat. Place the seasoned chops in the hot oil and cook for 3 minutes per side or until a meat thermometer reads 125°F when inserted in the center of one of the chops for medium-rare chops (or cook until done to your liking). Remove the chops from the pan and allow to rest while you make the sauce.

3. Leave the drippings in the skillet and reduce the heat to medium-low. Add the garlic and cook until fragrant, about 1 minute. Add the rest of the spice mixture, lime juice, and remaining 2 tablespoons of oil. Stir and taste for seasoning; add salt and pepper, if desired. Serve the sauce over the lamb chops. Garnish with fresh thyme.

4. Store in an airtight container in the refrigerator for up to 3 days. To reheat, place the chops in a lightly greased sauté pan over medium heat for 2 minutes per side or until warmed through.

nutritional info (per serving)				
calories	fat	protein	carbs	fiber
529	44g	31g	1g	0.3g

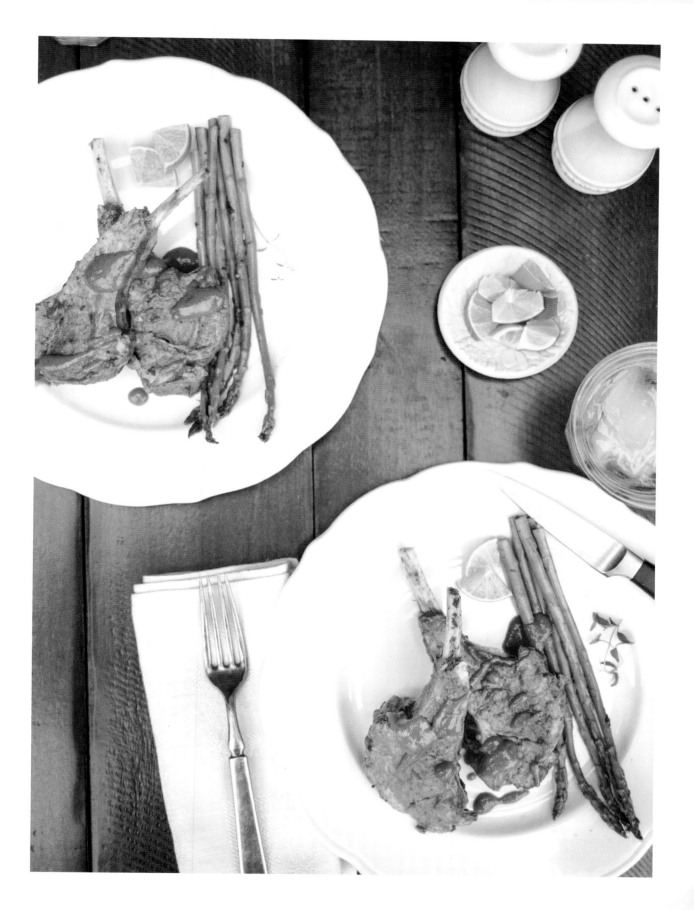

SLOW COOKER PHILLY STEAK SANDWICHES

Waffles make great "buns" for savory sandwiches like this one. All those delicious meat juices soak into the nooks and crannies of the waffles. What could be better?

prep time: **10 minutes** (not including time to cook eggs) *cook time:* **6 to 8 hours**
yield: **12 servings**

Philly Steak:

1 cup thinly sliced onions

2 green bell peppers, seeded and sliced

2 teaspoons fine sea salt

¼ teaspoon ground black pepper

2 pounds New York strip loin (aka top loin of beef)

1 cup beef bone broth, homemade (page 106) or store-bought

Waffles:

8 large eggs

4 hard-boiled eggs (see page 81), peeled

¼ cup unflavored egg white or beef protein powder

1 teaspoon onion powder (optional)

1 teaspoon baking powder

½ teaspoon fine sea salt

½ cup coconut oil, melted

1. Place the onions and bell peppers in a 4-quart slow cooker. Season with the salt and pepper. Top with the strip loin, then add the broth. Cover and cook on low for 6 to 8 hours, until the beef is fork-tender.

2. About an hour before the meat is done, make the waffles: Preheat a waffle iron to high heat. Place the raw eggs, hard-boiled eggs, protein powder, onion powder (if using), baking powder, and salt in a blender or food processor and pulse until the batter is smooth and thick. Add the melted coconut oil and combine well.

3. Grease the hot waffle iron. Place 2½ tablespoons of the batter in the center of the iron and close (the waffles should be small, about the size of hamburger buns). Cook for 3 to 4 minutes, until golden brown and crisp. Repeat with the rest of the batter to make a total of 24 waffles.

4. When the beef is fork-tender, remove it from the slow cooker and slice against the grain into very thin strips.

5. To assemble, place a waffle on a plate, top with a few slices of beef and a scoop of onions and peppers, then top with another waffle.

6. Store the waffles and Philly steak in separate airtight containers in the refrigerator for up to 3 days. To reheat the meat, place it in a lightly greased sauté pan over medium heat for about 2 minutes, stirring often, until warmed to your liking. Reheat the waffles in a toaster oven for 2 minutes or until warmed through. Then follow the assembly directions in Step 5.

Busy Family Tip: *The waffles can be made ahead and stored in the refrigerator for up to 3 days or frozen for up to a month. I often make a triple batch and store them in my freezer for easy sandwiches.*

nutritional info (per serving)				
calories	fat	protein	carbs	fiber
353	28g	23g	3g	1g

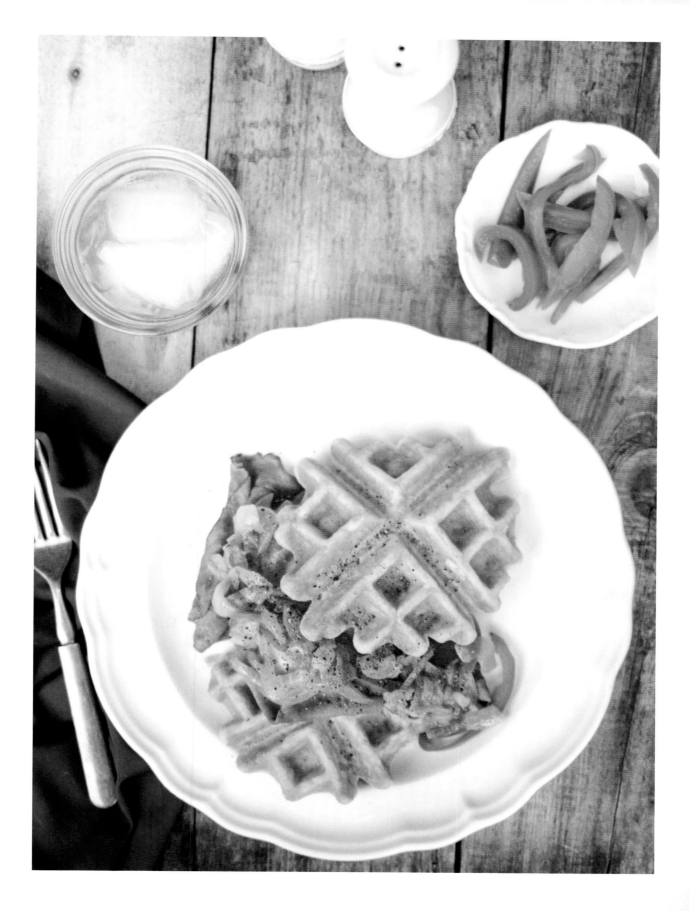

T-BONE STEAKS
with Romanesco Sauce

prep time: **2 minutes**   *cook time:* **6 minutes**   *yield:* **4 servings**

2 (1-pound) T-bone steaks, about 1 inch thick (see Note)

1 tablespoon fine sea salt

2 teaspoons ground black pepper

Melted coconut oil or lard, for the grill grates or pan

¼ cup Romanesco Sauce (page 42), for serving

Crushed red pepper, for garnish (optional)

1. Season the steaks generously with the salt and pepper. Preheat a grill to medium-high heat or set a large cast-iron skillet over medium-high heat. When hot, grease the grill grates with melted coconut oil or, if using a skillet, heat a teaspoon of coconut oil in the skillet. Place the steaks on the hot grill or in the hot skillet and cook for 3 minutes. Flip and cook for another 3 minutes for medium-rare (or cook the steaks to your liking, using the temperature chart below as a guide).

2. Remove the steaks from the heat and set on a cutting board to rest for 5 to 10 minutes before slicing. Slice and serve with the Romanesco sauce, garnished with crushed red pepper, if desired.

3. This dish is best served fresh; however, the steak and sauce can be stored in separate airtight containers in the refrigerator. The steak will keep for up to 3 days, and the sauce will keep for up to 5 days. To reheat the steak, place it in a baking dish in a preheated 350°F oven for 5 minutes or until warmed through.

Note: *If you can't find T-bone steaks, bone-in rib-eye steaks are another good option for this recipe.*

Rare: 120°F to 125°F

Medium-rare: 130°F to 135°F

Medium: 140°F to 145°F

Medium-well: 150°F to 155°F

Well-done: 160°F+

nutritional info (per serving, with 2 tablespoons of sauce)				
calories	fat	protein	carbs	fiber
591	43g	44g	2g	0.4g

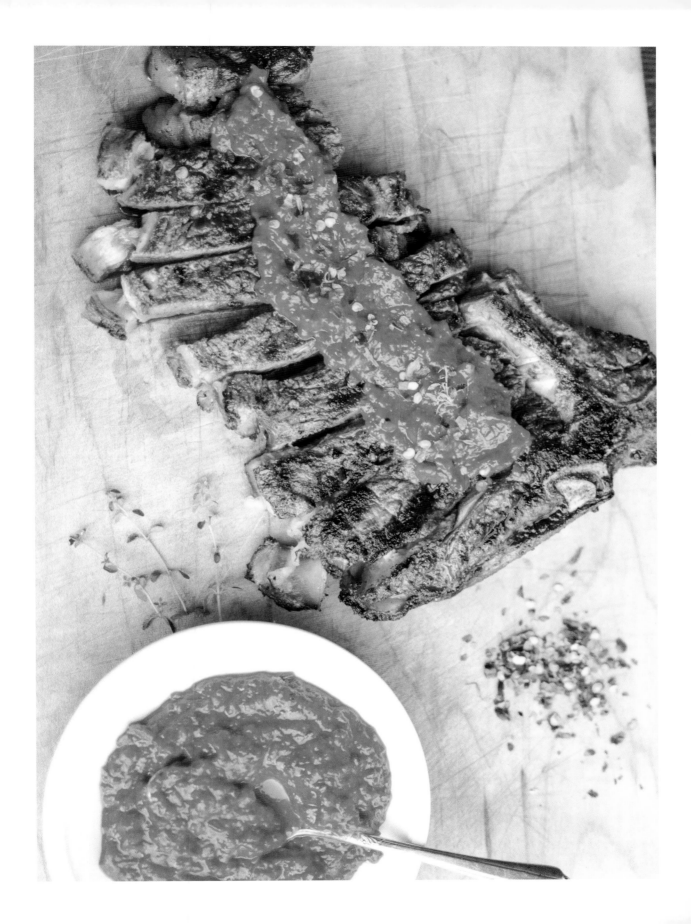

EASY BBQ BRISKET

KETO

We usually smoke our brisket, but if you don't have a smoker, you don't need to feel left out! This recipe is not only simple, but also gives the brisket an amazing smoky flavor.

prep time: **4 minutes**   *cook time:* **4 hours**   *yield:* **8 servings**

4 pounds brisket

6 tablespoons Swerve confectioners'-style sweetener or equivalent amount of powdered sweetener (see page 29)

2 tablespoons fine sea salt

1 tablespoon ground black pepper

1 tablespoon garlic powder

1 tablespoon onion powder

1 tablespoon dry mustard

1½ cups tomato sauce

1½ cups beef bone broth, homemade (page 106) or store-bought

2 teaspoons liquid smoke

Chopped fresh parsley, for garnish (optional)

1. Pat the brisket dry. Place in a large roasting pan that snugly fits the brisket and allow it to sit at room temperature for 10 to 15 minutes.

2. Preheat the oven to 350°F.

3. Place the sweetener, salt, pepper, garlic powder, onion powder, and dry mustard in a small bowl and stir to combine. Sprinkle the mixture all over the brisket, then use your hands to rub it into the meat.

4. Place the brisket in the oven and cook, uncovered, for 1 hour.

5. Meanwhile, place the tomato sauce, broth, and liquid smoke in a medium-sized bowl. Stir well to combine.

6. Remove the brisket from the oven and add the tomato-broth mixture to the pan. Lower the oven temperature to 300°F, cover the pan, and slow cook the brisket for 2½ hours or until fork-tender. If the brisket isn't tender enough after 2½ hours, cook, covered, for an additional 30 minutes.

7. Allow the meat to rest on a cutting board for 10 minutes while you make the sauce. Pour the juices from the roasting pan into a saucepan and boil for 7 minutes or until thickened to your liking.

8. Slice the meat across the grain into ⅛-inch slices. Serve with the sauce. Garnish with parsley, if desired.

9. Store in an airtight container in the refrigerator for up to 3 days. To reheat, place the brisket on a rimmed baking sheet in a preheated 350°F oven for 5 minutes or until warmed through.

nutritional info (per serving)				
calories	fat	protein	carbs	fiber
543	40g	39g	4g	1g

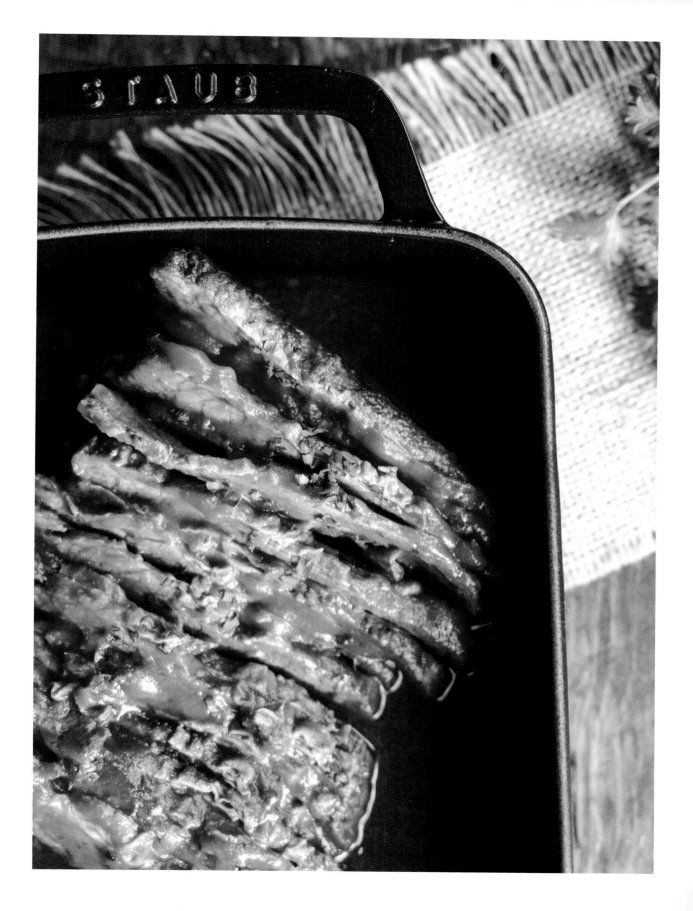

HERBY BROTH FONDUE

KETO   OPTION

A fondue pot makes this recipe super simple to prepare, but it's not required. You can heat up the broth in a saucepan on the stovetop. Then all you need is a way to keep the broth hot at the table. A hot plate works great for this purpose.

prep time: **8 minutes** (*not including time to make meatballs or dipping sauces*)
cook time: **5 minutes**   *yield:* **8 servings**

4 cups beef bone broth, homemade (page 106) or store-bought

1 sprig fresh rosemary

1 sprig fresh thyme

1 (⅛-inch-thick) slice red onion

Serving Suggestions:

(*Allow 4 ounces total per person*)

Boneless, skinless chicken thighs, cut into 1-inch chunks

Fillet of beef, cubed

Smoked sausage of choice, sliced

1 batch uncooked meatballs, any type

Button mushrooms, stemmed, halved if large

Cherry tomatoes

Fine sea salt and ground black pepper

Suggested Dipping Sauces:

½ cup Béarnaise Sauce (page 41)

½ cup Romanesco Sauce (page 42)

Special Equipment:

Fondue pot and set of fondue forks (optional)

1. Place the broth, herbs, and onion slice in a fondue pot and set the temperature to high (or 375°F). While the broth is heating, season the chicken and mushrooms with salt and pepper.

2. Once the broth is at a gentle simmer, place a piece of meat or a mushroom or tomato on a fondue fork and dip it into the broth until cooked through, 3 to 5 minutes for most of the suggested items but only 30 seconds for cherry tomatoes.

3. Serve the cooked items with one or more dipping sauces of your choice, if desired.

4. Store in an airtight container in the refrigerator for up to 3 days. To reheat, place the broth in the fondue pot and heat on high for 2 minutes or until warmed through, then lower the temperature to medium. If you cooked raw meat in the broth, be sure to bring the broth to a boil before reusing.

nutritional info (per serving for the broth)				
calories	fat	protein	carbs	fiber
9	0.3g	1g	0.1g	0g

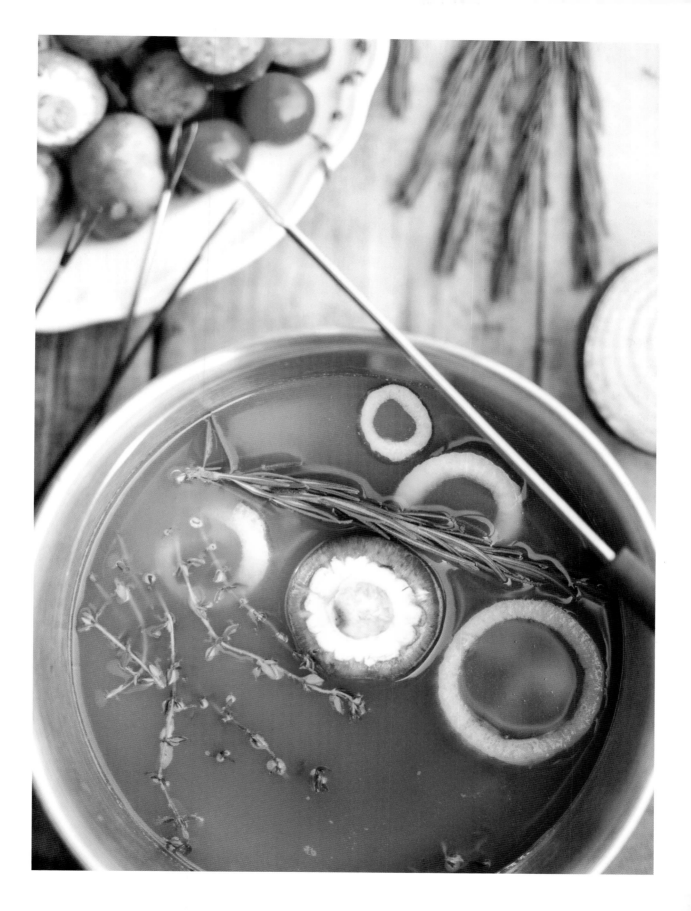

CURRY SHORT RIBS

These curry short ribs are a family favorite! My preferred way to eat them is over a bowl of Keto "Rice" (page 147) to soak up all the yummy sauce.

prep time: **5 minutes**   *cook time:* **8 hours**   *yield:* **8 servings**

1 cup beef bone broth, homemade (page 106) or store-bought

¼ cup chopped onions

¼ cup curry powder

2 tablespoons Swerve confectioners'-style sweetener or equivalent amount of liquid or powdered sweetener (see page 29)

1 tablespoon lime juice

2 cloves garlic, minced

4 beef short ribs (2 pounds total)

For Garnish:

Sliced scallions

Chopped fresh cilantro

1. Place the broth, onions, curry powder, sweetener, lime juice, and garlic in a 6-quart slow cooker and stir well to combine. Add the ribs and cook, covered, on low for 7 to 8 hours or until the meat is tender and easily pulls away from the bone.

2. To create a thicker sauce, pour the sauce from the slow cooker into a saucepan and boil while whisking for 2 minutes or until thickened to your liking. Taste and add more salt or lime juice, if desired.

3. Serve the ribs with the sauce. Garnish with scallions and cilantro.

4. Store in an airtight container in the refrigerator for up to 4 days. To reheat, place the ribs on a rimmed baking sheet in a preheated 400°F oven for a few minutes, until warmed to your liking.

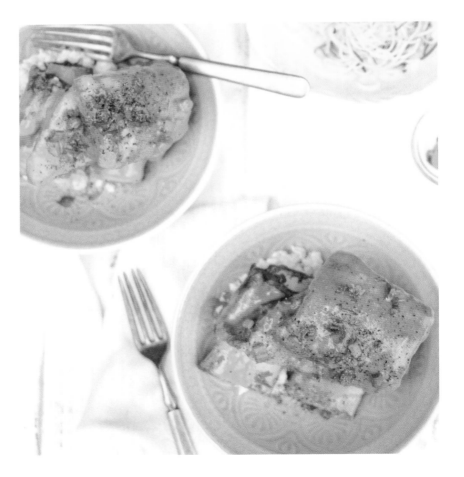

nutritional info (per serving)				
calories	fat	protein	carbs	fiber
528	47g	24g	1g	0.1g

SIMPLE SPAGHETTI

KETO

I serve this simple dish to my boys all the time. They devour it! It tastes great plain or over a bowl of very thin raw zucchini noodles.

prep time: **10 minutes**   *cook time:* **30 minutes**   *yield:* **8 servings**

1 tablespoon avocado oil or coconut oil

½ cup chopped onions

2 cloves garlic, minced

2 tablespoons Italian seasoning

1 teaspoon fine sea salt

½ teaspoon ground black pepper

2 pounds ground beef

2 cups tomato sauce

2 cups crushed tomatoes, drained

½ cup beef or chicken bone broth, homemade (page 106) or store-bought

2 medium zucchini, spiral-sliced into thin noodles, or 1 batch Cabbage Pasta (page 152)

Fresh herb of choice, for garnish (optional)

1. Heat the oil in a large pot over medium-high heat. Add the onions and cook for 4 minutes, stirring, until soft. Add the garlic, Italian seasoning, salt, and pepper and cook for 30 seconds, stirring.

2. Reduce the heat to medium-low, then add the beef. Cook for about 7 minutes, breaking up the clumps as it cooks, until the meat is no longer pink.

3. Add the tomato sauce, crushed tomatoes, and broth to the pot. Bring to a boil, then lower the heat and simmer lightly for 15 minutes to thicken the sauce. Serve over zucchini noodles or cabbage pasta. Garnish with the fresh herb of your choice, if desired.

4. Store in an airtight container in the refrigerator for up to 4 days. If using zucchini noodles, store the sauce and noodles separately; if using cabbage pasta, the pasta and sauce can be stored in the same container. To reheat, place the sauce and noodles or pasta in a pot over medium heat, stirring often, for a few minutes, until warmed to your liking.

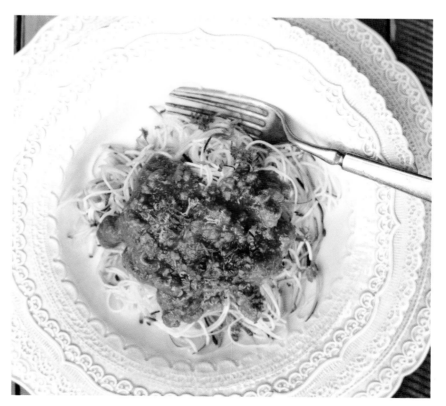

nutritional info (per serving)				
calories	fat	protein	carbs	fiber
347	25g	21g	8g	2g

SAUCY BBQ WRAPS

We adore BBQ night! One of my strategies for pulling our BBQ-themed dinner together quickly is to prepare the fixings for the next night's dinner while my husband, Craig, cleans up. That way, all I have to do is take the bowls of fixings out of the refrigerator and prepare the meat. Dinner is ready in minutes, and so much stress is eliminated from my day!

prep time: **10 minutes** *cook time:* **8 minutes** *yield:* **4 servings**

1 pound ground beef

2 tablespoons smoked paprika

2 teaspoons garlic powder

2 teaspoons onion powder

2 teaspoons fine sea salt

2 teaspoons liquid smoke (optional)

½ cup tomato sauce

For Serving:

Boston lettuce leaves

¼ cup Simple BBQ Sauce (page 43)

Topping Suggestions:

¼ cup prepared yellow mustard

½ cup baby dill pickles

About ⅓ cup sliced red onions

About ⅓ cup chopped fresh chives

Cherry tomatoes

1. Place the ground beef in a large skillet over medium heat. Sprinkle the spices, salt, and liquid smoke, if using, over the meat. Brown the beef, stirring to break up the clumps as it cooks, until it is cooked through, about 6 minutes.

2. While the meat is browning, place the lettuce leaves in a large bowl and place the BBQ sauce and any additional toppings of your choice in serving dishes.

3. When the meat is browned, add the tomato sauce to the skillet, stir well, and heat just long enough to warm the sauce. Transfer the meat to a serving dish.

4. To assemble the wraps, fill the lettuce leaves with a spoonful of the meat filling and garnish with desired toppings.

5. Store the meat filling and toppings in separate airtight containers in the refrigerator for up to 4 days. To reheat the meat, place it in a pot over medium heat, stirring often, for a few minutes, until warmed to your liking.

nutritional info (per serving)				
calories	fat	protein	carbs	fiber
322	23g	21g	7g	2g

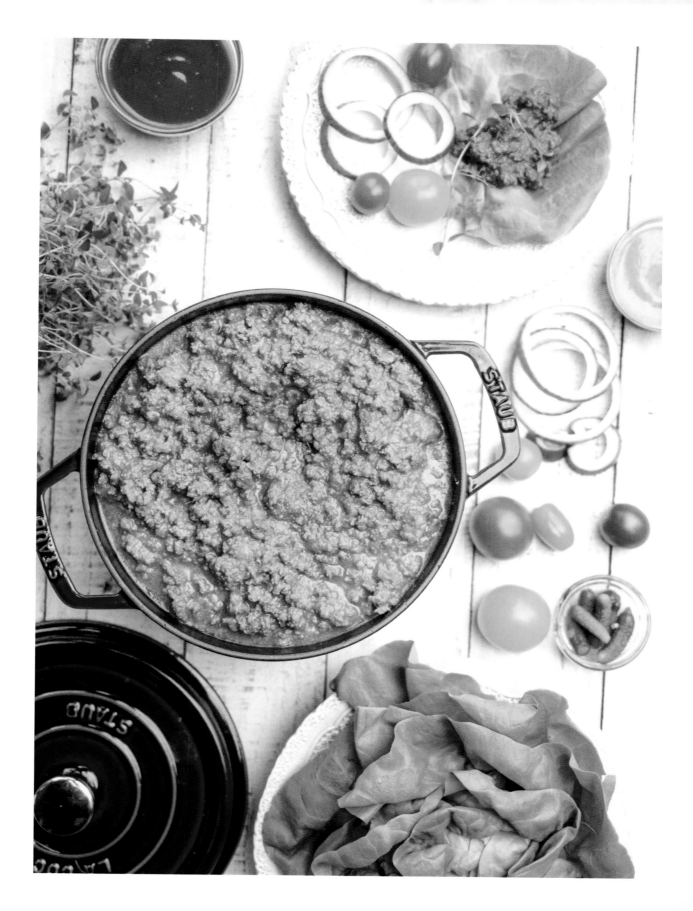

HUNGARIAN GOULASH

prep time: **8 minutes**   *cook time:* **48 minutes**   *yield:* **4 servings**

1 pound ground beef

½ cup diced onions

2 shallots, diced

2 cloves garlic, smashed to a paste

4 sprigs fresh thyme

2 sprigs fresh rosemary

1 (7-ounce) jar tomato paste

1 cup beef bone broth, homemade (page 106) or store-bought

¼ cup smoked paprika

1½ teaspoons fine sea salt

4 cups cauliflower florets, cut into ½-inch pieces

2 cups sliced mushrooms

For Garnish:

Drizzle of avocado oil or extra-virgin olive oil

Freshly ground black pepper

Fresh thyme leaves

1. Place the ground beef, onions, shallots, and garlic in a Dutch oven or soup pot over medium heat. Cook, stirring frequently to break up the large clumps, until the meat is cooked through, about 8 minutes. Meanwhile, tie the sprigs of thyme and rosemary together with kitchen twine.

2. Add the tomato paste, broth, paprika, salt, and tied herbs to the pot. Cover and simmer for 30 minutes. Add the cauliflower and mushrooms and cook for another 10 minutes or until the cauliflower is soft. Taste and adjust the seasoning, if desired. Remove the tied herbs. Serve the goulash in bowls, garnished with a drizzle of oil and a sprinkle of freshly ground pepper and thyme leaves.

3. Store in an airtight container in the refrigerator for up to 3 days. To reheat, place the goulash in a saucepan over medium heat for 3 minutes or until warmed through.

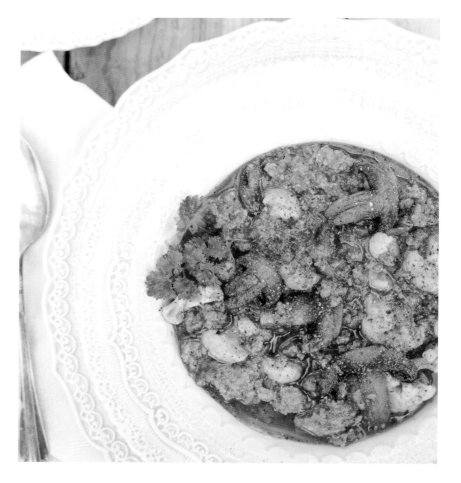

nutritional info (per serving)				
calories	fat	protein	carbs	fiber
381	23g	25g	17g	5g

JAMAICAN JERK POT ROAST

prep time: 10 minutes, plus time to marinate   cook time: 8 hours
yield: 8 servings

6 scallions, chopped

1 onion, chopped

1 jalapeño pepper, seeded and minced

½ cup coconut vinegar or apple cider vinegar

¼ cup MCT oil

3 tablespoons wheat-free tamari, or ¾ cup coconut aminos

2 tablespoons paprika

2 tablespoons Swerve confectioners'-style sweetener or equivalent amount of liquid or powdered sweetener (see page 29)

1 tablespoon chopped fresh thyme

½ teaspoon ground allspice

½ teaspoon ground cloves

½ teaspoon ground nutmeg

2 pounds boneless beef roast, cut into 4 equal chunks

4 cups shredded red cabbage, for serving

Pickled jalapeño slices, for garnish

Fresh thyme, for garnish

1. In a food processor or blender, combine the scallions, onion, jalapeño, vinegar, oil, tamari, paprika, sweetener, thyme, allspice, cloves, and nutmeg. Pulse until the ingredients are well combined and the mixture resembles a coarse paste.

2. Place the chunks of pot roast in a medium-sized bowl and coat with the marinade. Refrigerate for 4 to 6 hours or overnight.

3. Place the pot roast pieces and marinade in a 4-quart or larger slow cooker. Cover and cook on low for 7 to 8 hours, until the meat is tender and falls apart easily when pierced with a fork.

4. Remove the meat from the slow cooker and shred with 2 forks. Serve over shredded purple cabbage, garnished with pickled jalapeño and fresh thyme.

5. Store in an airtight container in the refrigerator for up to 4 days. To reheat, place the meat on a rimmed baking sheet in a 400°F oven for a few minutes, until warmed to your liking.

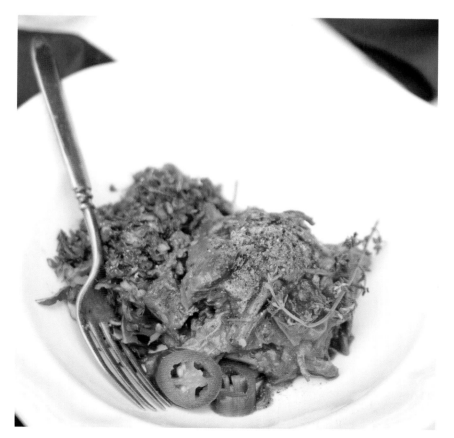

nutritional info (per serving)				
calories	fat	protein	carbs	fiber
411	27g	33g	8g	2g

FAJITA KABOBS

prep time: **10 minutes, plus time to marinate beef** *cook time:* **6 minutes**
yield: **4 servings**

¼ cup avocado oil or MCT oil

¼ cup lime juice

2 cloves garlic, minced

1 teaspoon fine sea salt

1 teaspoon chili powder

¾ teaspoon cayenne pepper

½ teaspoon ground cumin

½ teaspoon paprika

2 (8-ounce) boneless rib-eye steaks, about 1 inch thick

2 green bell peppers

1 red onion

8 grape tomatoes

½ cup Citrus Avocado Salsa (page 86), for serving

Boston lettuce leaves, for serving (optional)

Special Equipment:

8 wood skewers, soaked in water for 15 minutes

1. Make the marinade: Place the oil, lime juice, garlic, salt, and spices in a large bowl.

2. Cut the steaks into 1-inch cubes. Add the meat to the marinade and stir to coat well. Cover and refrigerate for at least 1 hour or overnight.

3. Preheat a grill to high heat. While the grill is heating up, cut the bell peppers and onion into 1-inch squares. Remove the meat from the marinade; reserve the marinade for basting.

4. Place 2 cubes of steak on a skewer, followed by an onion piece, a steak piece, a bell pepper piece, a steak piece, and a grape tomato, then repeat the sequence with another piece of steak, then onion, steak, and bell pepper, ending with 2 pieces of steak. Repeat with the remaining skewers and ingredients.

5. Lightly brush the hot grill grates with oil. Place the skewers on the grill for 3 minutes, basting every minute with the reserved marinade. Flip and cook, basting, for another 3 minutes for medium-rare steak (or cook longer for more well-done steak). Serve with the salsa and lettuce leaves for wrapping, if desired.

6. Store in an airtight container in the refrigerator for up to 4 days. To reheat, place in a skillet over medium heat, stirring often, for a few minutes, until warmed to your liking.

nutritional info (per serving)				
calories	fat	protein	carbs	fiber
370	28g	21g	10g	2g

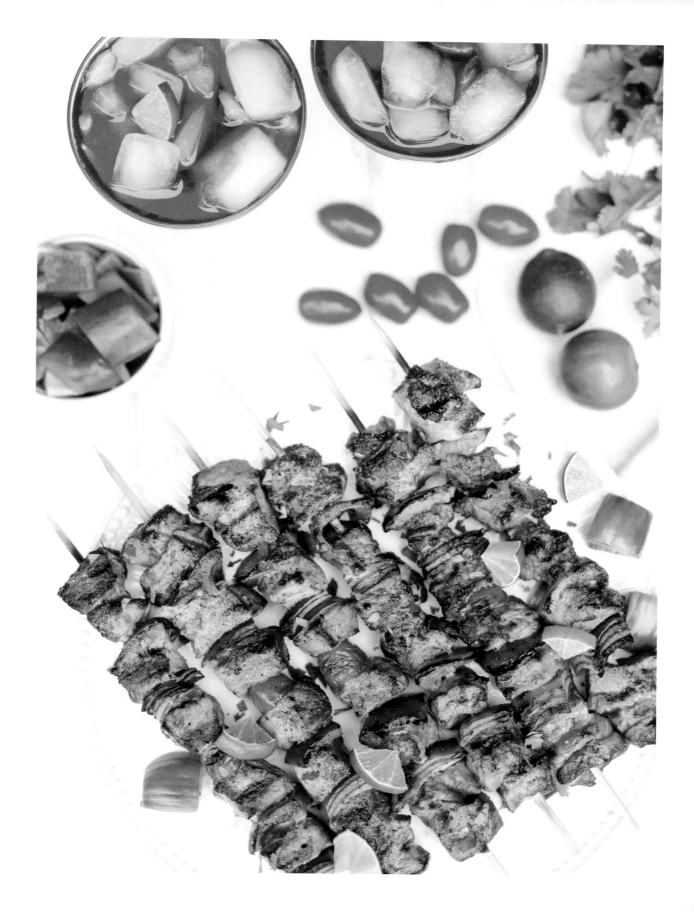

SIMPLE LAMB CHOPS
with Lemon Mustard Gravy

prep time: **3 minutes**   *cook time:* **10 minutes**   *yield:* **4 servings (2 chops per serving)**

8 (½-inch-thick) lamb chops

1½ teaspoons fine sea salt

1 teaspoon ground black pepper

1 tablespoon lard or coconut oil

1 clove garlic, smashed to a paste

1 teaspoon fresh thyme leaves, plus more for garnish

½ cup beef or chicken bone broth, homemade (page 106) or store-bought

2 tablespoons Dijon mustard

1 tablespoon lemon juice

1 tablespoon Swerve confectioners'-style sweetener or equivalent amount of liquid or powdered sweetener (see page 29)

1. Season the lamb chops with the salt and pepper.

2. Heat the lard in a large cast-iron skillet over medium-high heat. Sear the chops for 4 minutes or until golden brown, then flip and cook for another 4 minutes for medium-done chops (or cook longer if you prefer more well-done chops, adjusting the cook time if your chops are thicker than ½ inch). Remove the chops from the pan and set aside while you make the sauce; leave the drippings in the skillet.

3. Lower the heat to medium, then add the garlic and thyme to the skillet and cook for 30 seconds. Add the broth and use a whisk to scrape up the bits stuck to the bottom of the skillet. Whisk in the mustard, lemon juice, and sweetener. Bring to a boil and cook for 2 minutes or until thickened a little. To serve, spoon the sauce over the chops and garnish with additional thyme.

4. Store in an airtight container in the refrigerator for up to 3 days. To reheat, place the chops in a preheated 350°F oven for 4 minutes or until warmed through.

nutritional info (per serving)				
calories	fat	protein	carbs	fiber
730	57g	48g	1g	0.4g

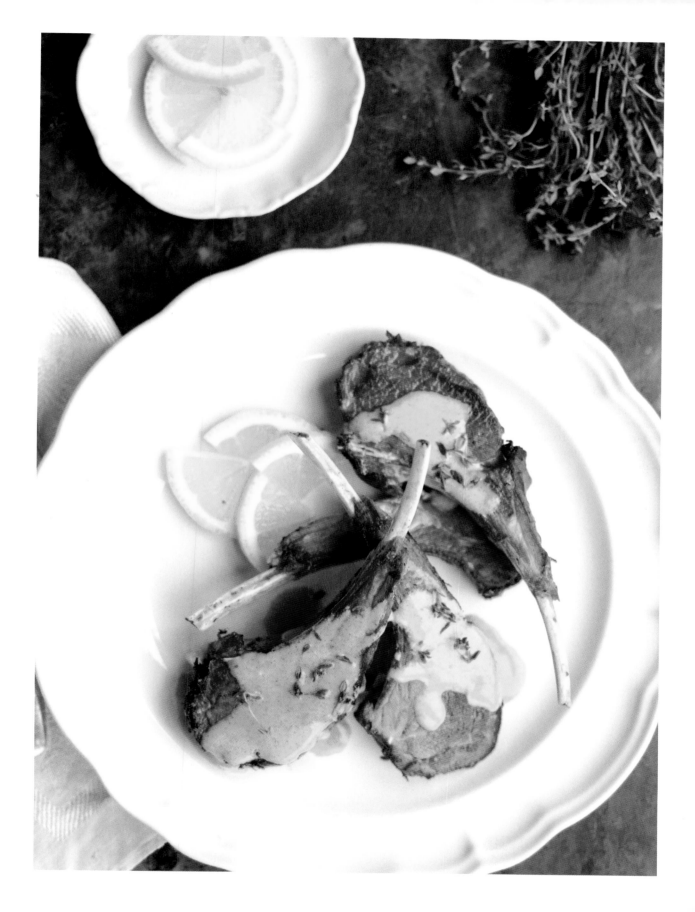

KUNG PAO MEATBALLS IN LETTUCE CUPS

Meatballs:

2 pounds ground beef

2 large eggs, beaten

¾ cup finely chopped button mushrooms

¼ cup finely chopped scallions

2 tablespoons Swerve confectioners'-style sweetener or equivalent amount of liquid or powdered sweetener (see page 29)

2 teaspoons peeled and grated fresh ginger

1½ teaspoons wheat-free tamari, or 2 tablespoons coconut aminos

1 teaspoon toasted (dark) sesame oil

1 teaspoon crushed red pepper

1 clove garlic, smashed to a paste

Boston lettuce leaves, for serving

For Garnish (optional):

Crushed pili nuts or macadamia nuts

Crushed red pepper

1. Preheat the oven to 400°F.

2. Place the ingredients for the meatballs in a large bowl. Using your hands, mix together until well combined. Shape into 1½-inch meatballs and place on a rimmed baking sheet.

3. Bake the meatballs for 20 minutes or until browned. To serve, place the meatballs in the lettuce leaves. Garnish with crushed nuts and/ or crushed red pepper, if desired.

4. Store in an airtight container in the refrigerator for up to 4 days or in the freezer for up to a month. To reheat, place the meatballs in a baking dish in a preheated 350°F oven for 5 minutes or until warmed through.

nutritional info (per serving)				
calories	fat	protein	carbs	fiber
373	29g	22g	5g	3g

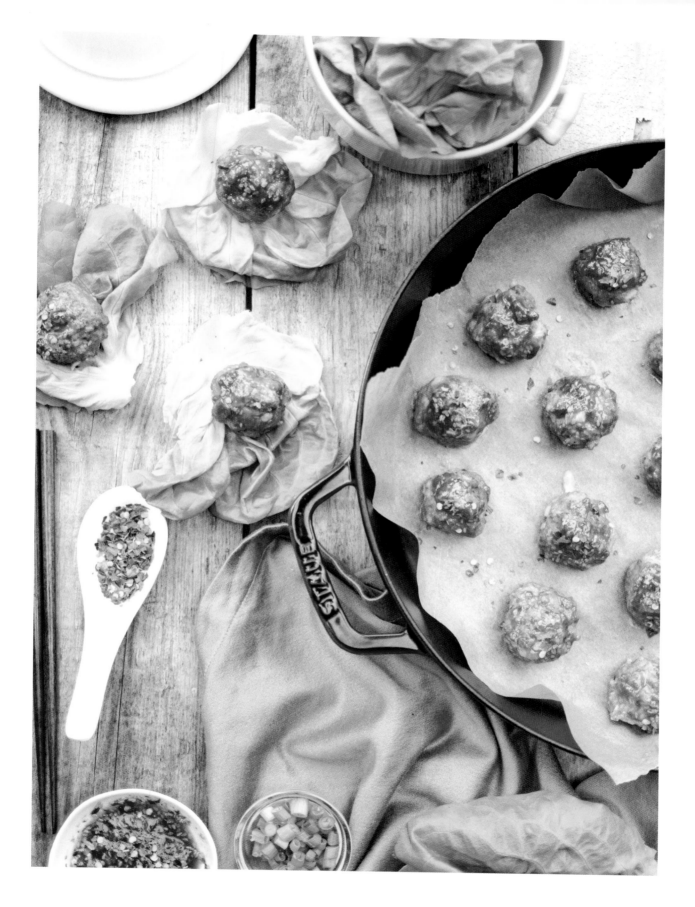

CHINESE FIVE-SPICE ROAST BEEF

If you're in a hurry, you can make this recipe in a pressure cooker. If you have time to spare, a slow cooker is an excellent option as well. Both methods are included below. The shredded meat makes a delicious filling for wraps.

prep time: 5 minutes   *cook time:* 30 minutes in a pressure cooker; 8 hours in a slow cooker   *yield:* 12 servings

1 (4-pound) boneless beef roast

Fine sea salt and ground black pepper

1 cup beef bone broth, homemade (page 106) or store-bought

2 tablespoons wheat-free tamari, or ½ cup coconut aminos

½ cup diced onions

2 tablespoons Chinese five-spice powder

4 cloves garlic, minced

For Garnish:

Sliced scallions

Fresh cilantro

1. Generously season the roast on all sides with salt and pepper. Place the roast in a pressure cooker or 4-quart or larger slow cooker, then add the rest of the ingredients.

2. If using a pressure cooker, cover and cook for 30 minutes, then slowly release the pressure before removing the lid. If using a slow cooker, cover and cook on low for 6 to 8 hours or until the meat is fork-tender and falls apart easily when pierced with a fork.

3. Shred the meat with 2 forks. Toss with the accumulated juices in the cooker to moisten the meat. Garnish with scallions and cilantro and serve.

4. Store in an airtight container in the refrigerator for up to 4 days. To reheat, place the roast beef in a pot over medium heat, stirring often, for a few minutes, until warmed to your liking.

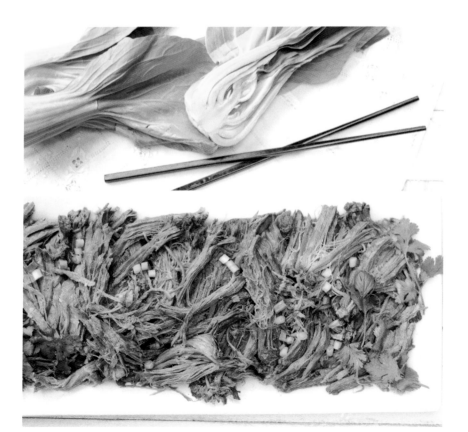

nutritional info (per serving)				
calories	fat	protein	carbs	fiber
418	26g	41g	2g	0.1g

COWBOY STEAK FOR TWO

1 (1½-pound) bone-in rib-eye steak, about 1½ inches thick

2 teaspoons fine sea salt

1 teaspoon ground black pepper

½ cup Steak Sauce (page 36), for serving (optional)

You can use a different cut of steak, such as porterhouse, if you prefer. The timing will depend on how well-done you like your steak and how thick the steak is. Leftovers taste great over greens!

prep time: **3 minutes, plus time to let steak come to room temperature and rest**
cook time: **10 minutes** *yield:* **2 servings**

1. Preheat a grill to high heat. Pat the steaks dry and season with the salt and pepper. Allow to sit at room temperature for 15 minutes.

2. Place the steak on the hot grill and cook for 5 minutes, then flip and cook for another 5 minutes for a rare steak, or continue to cook to your liking.

3. Allow the steak to rest for 10 minutes before serving. Serve with steak sauce, if desired.

4. Store in an airtight container in the refrigerator for up to 4 days. To reheat, place the steak in a cast-iron skillet over medium heat, turning often, for a few minutes on each side or until warmed through.

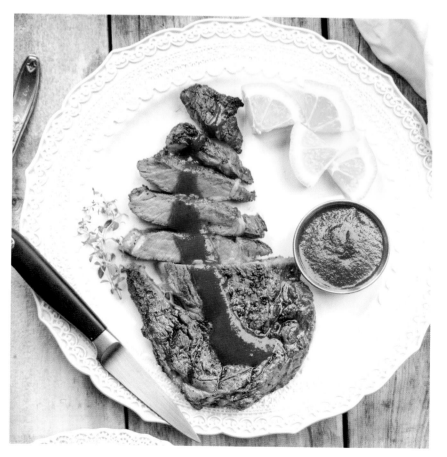

nutritional info (per serving)				
calories	fat	protein	carbs	fiber
823	64g	61g	1g	0.3g

SHAN BEEF STIR-FRY

KETO

Shan-style cooking comes from Myanmar, where the food is often made with delicious spices and is served with rice. This tasty Shan-inspired beef is served over keto "rice."

prep time: **4 minutes** *cook time:* **18 minutes** *yield:* **4 servings**

2 tablespoons coconut oil

1 cup thinly sliced shallots

1½ teaspoons turmeric powder

½ teaspoon crushed red pepper, plus more for garnish (optional)

1 pound ground beef

2 teaspoons fine sea salt, divided

8 large eggs

¼ cup beef bone broth, homemade (page 106) or store-bought

1. Heat the oil in a wok or large cast-iron skillet over medium-high heat. When hot, add the shallots, turmeric, and crushed red pepper and stir-fry for 2 minutes.

2. Add the beef and season with 1½ teaspoons of the salt. Stir-fry, while breaking up the clumps, until the beef is cooked through, about 4 minutes. Meanwhile, beat the eggs with the broth and the remaining ½ teaspoon of salt. Remove the beef from the wok and set aside on a warm plate, leaving the drippings in the wok.

3. Set the wok over medium heat. Pour the egg-broth mixture into the wok and cook, whisking constantly, until the eggs are set and whisked into small ricelike pieces.

4. Divide the "rice" among 4 serving bowls. Add one-quarter of the beef mixture to each bowl. Garnish with additional crushed red pepper, if desired.

5. Store in an airtight container in the refrigerator for up to 4 days. To reheat, place the stir-fry in a pot over medium heat, stirring often, for a few minutes, until warmed to your liking.

nutritional info (per serving)				
calories	fat	protein	carbs	fiber
581	48g	34g	5g	1g

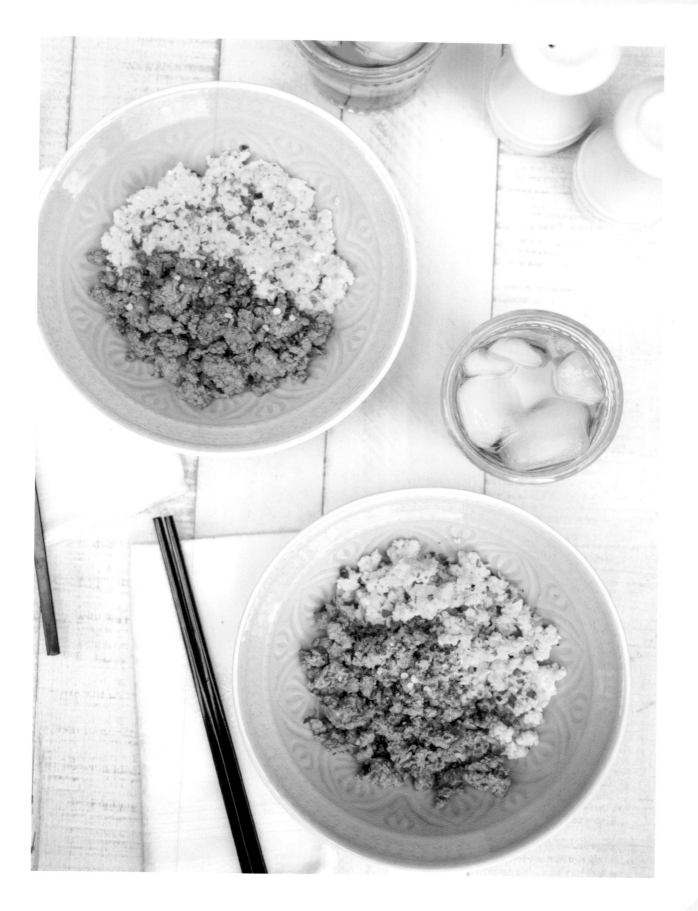

LAMB CHOPS
with Gyro Salad

To make this flavorful meal even easier, I chop up the ingredients for the salad and make the vinaigrette the night before. All I have to do come mealtime is grill the chops for 4 minutes, and dinner is served!

prep time: **8 minutes** *(not including time to make vinaigrette)*
cook time: **4 minutes**   *yield:* **8 servings**

8 lamb loin chops, about 1¼ inches thick

2 teaspoons fine sea salt

½ teaspoon ground black pepper

Gyro Salad:

2 cups Greek olives, pitted

¼ cup diced red onions

1 medium cucumber, diced

1 medium tomato, diced

4 sprigs fresh oregano

1 batch Greek Vinaigrette (page 46)

1. Preheat a grill to high heat.

2. While the grill is heating up, season the chops with the salt and pepper and allow to sit at room temperature.

3. When the grill is hot, place the chops on the grill and cook for 2 minutes per side for medium-rare chops, or cook longer if you prefer more well-done meat. (*Note:* If the chops are thicker than 1¼ inches, you will need to cook them longer.) Place on a platter and allow to rest for a few minutes before slicing.

4. Make the salad: Toss the olives, onions, cucumber, tomato, and oregano in the vinaigrette; dress only the amount of salad you plan to eat right away. Serve the salad with the chops.

5. Store the chops and salad in separate airtight containers in the refrigerator for up to 4 days. To reheat the chops, place them in a cast-iron skillet over medium heat for a few minutes, turning often, until warmed through.

Note: *A full batch of the Greek Vinaigrette is more than you will need for this recipe, but it keeps for up to 2 weeks in the refrigerator and is wonderful to have on hand for easy salads. You can also use the leftover dressing to make Greek Chicken Thighs (page 186).*

nutritional info (per serving)				
calories	fat	protein	carbs	fiber
596	53g	27g	5g	3g

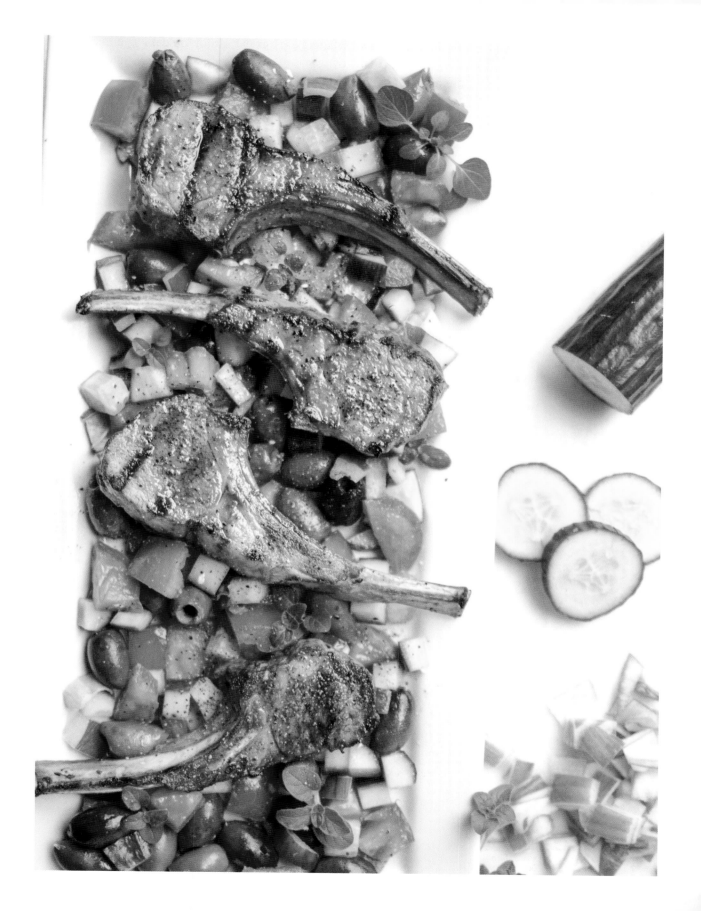

ITALIAN BEEF TIPS

KETO

Craig and I got married in the Northwoods of Wisconsin at High Point Village. One of the things we served for dinner was beef tips, which are a standard at Wisconsin weddings. If I were able to do it over again, I would certainly make the beef tips like this instead! Low and slow creates tender and juicy meat.

prep time: 5 minutes *cook time:* 6 hours *yield:* 10 servings

2 cups marinara sauce

1 cup beef bone broth, homemade (page 106) or store-bought

¼ cup diced onions

4 cloves garlic, minced

2 teaspoons dried basil leaves

2 teaspoons ground dried oregano

1 teaspoon fine ground sea salt

1 teaspoon ground black pepper

1 (5-pound) boneless top sirloin or rump roast, cut into 1-inch cubes

Fresh thyme or oregano leaves, for garnish (optional)

1. Place the marinara sauce, broth, onions, garlic, basil, oregano, salt, and pepper in a 4-quart or larger slow cooker. Place the cubed roast on top of the broth mixture. Cook, covered, on low for 6 hours. The roast is done when the meat is very tender and falls apart easily.

2. Serve the meat with the sauce from the slow cooker. Garnish with fresh thyme or oregano, if desired.

3. Store in an airtight container in the refrigerator for up to 3 days. To reheat, place the meat in a large cast-iron skillet over medium heat, stirring occasionally, for 5 minutes or until warmed through.

nutritional info (per serving)				
calories	fat	protein	carbs	fiber
667	51g	39g	2g	1g

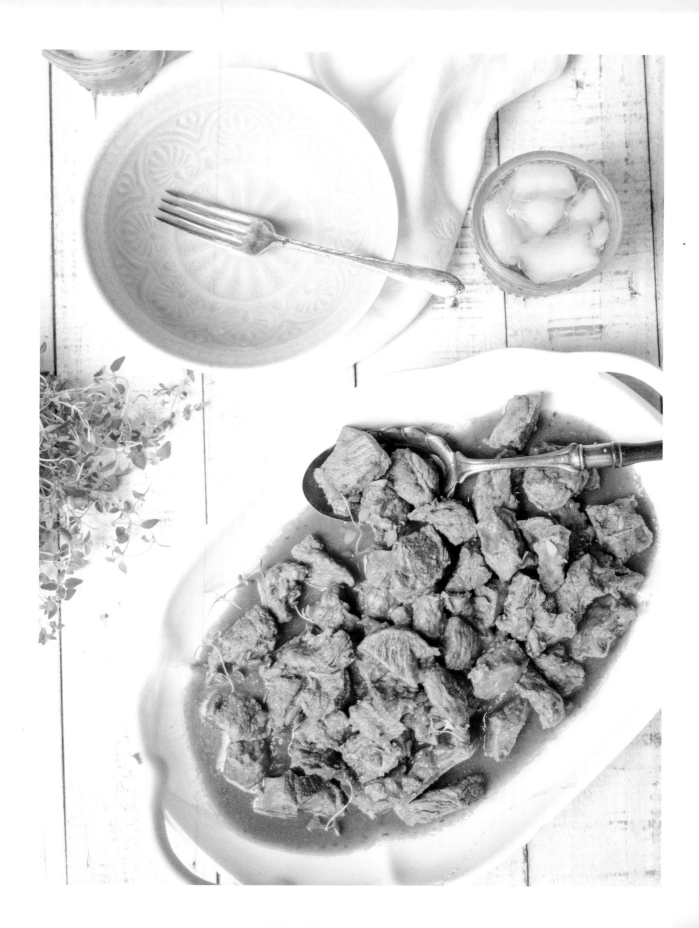

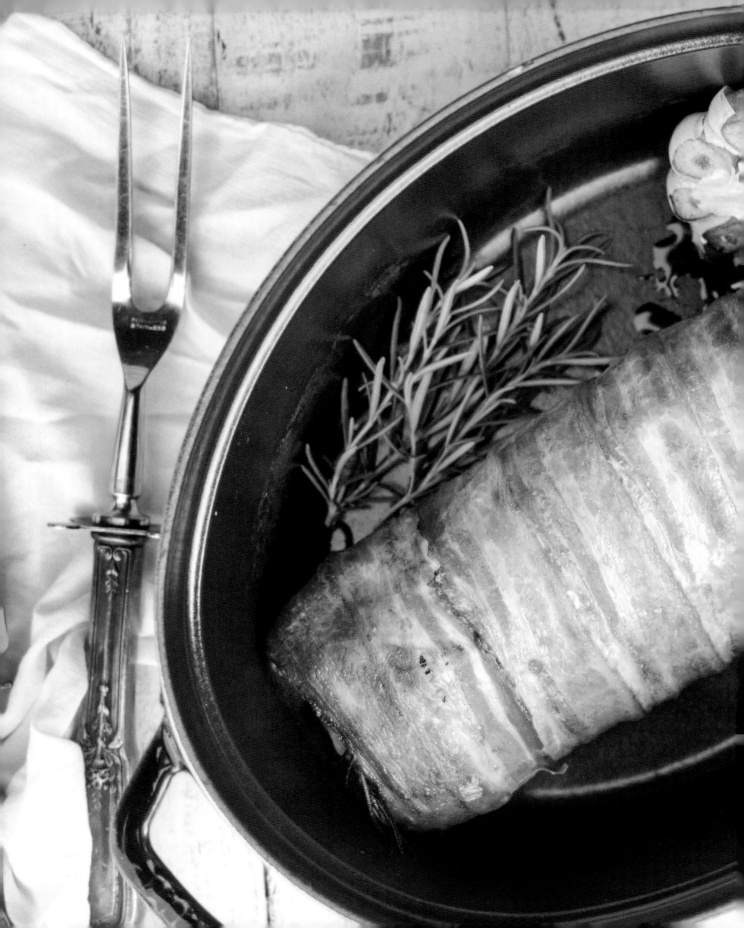

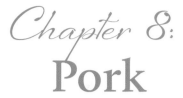

Chapter 8:
Pork

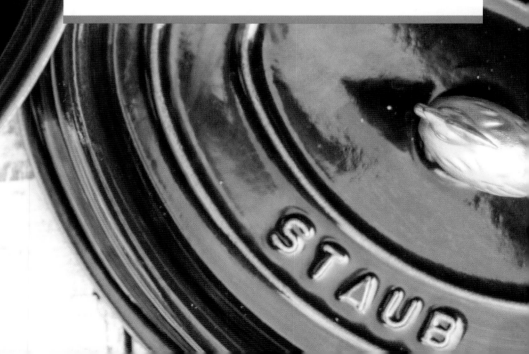

CITRUS PORK SHOULDER
with Spicy Cilantro-Ginger Sauce

prep time: **10 minutes**   *cook time:* **8 hours**   *yield:* **8 servings**

¼ cup diced onions

8 cloves garlic, minced

¼ cup melted lard or avocado oil

¼ cup Swerve confectioners'-style sweetener or equivalent amount of liquid or powdered sweetener (see page 29) (optional)

2 tablespoons fine sea salt

2 teaspoons ground black pepper

2 teaspoons smoked paprika

Juice of 2 limes

4 drops orange oil

1 (6-pound) boneless pork shoulder

Spicy Cilantro-Ginger Sauce:

1 cup mayonnaise, homemade (page 34 or 35) or store-bought

¼ cup chopped fresh cilantro

¼ cup lime juice

2 tablespoons peeled and grated fresh ginger

2 tablespoons chopped fresh chives

1 teaspoon chopped garlic

1 jalapeño pepper, seeded and coarsely chopped

½ teaspoon fine sea salt

For Garnish:

Lime wedges

Freshly ground black pepper

1. Place the onions, garlic, melted lard, sweetener, salt, pepper, paprika, lime juice, and orange oil in a slow cooker. Stir to combine, then place the pork shoulder on top of the other ingredients. Turn the pork in the seasonings to coat it on all sides, then cover the slow cooker and cook on low for 8 hours or until the pork shreds easily.

2. Meanwhile, make the sauce: Place all the ingredients for the sauce in a food processor and puree until very smooth. Set aside in the refrigerator until ready to serve.

3. When the meat is done, shred it with 2 forks and toss the meat in the juices from the slow cooker. Garnish with lime wedges and freshly ground pepper. Serve each portion of meat with 3 tablespoons of the sauce.

4. Store in an airtight container in the refrigerator for up to 3 days. To reheat, place the pork on a rimmed baking sheet in a preheated 350°F oven for 5 minutes or until warmed through.

Busy Family Tip: *The sauce can be made up to a week ahead and stored in an airtight container in the refrigerator. Shake well before using.*

nutritional info (per serving)				
calories	fat	protein	carbs	fiber
713	59g	39g	3g	1g

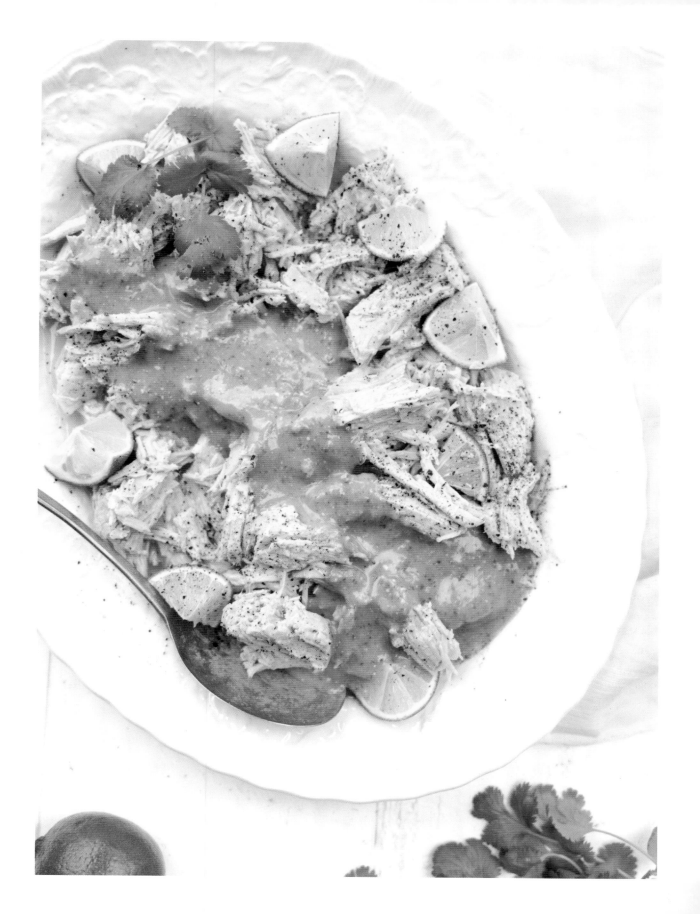

SPRING HAM BAKE
with Dijon Sauce

KETO

If you have a large crew coming over for brunch, this tasty recipe can easily be doubled. The presentation is so lovely that your guests will think that you slaved over it, but nothing could be further from the truth. I often prepare the dish the night before so that all I have to do is throw it in the oven before guests arrive. To make this recipe even easier, you can purchase premade and peeled hard-boiled eggs at your local grocery store.

prep time: **8 minutes (not including time to boil egg)** *cook time:* **20 minutes**
yield: **4 servings (2 bundles per serving)**

Fine sea salt

16 thick asparagus spears, ends trimmed

1 tablespoon avocado oil

8 slices ham

½ cup mayonnaise, homemade (page 34) or store-bought, or Baconnaise (page 34), or more to taste

2 tablespoons Dijon mustard

1 hard-boiled egg (see page 81), peeled and thinly sliced

For Garnish:

Freshly ground black pepper

Fresh thyme leaves

1. Preheat the oven to 375°F.

2. Bring a large pot of water to a boil. When it reaches a boil, salt it well with about 2 tablespoons of salt. Add the asparagus and boil for 5 minutes or until crisp-tender. Drain and rinse the asparagus with cold water; this helps retain the bright green color. Sprinkle the asparagus with salt and rub some oil over each spear using your hands.

3. Wrap a slice of ham around 2 asparagus spears to form a bundle. Repeat with the remaining ham and asparagus. Place in a 13 by 9-inch baking dish. (*Note:* This can be done the night before.)

4. Bake for 12 to 15 minutes, until the ham is warm and the asparagus is tender.

5. Meanwhile, make the Dijon sauce: Place the mayonnaise and mustard in a small bowl and stir well to combine. Season with salt to taste. Add more mayo if the sauce is too spicy for you.

6. Remove the baking dish from the oven and pour the sauce down the middle of the ham-wrapped asparagus. Arrange the sliced hard-boiled egg on top. Sprinkle with additional salt, some freshly ground pepper, and thyme leaves.

7. This dish is best served fresh; however, you can store leftovers in an airtight container in the refrigerator for up to 3 days. To reheat, place in a baking dish in a preheated 375°F oven for 5 minutes or until warmed through.

nutritional info (per serving)				
calories	fat	protein	carbs	fiber
356	31g	15g	2g	1g

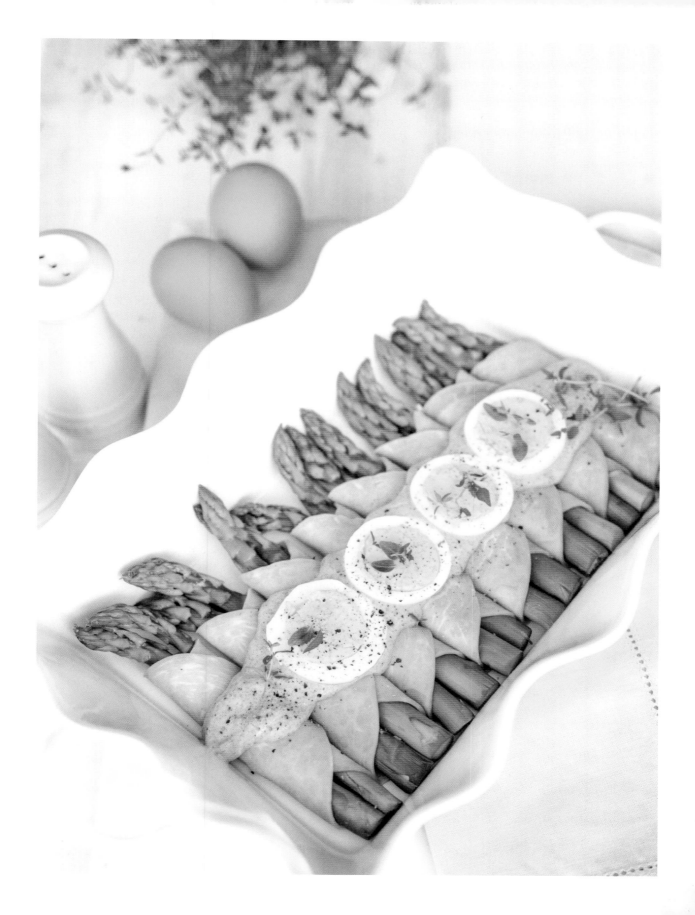

EASY BARBECUE RIBS

KETO

⅓ cup Swerve confectioners'-style sweetener or equivalent amount of powdered sweetener (see page 29)

1½ teaspoons fine sea salt

1 tablespoon paprika

1½ teaspoons chili powder

1 teaspoon ground black pepper

¾ teaspoon onion powder

4 pounds country-style pork ribs

2 cups tomato sauce

1 teaspoon liquid smoke (optional)

When Craig and I first started dating, he took me to a restaurant called Famous Dave's that specializes in smoked meats and ribs. Their ribs are amazing, but they're also loaded with sugar. I love barbecue sauce, and the amount of sauce I would use at Famous Dave's probably contained ½ cup of sugar! I still love BBQ ribs; I just make my own now.

prep time: **5 minutes**   *cook time:* **8 hours**   *yield:* **12 servings**

1. In a small bowl, combine the sweetener, salt, and spices. Rub the mixture all over the surface of the ribs.

2. Place the ribs in a 4-quart (or larger) slow cooker standing on their ends with the meaty side facing out. Pour the tomato sauce into the slow cooker and add the liquid smoke, if using. Cover the slow cooker and cook on low for 7 to 8 hours, until the meat is fork-tender and falls off the bone. Serve topped with the flavorful barbecue sauce from the slow cooker.

3. Store in an airtight container in the refrigerator for up to 3 days. To reheat, place the ribs on a rimmed baking sheet in a preheated 350°F oven for 5 minutes or until warmed through.

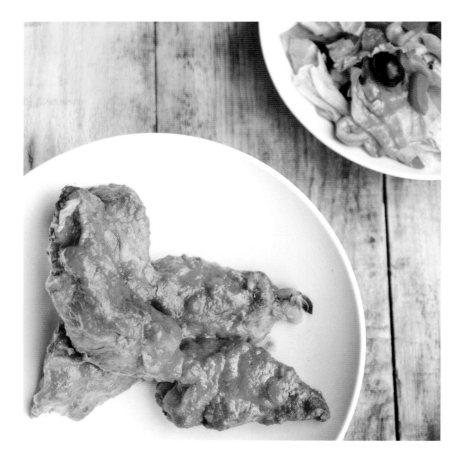

nutritional info (per serving)				
calories	fat	protein	carbs	fiber
602	46g	44g	2g	0.5g

SAUCY BARBECUE PORK CHOPS

prep time: **5 minutes**   *cook time:* **15 minutes**   *yield:* **4 servings**

2 tablespoons lard or coconut oil, plus more for drizzling

¼ cup diced onions

4 (¾-inch-thick) bone-in pork chops (about 8 ounces each)

½ teaspoon fine sea salt

¼ teaspoon ground black pepper

2 cups tomato sauce

½ cup Swerve confectioners'-style sweetener or equivalent amount of liquid or powdered sweetener (see page 29)

1 clove garlic, smashed to a paste

1 teaspoon liquid smoke (optional)

For Garnish (optional):

Fresh parsley or sliced scallions

Freshly ground black pepper

1. Heat the lard in a large cast-iron skillet over medium-high heat. Add the onions and sauté for 2 minutes or until soft.

2. Sprinkle the pork chops with the salt and pepper. Move the onions to the side of the skillet and sear the chops on one side for 3 minutes, then flip and sear on the other side for 3 minutes.

3. Add the tomato sauce, sweetener, garlic, and liquid smoke, if using, to the skillet and stir well. Cook for another 7 minutes or until the pork chops are cooked through. The internal temperature of the chops should reach 135°F.

4. To serve, place the pork chops on a platter and pour the sauce on top. Garnish with parsley, freshly ground pepper, and a drizzle of melted lard.

5. Store in an airtight container in the refrigerator for up to 3 days. To reheat, place the chops in a greased skillet over medium-high heat for a few minutes, until warmed through.

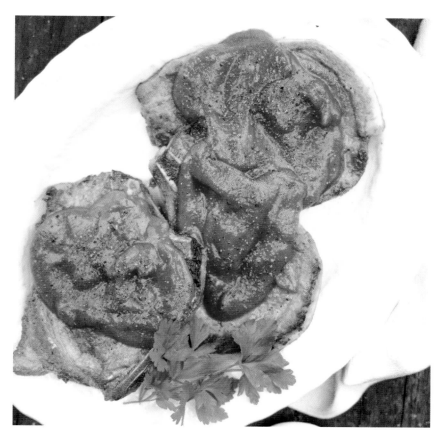

nutritional info (per serving)				
calories	fat	protein	carbs	fiber
756	63g	37g	7g	1g

GINGER LIME PORK LETTUCE CUPS

prep time: **8 minutes**   *cook time:* **8 minutes**   *yield:* **4 servings**

Pork Filling:

1 tablespoon coconut oil or avocado oil

½ cup chopped onions

2 cloves garlic, minced

1 pound ground pork

Fine sea salt

2 teaspoons peeled and grated fresh ginger

1 tablespoon coconut vinegar or rice wine vinegar

2 teaspoons toasted (dark) sesame oil

1 teaspoon fish sauce (optional, for umami flavor)

¾ teaspoon wheat-free tamari, or 1 tablespoon coconut aminos

Dipping Sauce:

½ cup lime juice

2 tablespoons fish sauce

¼ cup Swerve confectioners'-style sweetener or equivalent amount of liquid or powdered sweetener (see page 29)

1 clove garlic, crushed

1 teaspoon peeled and grated fresh ginger

1 teaspoon Asian chile sauce, such as sambal oelek

½ teaspoon fine sea salt

For Serving:

1 head butter lettuce, leaves separated

½ bunch fresh basil

½ bunch fresh cilantro

½ bunch fresh mint

1 jalapeño pepper, seeded and thinly sliced (optional)

Lime slices or wedges (optional)

1. Make the pork filling: Heat the oil in a large cast-iron skillet over medium-high heat. Add the onions and sauté for 1 minute or until softened. Add the garlic and cook for another minute, stirring often. Add the ground pork and season with a few pinches of salt. Cook while crumbling for 4 minutes or until the pork is cooked through and no longer pink. Add the ginger, vinegar, sesame oil, fish sauce (if using), and tamari and stir to coat the meat well. Slide the pan off the heat.

2. Make the dipping sauce: Place the ingredients for the sauce in a medium-sized bowl and stir well to combine.

3. To serve, spoon the pork filling into lettuce leaves. (Make only the number of lettuce cups that will be eaten right away.) If desired, top with fresh herbs and jalapeño slices. Wrap the lettuce around the fillings and serve with the dipping sauce, with lime slices or wedges on the side, if desired.

4. Store in an airtight container in the refrigerator for up to 4 days. To reheat, place the pork filling in a cast-iron skillet over medium heat for 3 minutes or until warmed through.

nutritional info (per serving)				
calories	fat	protein	carbs	fiber
353	27g	23g	8g	3g

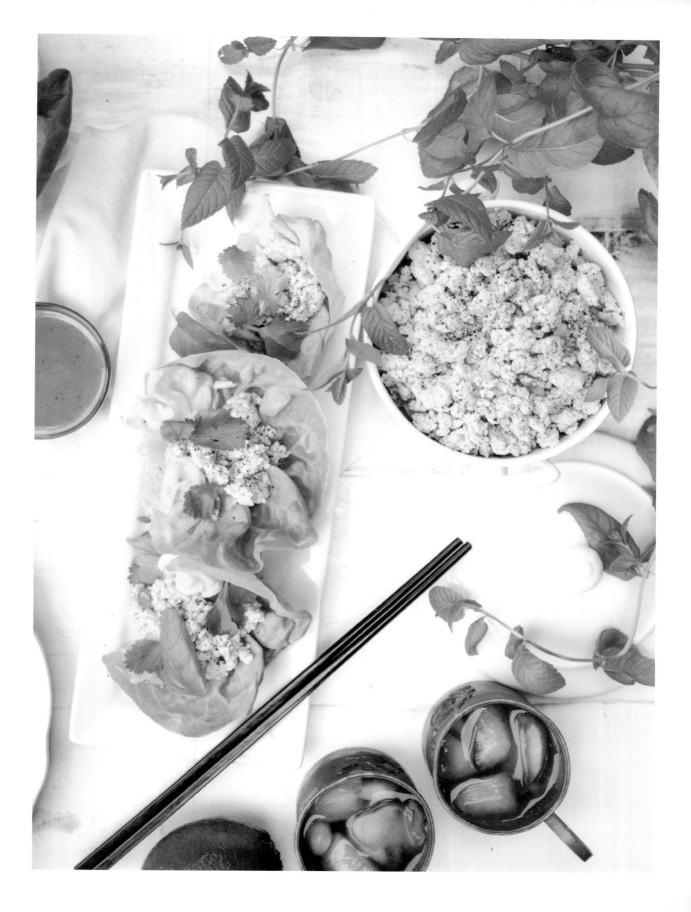

PORK CHOPS
with Dijon Gravy

prep time: **4 minutes**   *cook time:* **16 minutes**   *yield:* **4 servings**

1 tablespoon coconut oil or avocado oil

¼ cup diced onions

4 (¾-inch-thick) bone-in pork chops (about 8 ounces each)

1 teaspoon fine sea salt

½ teaspoon ground black pepper

¾ cup chicken bone broth, homemade (page 106) or store-bought

¼ cup plus 2 tablespoons Dijon mustard

Sprigs of fresh oregano or other herb of choice, for garnish (optional)

2 teaspoons avocado oil, for drizzling (optional)

1. Heat the oil in a large cast-iron skillet over medium heat. Add the onions and sauté for 2 minutes.

2. Season the pork chops on all sides with the salt and pepper. Place the chops in the skillet and sear on one side for 6 minutes. Flip and cook for another 6 minutes or until cooked through. (The internal temperature of the chops should reach 135°F.)

3. Add the broth and mustard to the skillet. Whisk until well combined, then bring to a boil for 2 minutes to thicken slightly.

4. Serve the chops smothered in the mustard gravy. Garnish with fresh herbs and a drizzle of avocado oil, if desired.

5. Store in an airtight container in the refrigerator for up to 3 days. To reheat, place the chops in a greased skillet over medium-high heat for a few minutes, until warmed through.

nutritional info (per serving)				
calories	fat	protein	carbs	fiber
287	17g	25g	1g	0.3g

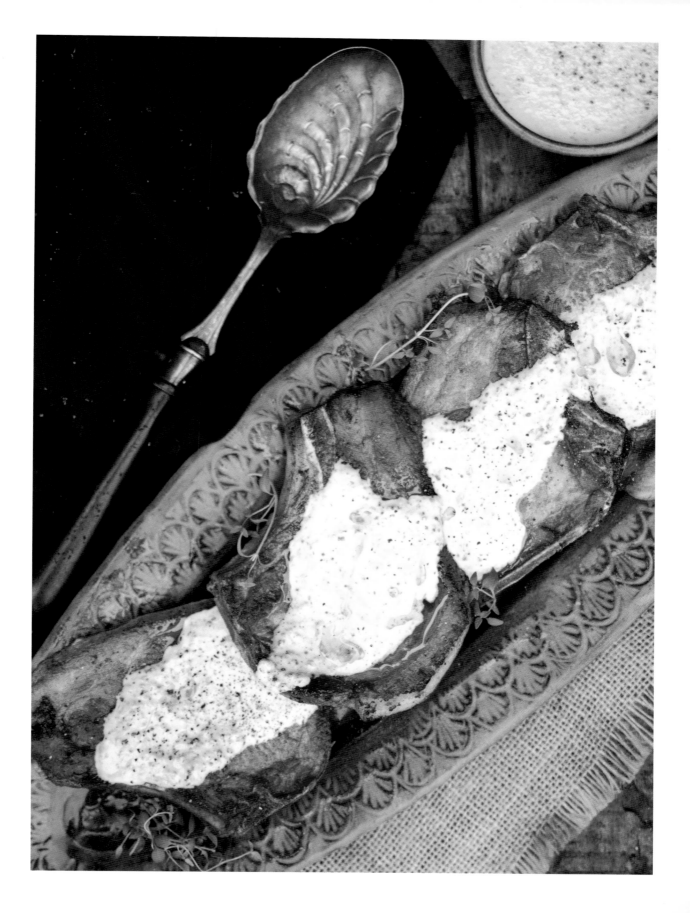

SAUSAGE ZUCCHINI RAVIOLI

prep time: **7 minutes, plus time to sweat zucchini** *cook time:* **14 minutes**

yield: **2 servings (4 ravioli per serving)**

2 medium zucchini, about 8 inches long by 1½ inches wide

1½ teaspoons fine sea salt, divided

4 ounces bulk Italian sausage

¼ teaspoon ground black pepper

2 cups marinara sauce, warmed

Chopped fresh basil, for garnish

1. Preheat the oven to 350°F.

2. Very thinly slice the zucchini lengthwise into 16 lasagna-like "noodles." (You will need 16 noodles to make 8 ravioli.) Place the slices of zucchini in a colander in the sink. Sprinkle with 1¼ teaspoons of the salt and let sit for 5 minutes to allow the excess water to drain from the zucchini. Squeeze the zucchini slices gently to release the excess moisture.

3. Place the sausage in a medium-sized sauté pan over medium heat. Season with the remaining ¼ teaspoon of salt and the pepper and sauté, breaking up the meat with a spatula, until cooked through, about 4 minutes. Slide the pan off the heat.

4. To make the ravioli, place 2 slices of zucchini on a work surface in a cross shape, overlapping in the center. Spoon 1 tablespoon of the sausage into the center of the cross of zucchini slices. Fold the edges over to make a tight ravioli-shaped "pocket." Repeat with the remaining zucchini and sausage. Place the ravioli, edges side down, in a 13 by 9-inch baking dish. Bake for 10 minutes or until the zucchini is soft.

5. To serve, place 4 ravioli on each plate, cover with marinara sauce, and garnish with basil.

6. Store in an airtight container in the refrigerator for up to 4 days. To reheat, place the ravioli on a rimmed baking sheet in a preheated 350°F oven for about 3 minutes, until warmed through.

nutritional info (per serving)				
calories	fat	protein	carbs	fiber
217	15g	12g	9g	3g

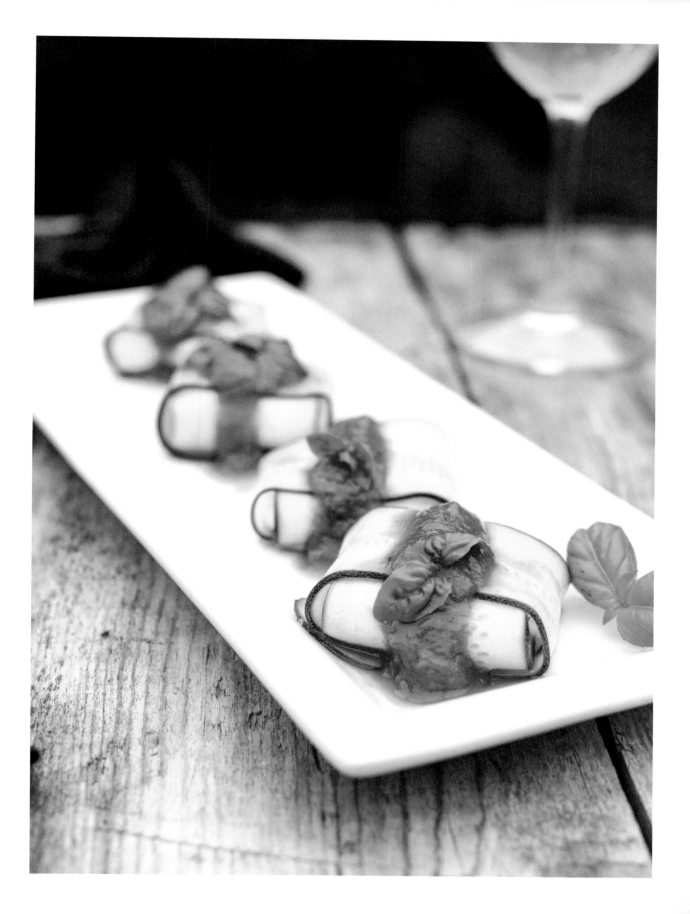

JUICY PORK TENDERLOIN

KETO

Pork tenderloins are often sold in packages of two small tenderloins rather than one large tenderloin. I like purchasing these smaller loins because they cook faster—and that makes getting dinner on the table that much quicker!

prep time: **5 minutes**   *cook time:* **40 minutes**   *yield:* **12 servings**

2 (2-pound) pork tenderloins

Coconut oil, for the baking dish

8 cloves garlic, sliced in half lengthwise

¼ cup Swerve confectioners'-style sweetener or equivalent amount of liquid or powdered sweetener (see page 29)

2 tablespoons wheat-free tamari, or ½ cup coconut aminos

2 tablespoons lime juice

1 tablespoon peeled and grated fresh ginger

4 drops orange oil (optional)

For Garnish (optional):

Chopped fresh cilantro

Lime slices

1. Preheat the oven to 350°F. Grease a baking dish large enough to fit both tenderloins with coconut oil.

2. Place the tenderloins in the baking dish, then cut 8 small slits into the top of each loin, just deep enough to fit half a clove of garlic. Push the garlic into the slits.

3. Place the sweetener, tamari, lime juice, ginger, and orange oil, if using, in a small bowl and stir well to combine. Pour over the pork in the baking dish.

4. Bake for 40 minutes or until the pork is cooked through and no longer pink inside. (A meat thermometer should read 140°F when inserted into the middle of one of the tenderloins.)

5. Place the pork on a cutting board to rest for 10 minutes before slicing. Cut into ½-inch slices and pour the sauce from the pan over the pork. Garnish with cilantro and lime slices, if desired.

6. Store in an airtight container in the refrigerator for up to 4 days. To reheat, place the pork in a baking dish in a preheated 350°F oven for 4 minutes or until warmed through.

nutritional info (per serving)				
calories	fat	protein	carbs	fiber
216	8g	32g	1g	0.1g

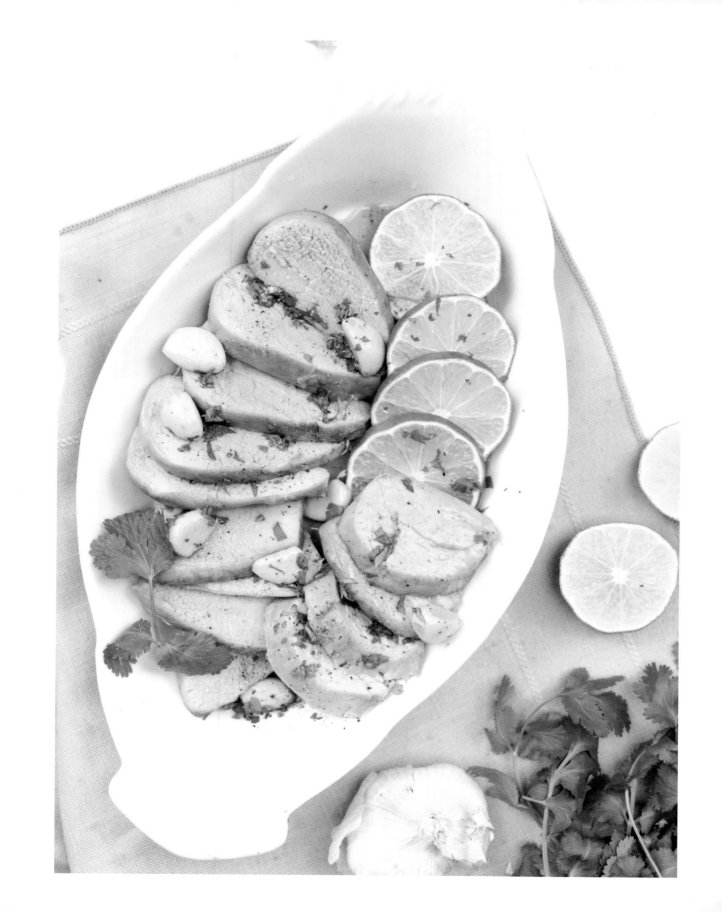

THAI PULLED PORK
with Keto Fried "Rice"

KETO · OPTION

prep time: **5 minutes** *cook time:* **4 to 8 hours** *yield:* **12 servings**

3 pounds boneless pork shoulder

2 cups full-fat coconut milk

¼ cup fish sauce, or 2 teaspoons fine sea salt

½ cup chopped fresh cilantro

½ cup chopped scallions

2 batches Keto Fried "Rice" (page 148) or Cauliflower Rice (page 149), for serving

For Garnish:

Lime wedges

Fresh cilantro

Sliced scallions

1. Place the pork shoulder in a 4-quart or larger slow cooker. Add the coconut milk, fish sauce, cilantro, and scallions. Cover the slow cooker and cook on low for 8 hours or on high for 4 to 5 hours, until the pork is tender and falls apart easily when pierced with a fork.

2. Remove the pork from the slow cooker and shred the meat with 2 forks. Toss to coat with the juices from the slow cooker. Serve the pulled pork over rice, garnished with lime wedges, cilantro, and scallions.

3. Store in an airtight container in the refrigerator for up to 3 days. To reheat, place the pulled pork in a greased skillet over medium-high heat for a few minutes, until warmed through.

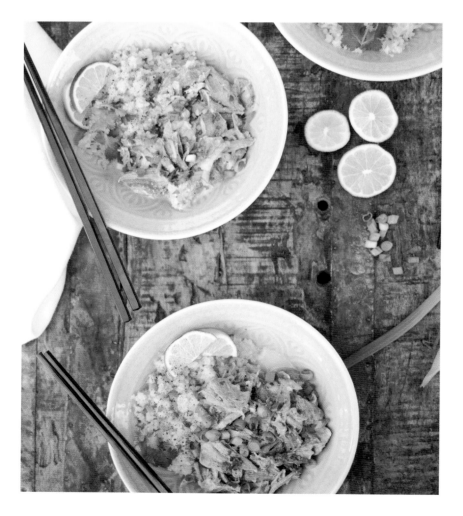

nutritional info (per serving)				
calories	fat	protein	carbs	fiber
442	34g	29g	2g	0.2g

30-MINUTE PORCHETTA

KETO

Porchetta is traditionally made with pork belly and stuffed with herbs, which typically takes a long time to prepare. Using a bacon-wrapped tenderloin rubbed with herbs cuts the time down to only 30 minutes.

prep time: **8 minutes** *cook time:* **30 minutes** *yield:* **4 servings**

2½ tablespoons avocado oil, MCT oil, or melted coconut oil

6 cloves roasted garlic, or 3 cloves raw garlic, smashed to a paste

1½ tablespoons finely chopped fresh rosemary

1 tablespoon finely diced fresh fennel bulb

1½ teaspoons fine sea salt

1 teaspoon ground black pepper

1 (1-pound) pork tenderloin

6 strips thin-cut bacon

1. Preheat the oven to 425°F. Place the oil, garlic, rosemary, fennel, salt, and pepper in a small bowl and stir well to combine. Using your hands, rub the seasoning all over the tenderloin. Starting at one end of the loin, wrap one piece of bacon at a time to cover the whole tenderloin. Secure the ends of the bacon to the loin with toothpicks.

2. Place the bacon-wrapped tenderloin in a roasting pan and roast for 28 to 30 minutes, until the pork is cooked through. (The internal temperature in the center should read 145°F.) Allow to rest for 10 minutes before slicing and serving.

3. Store in an airtight container in the refrigerator for up to 4 days. To reheat, place the porchetta on a rimmed baking sheet in a preheated 425°F oven for 4 minutes or until warmed through.

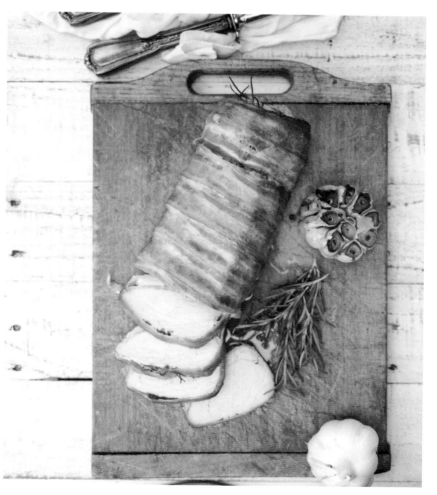

nutritional info (per serving)				
calories	fat	protein	carbs	fiber
341	24g	30g	1g	0.3g

SWEET 'N' SOUR PORK MEATBALLS

prep time: **10 minutes**   *cook time:* **20 minutes**   *yield:* **8 servings**

Meatballs:

2 pounds ground pork

2 large eggs, beaten

¾ cup finely chopped button mushrooms

¼ cup finely chopped scallions

2 tablespoons Swerve confectioners'-style sweetener or equivalent amount of liquid or powdered sweetener (see page 29)

1 tablespoon wheat-free tamari, or ¼ cup coconut aminos

2 teaspoons peeled and grated fresh ginger

1 clove garlic, smashed to a paste

Sweet 'n' Sour Sauce:

1 (6-ounce) can tomato paste

1½ cups chicken bone broth, homemade (page 106) or store-bought (see Notes)

⅓ cup Swerve confectioners'-style sweetener or equivalent amount of liquid or powdered sweetener (see page 29)

¼ cup coconut vinegar

¾ tablespoon lime or lemon juice

¾ teaspoon fish sauce

½ teaspoon fine sea salt

½ teaspoon garlic powder

⅛ teaspoon peeled and grated fresh ginger

¼ teaspoon guar gum (if using store-bought broth)

2 batches Keto Fried "Rice" (page 148), for serving

Sliced scallions, for garnish

Sesame seeds, for garnish

1. Preheat the oven to 400°F.

2. Make the meatballs: In a large bowl, mix together the ingredients for the meatballs with your hands until well combined. Shape into 1½-inch balls and place on a rimmed baking sheet. Bake for 20 minutes or until browned.

3. Meanwhile, make the sauce: Place the ingredients for the sauce in a medium-sized saucepan. Bring to a boil over medium heat, stirring often. Reduce the heat and simmer for 20 minutes, stirring occasionally. Add the guar gum to thicken, if using.

4. When the meatballs are done, add them to the saucepan and turn gently to coat in the sauce. Serve the sauced meatballs over fried "rice." Drizzle more sauce on top of the meatballs and garnish with sliced scallions and sesame seeds.

5. Store in an airtight container in the refrigerator for up to 5 days or in the freezer for up to a month. To reheat, place the sauced meatballs in a baking dish in a preheated 350°F oven for 5 minutes or until warmed through.

Notes: *These meatballs are equally delicious when made with ground chicken.*

If you opt for homemade bone broth, which is naturally thick, you won't need to use guar gum to thicken the sauce.

nutritional info (per serving)				
calories	fat	protein	carbs	fiber
351	26g	23g	5g	2g

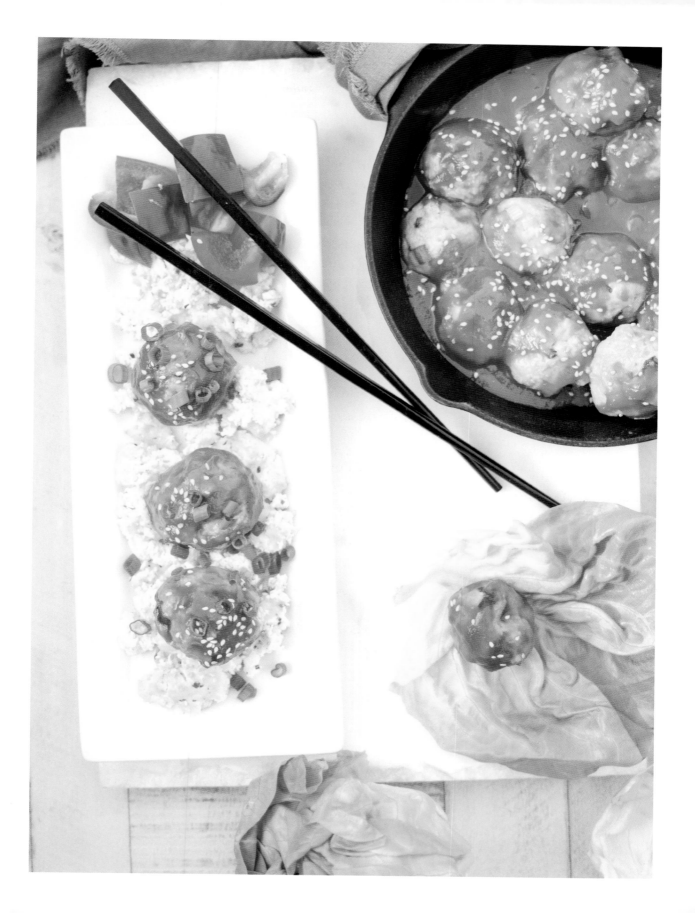

DEVILED HAM

In every book of mine, I try to sneak in a *Green Eggs and Ham*–themed recipe. I have always been a fan of Dr. Seuss, and on March 2, which is his birthday, we always celebrate with my Green Eggs and Ham dish. Here, the eggs are not green, but they are *on* greens. This deviled ham tastes great wrapped in lettuce and topped with a fried egg!

prep time: **15 minutes** *yield:* **6 servings**

3 cups diced cooked ham

1 cup mayonnaise, homemade (page 34 or 35) or store-bought

1 tablespoon Dijon mustard

½ teaspoon hot sauce, or more to taste

Serving Suggestions:

Butter lettuce leaves, for wrapping

Fried eggs

1. Place the ham in a food processor and pulse until very fine. Transfer to a medium-sized bowl.

2. In a separate bowl, combine the mayonnaise, mustard, and hot sauce. Pour the mixture over the ham and stir to coat.

3. If desired, serve the deviled ham in lettuce leaves, with fried eggs.

4. Store in an airtight container in the refrigerator for up to 3 days.

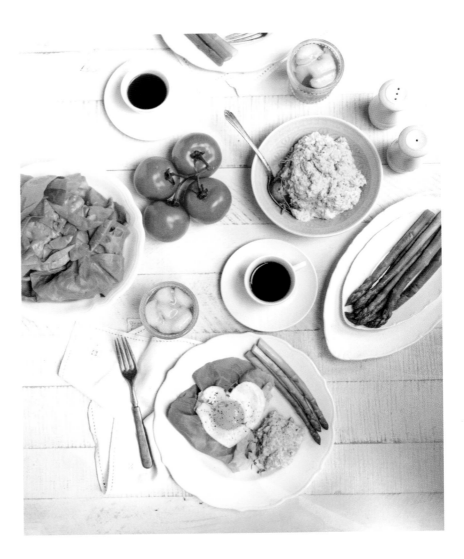

nutritional info (per serving)				
calories	fat	protein	carbs	fiber
531	46g	24g	0g	0g

MUSTARD-GLAZED HAM

KETO

This recipe is a perfect Christmas or Easter main dish. It is super easy to prepare and makes yummy leftovers for days!

prep time: **5 minutes** *cook time:* **2 hours** *yield:* **20 servings**

1 (10-pound) spiral-cut smoked ham

⅔ cup Swerve confectioners'-style sweetener or equivalent amount of liquid or powdered sweetener (see page 29)

½ cup Dijon mustard

1 teaspoon maple extract (optional)

1. Preheat the oven to 300°F.

2. Place the ham in roasting pan. Cover tightly with parchment paper, then aluminum foil. Bake for 1 hour 40 minutes.

3. Meanwhile, make the glaze: In a small bowl, stir together the sweetener, mustard, and maple extract, if using.

4. After 1 hour 40 minutes, remove the ham from the oven and rub the glaze all over the ham. Increase the oven temperature to 400°F. Place the ham back in the oven and bake, uncovered, for 15 more minutes. Remove from the oven and allow to rest for 10 minutes before slicing and serving.

5. Store in an airtight container in the refrigerator for up to 3 days. To reheat, place the ham in a roasting pan in a preheated 300°F oven for 15 minutes or until warmed through.

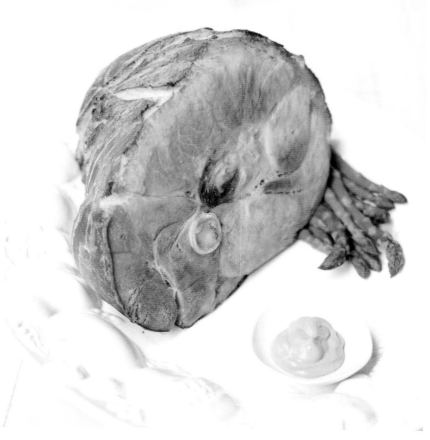

nutritional info (per serving)				
calories	fat	protein	carbs	fiber
558	38g	49g	0g	0g

HAWAIIAN LUAU PORK

KETO OPTION

Craig and I went to Hawaii for our honeymoon and enjoyed a traditional Hawaiian luau in Lahaina on the island of Maui. A lot of shredded pork was served at that meal, and this fantastic dish brings up such amazing memories of that trip.

I love to serve this dish with a simple side of shredded purple cabbage drizzled with Creamy Lime Sauce (page 38).

prep time: **4 minutes** *cook time:* **1 hour if using a pressure cooker; 6 to 8 hours if using a slow cooker** *yield:* **4 servings**

2 pounds boneless pork shoulder, cut into 4 equal chunks

1½ teaspoons fine sea salt

3 cloves garlic, minced

½ cup chicken or pork bone broth, homemade (page 106) or store-bought

2 tablespoons Swerve confectioners'-style sweetener or equivalent amount of liquid or powdered sweetener (see page 29) (optional; see Note)

1½ tablespoons liquid smoke

1 tablespoon wheat-free tamari, or ¼ cup coconut aminos

1 lime, quartered, for garnish

1 batch Keto "Rice" (page 147) or Cauliflower Rice (page 149), for serving (optional)

1. Season the pork on all sides with the salt. Place the pork in a 4-quart or larger slow cooker or pressure cooker. Add the garlic, broth, sweetener (if using), liquid smoke, and tamari to the cooker.

2. If using a slow cooker, cover and cook on low for 6 to 8 hours, until the pork is fork-tender and shreds easily. If using a pressure cooker, seal the lid and select high pressure, then set the timer for 60 minutes. After 60 minutes, select the natural pressure release to gently release the pressure.

3. Using 2 forks, shred the pork. Garnish with lime quarters and serve over "rice," if desired.

4. Store in an airtight container in the refrigerator for up to 4 days. To reheat, place the pork on a rimmed baking sheet in a preheated 425°F oven for 4 minutes or until warmed through.

Note: *Hawaiian pork is traditionally made with sugar or brown sugar for sweetness. If you prefer a more traditional kalua pig flavor, I suggest that you add the sweetener.*

nutritional info (per serving)				
calories	fat	protein	carbs	fiber
567	42g	40g	6g	4g

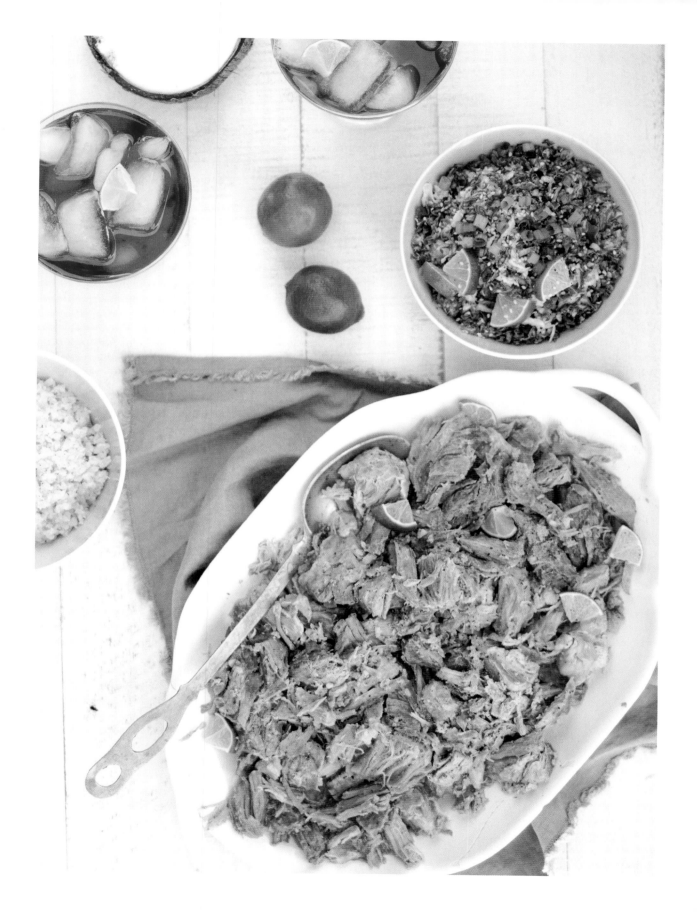

CILANTRO LIME SLOW COOKER RIBS

KETO

I love the creamy cilantro sauce in this dish. It pairs wonderfully with almost any preparation of pork. (In fact, I use a variation of it in my Citrus Pork Shoulder recipe on page 234.) Here, baconnaise adds a unique flavor that goes particularly well with ribs. If you don't have baconnaise, you can always make the sauce with plain mayo, but I recommend that you give it a try!

prep time: **10 minutes**   *cook time:* **4 to 8 hours**   *yield:* **8 servings**

Ribs:

4 pounds pork ribs

2 cups chicken or beef bone broth, homemade (page 106) or store-bought

¼ cup lime juice

1 teaspoon minced garlic

1 teaspoon fine sea salt

Sauce:

1 cup Baconnaise (page 34)

¼ cup lime juice

¼ cup chopped fresh cilantro

2 tablespoons chopped fresh chives

2 tablespoons peeled and grated fresh ginger

1 teaspoon chopped garlic

1 jalapeño pepper, seeded and coarsely chopped

½ teaspoon fine sea salt

1. Place the ribs in a 4-quart or larger slow cooker. Add the broth, lime juice, garlic, and salt to the cooker.

2. Cover and cook on high for 4 to 5 hours or on low for 7 to 8 hours, until the ribs are fork-tender and the meat is falling off the bone.

3. Meanwhile, make the sauce: Place the ingredients for the sauce in a food processor and puree until very smooth.

4. Preheat the oven to broil. Remove the ribs from the slow cooker (discard the cooking liquid) and place the ribs on a rimmed baking sheet. Baste the ribs with a few tablespoons of the sauce. Broil for about 2 minutes, until the sauce is bubbling and the ribs are slightly crispy on the edges. Serve the ribs topped with extra sauce.

5. Store in an airtight container in the refrigerator for up to 4 days. To reheat, place the ribs in a greased skillet over medium-high heat for a few minutes, until warmed through.

Busy Family Tip: *Make extra ribs and store them in an airtight container in the refrigerator for up to 3 days. Then simply run them under the broiler, as described in Step 4. The sauce can be made up to a week ahead and stored in an airtight container in the refrigerator. Shake well before using.*

nutritional info (per serving)				
calories	fat	protein	carbs	fiber
623	53g	31g	2g	0.3g

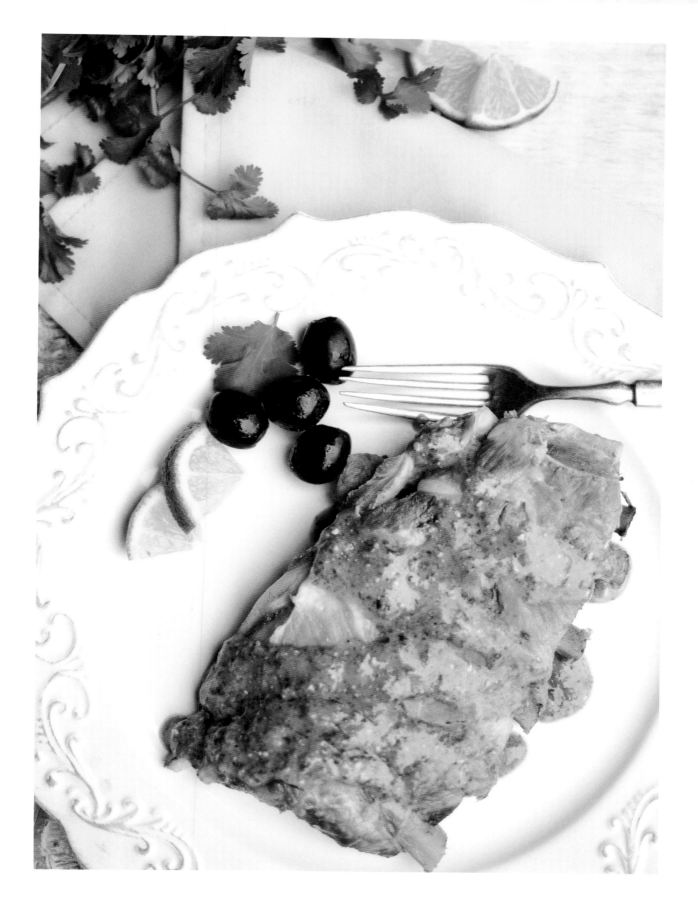

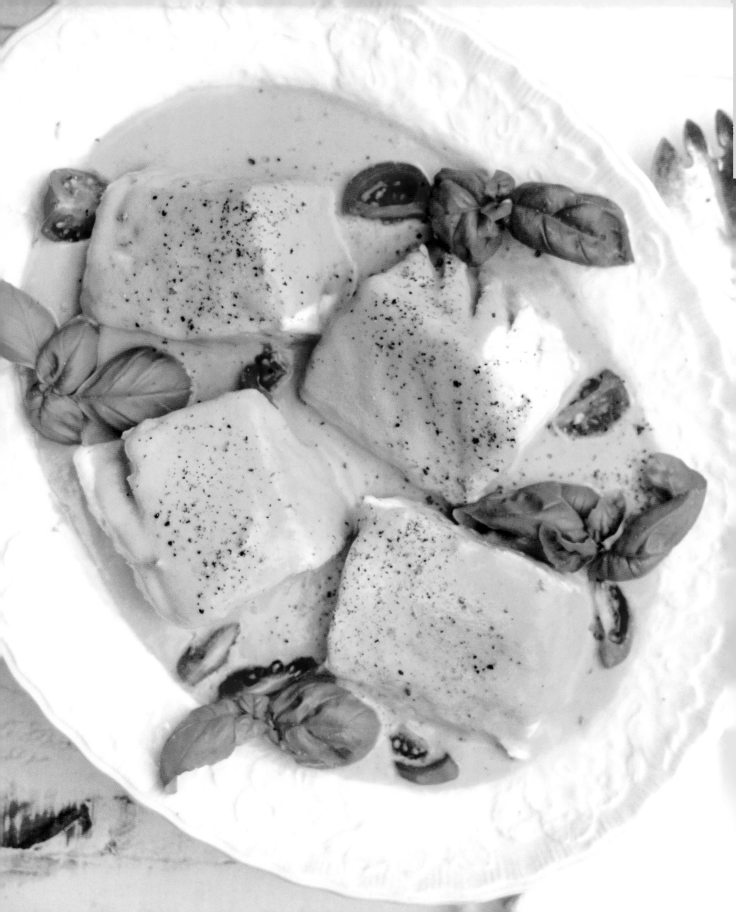

Chapter 9:
Fish and Seafood

BACON-WRAPPED SCALLOPS
with Avocado Cream

KETO

prep time: **8 minutes** cook time: **20 minutes**
yield: **4 main dish servings or 8 appetizer servings**

Avocado Cream:

¼ cup avocado oil

¼ cup chicken bone broth, homemade (page 106) or store-bought

Juice of 1 lime

1 ripe avocado, peeled and pitted

¼ cup fresh cilantro leaves

½ to 1 small jalapeño pepper (depending on how hot you want the dish to be)

1 teaspoon minced garlic

½ teaspoon ground cumin

¼ teaspoon dried oregano leaves

Bacon-Wrapped Scallops:

½ pound sea scallops

½ teaspoon fine sea salt

½ teaspoon ground black pepper

6 ounces bacon, each strip cut in half lengthwise

Sliced fresh chives, for garnish (optional)

Limes, quartered, for serving

Special Equipment:

4 wood skewers, about 8 inches long, or toothpicks, soaked in water for 15 minutes

1. Make the sauce: Place the ingredients for the sauce in a food processor and puree until smooth. Set aside in the refrigerator until ready to serve.

2. Preheat the oven to 400°F. Sprinkle the tops and bottoms of the scallops with the salt and pepper, then wrap a half-strip of bacon around each scallop. Thread the bacon-wrapped scallops onto the skewers, 4 to a skewer, or secure each bacon-wrapped scallop with a toothpick.

3. Place the wrapped scallops on a rimmed baking sheet and bake for 10 minutes. Flip the scallops over and bake for another 8 to 10 minutes, until the bacon is cooked through and the scallops are no longer translucent.

4. To serve as a meal, divide the scallops among 4 plates, then drizzle with the sauce. To serve as an appetizer, place the scallops on a platter and drizzle with the sauce. If desired, garnish with chives and serve with lime wedges for an extra hit of lime. For a fancier presentation, as pictured, place ½ tablespoon of the sauce in a serving spoon, place a scallop in the spoon, and then garnish with chives and serve with lime wedges.

5. Store in an airtight container in the refrigerator for up to 3 days. To reheat, place the scallops in a lightly greased skillet over medium heat until warmed through.

Busy Family Tips: *The sauce can be made up to a week ahead and stored in an airtight container in the refrigerator.*

The scallops can be marinated and then wrapped in bacon the day before serving for an easy party appetizer.

nutritional info (per serving)				
calories	fat	protein	carbs	fiber
461	44g	14g	6g	4g

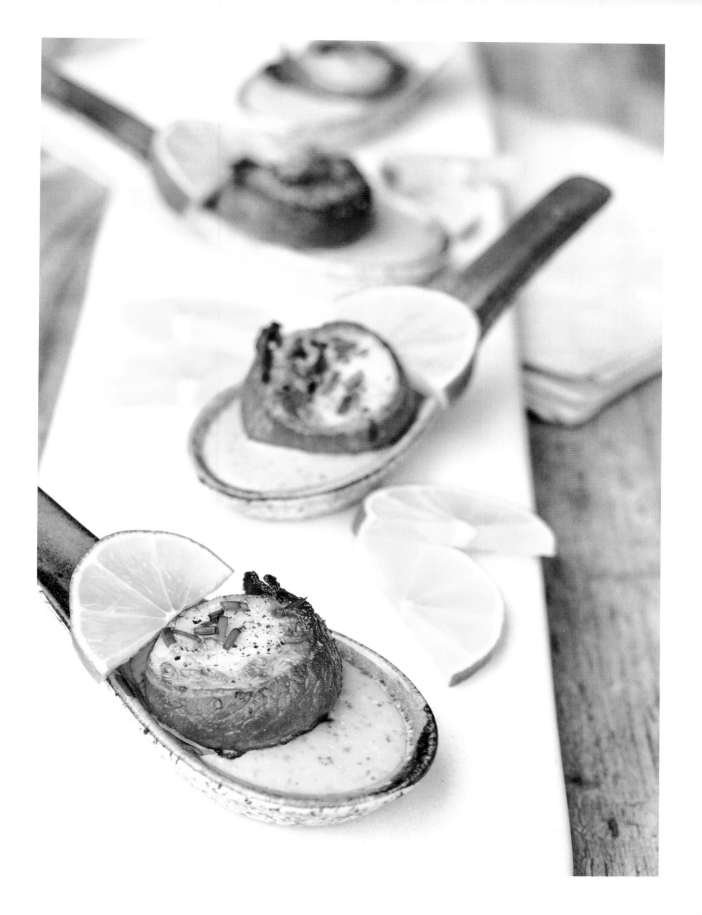

HALIBUT CONFIT

KETO

1 lemon or lime, thinly sliced

½ onion, diced

¼ cup chopped fresh cilantro

1 (1-pound) skinless halibut fillet, cut into 4 (4-ounce) pieces

1½ teaspoons fine sea salt

1½ teaspoons ground coriander

1 cup avocado oil or extra-virgin olive oil

For Garnish (optional):

Fresh cilantro leaves

Whole coriander seeds

Coarse sea salt

Freshly ground black pepper

Lemon or lime wedges

1. Preheat the oven to 275°F.

2. Place the lemon slices in a large cast-iron skillet or an 8-inch square baking dish. Top with the onion and cilantro. Season the halibut with the salt and coriander. Place the pieces of fish on top of the onion and cilantro.

3. Pour the oil over the fish. Bake for 20 minutes or until the fish flakes easily and is no longer translucent in the center.

4. Garnish with additional cilantro leaves, coriander seeds, coarse sea salt, freshly ground pepper, and lemon wedges, if desired.

5. Store in an airtight container in the refrigerator for up to 4 days. To reheat, place the fish in a cast-iron skillet or baking dish in a pre-heated 275°F oven for 5 minutes or until warmed through.

nutritional info (per serving)				
calories	fat	protein	carbs	fiber
375	31g	23g	1g	0.5g

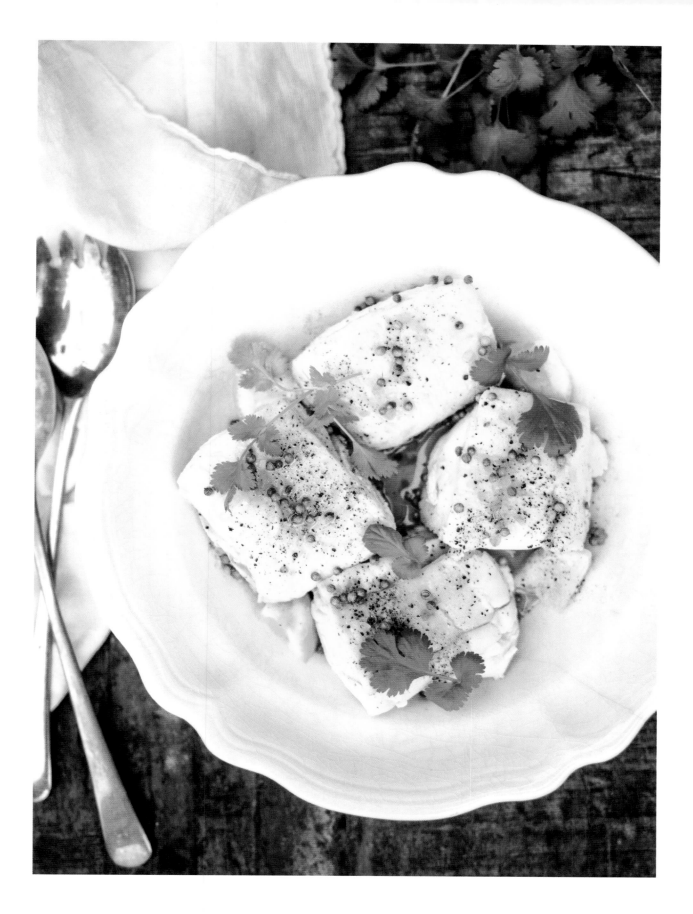

BAKED SOLE
with Zucchini

prep time: **5 minutes**   *cook time:* **6 minutes**   *yield:* **4 servings**

1 medium zucchini, cut into ¼-inch dice

Fine sea salt and ground black pepper

4 (4-ounce) sole fillets

2 lemons, thinly sliced

4 sprigs fresh thyme or dill, plus extra for garnish (optional)

4 tablespoons avocado oil or extra-virgin olive oil, divided, plus extra for garnish (optional)

1. Preheat the oven to 350°F. Lay four 12-inch square pieces of aluminum foil on a work surface, then lay four 12-inch square pieces of parchment paper on top of the pieces of foil.

2. Spread out ½ cup of the zucchini in the center of each piece of parchment, roughly the size and shape of the fish fillets. Sprinkle with salt and pepper. Season both sides of the fish fillets with salt and pepper, then place the fillets on top of the zucchini, in the center of the parchment. Top with lemon slices and thyme. Drizzle each fillet with a tablespoon of oil.

3. To form a packet, wrap the ends of the parchment and foil tightly around the fish and fold them over twice to secure. Twist the ends and fold them under the fish (or secure with tape). Place on a rimmed baking sheet and bake for 6 minutes or until the fish is flaky and the zucchini is crisp-tender. (Be careful when opening the packet to check for doneness; a lot of piping-hot steam will escape.) If desired, drizzle the fish with more oil and garnish with additional fresh thyme.

4. Store in an airtight container in the refrigerator for up to 4 days. To reheat, place the fish in a cast-iron skillet or baking dish in a preheated 350°F oven for 5 minutes or until warmed through.

Busy Family Tip: *You can prepare all four packets but bake them one at a time for an easy dinner for one! Prepped packets will keep for up to 3 days in the refrigerator.*

nutritional info (per serving)				
calories	fat	protein	carbs	fiber
239	16g	22g	5g	2g

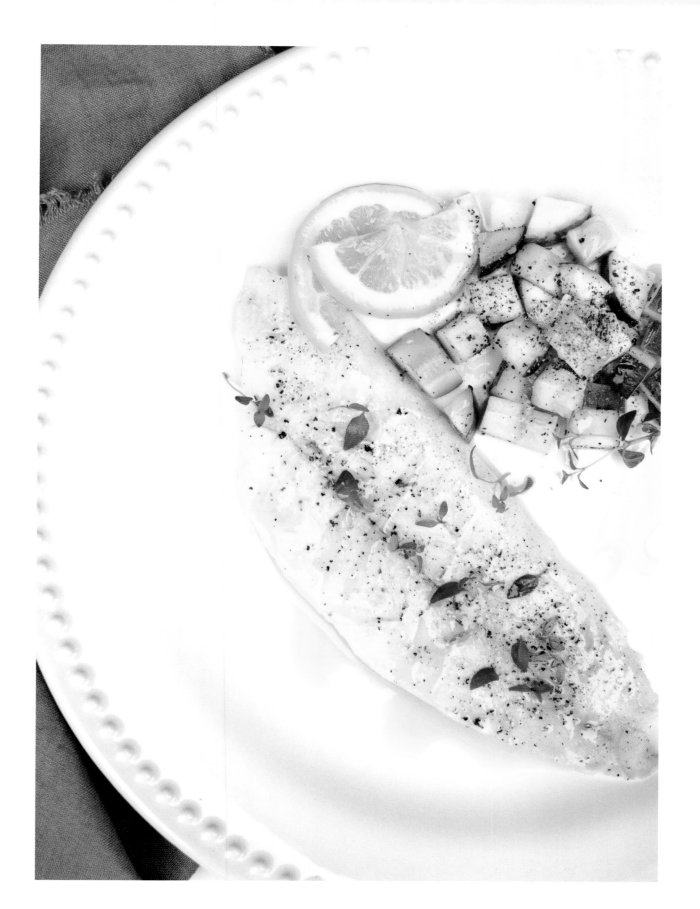

PAN-FRIED FISH
with Tartar Sauce

prep time: 5 minutes (not including time to make tartar sauce)
cook time: 11 minutes   *yield:* 4 servings

4 (5-ounce) skin-on halibut fillets

Fine sea salt and ground black pepper

2 tablespoons coconut oil

½ batch Tartar Sauce (page 40), for serving

For Garnish (optional):

Capers

Drizzle of avocado oil or extra-virgin olive oil

Chopped fresh parsley

Freshly ground black pepper

Lemon slices

1. Season the fish fillets on both sides with salt and pepper.

2. Heat the oil in a cast-iron skillet over medium-high heat. Sear the fillets skin side down for 8 minutes; do not move them. Flip the fillets and turn off the heat. Continue to cook for 3 more minutes or until the fish flakes easily and is opaque in the center; the exact timing will depend on the thickness of the fillets.

3. Serve each fillet with 2 tablespoons of tartar sauce and garnish as desired.

4. Store in an airtight container in the refrigerator for up to 4 days. To reheat, place the fish in a cast-iron skillet or baking dish in a pre-heated 375°F oven for 5 minutes or until warmed through.

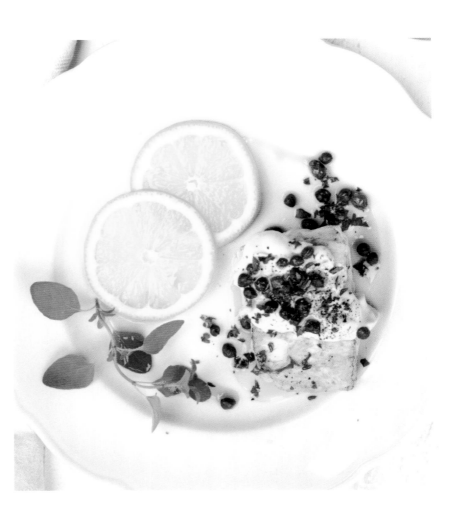

nutritional info (per serving)				
calories	fat	protein	carbs	fiber
402	31g	29g	0g	0g

HALIBUT SMOTHERED
in Tomato Basil Cream

prep time: **5 minutes**   *cook time:* **12 minutes**   *yield:* **4 servings**

2 tablespoons lard or coconut oil

½ cup diced onions

1 clove garlic, smashed to a paste

4 (4-ounce) skinless halibut fillets

1 teaspoon fine sea salt

¼ teaspoon ground black pepper

¾ cup tomato sauce

¼ cup fish bone broth or chicken bone broth, homemade (page 106) or store-bought

¼ cup full-fat coconut milk

1 tablespoon chopped fresh basil leaves

For Garnish:

Fresh basil leaves

Cherry tomatoes, quartered

Freshly ground black pepper

1. Melt the lard in a cast-iron skillet over medium heat. Add the onions and garlic and sauté for 2 minutes.

2. Season the fish fillets on both sides with the salt and pepper. Place the fish in the skillet and top with the tomato sauce. Add the broth, coconut milk, and basil to the skillet, around the fish, and cook, uncovered, for 10 minutes or until the fillets flake easily and are opaque in the center.

3. If you prefer a thicker sauce, remove the fish from the pan and continue to boil the sauce for 10 minutes or until thickened to your liking.

4. Place the fish on a platter, cover the fillets with the sauce, and garnish with basil leaves, cherry tomatoes, and freshly ground pepper.

5. Store in an airtight container in the refrigerator for up to 3 days. To reheat, place the fish in a lightly greased skillet over medium heat until warmed through.

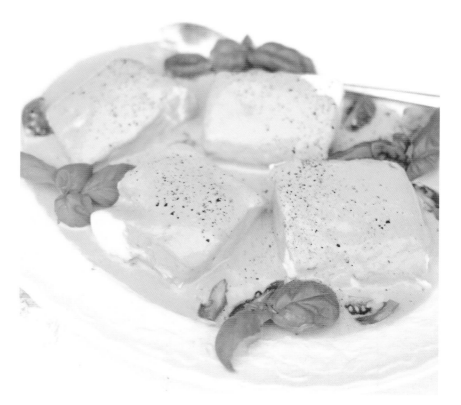

nutritional info (per serving)				
calories	fat	protein	carbs	fiber
233	12g	24g	5g	1g

SALMON BURGERS
with Dill Sauce

These are not your average salmon burgers. The addition of smoked salmon takes these patties to a whole new level of tastiness!

prep time: **7 minutes**   *cook time:* **6 minutes**   *yield:* **6 burgers (1 per serving)**

Burgers:

1 (14-ounce) can pink salmon, drained

2 ounces smoked salmon, chopped

⅓ cup pork dust (powdered pork rinds)

1 large egg

2 tablespoons Baconnaise (page 34) or mayonnaise, homemade (page 34 or 35) or store-bought

2 tablespoons chopped scallions

1 teaspoon fine sea salt

1 teaspoon lemon juice

1 tablespoon coconut oil or avocado oil, for frying

Dill Sauce:

¾ cup Baconnaise (page 34) or mayonnaise, homemade (page 34 or 35) or store-bought

2 tablespoons lemon or lime juice

2 tablespoons chopped fresh dill, or 2 teaspoons dried dill weed

Fine sea salt (optional)

For Serving:

6 romaine lettuce leaves

1 avocado, pitted and sliced

¼ red onion, sliced into thin rings

1. Place the ingredients for the burgers in a medium-sized bowl and use your hands to combine well. Form into six 3½-inch round patties.

2. Heat the oil in a large cast-iron skillet over medium heat. When hot, add the patties and cook for 3 minutes or until they turn a touch golden. Flip and cook for another 3 minutes or until light golden brown on both sides.

3. Meanwhile, make the dill sauce: Place the baconnaise, lemon juice, and dill in a small bowl. Stir well to combine, then taste and add salt, if desired. Serve the burgers with lettuce leaves for wrapping. Top with slices of avocado, onion, and the dill sauce.

4. Store in an airtight container in the refrigerator for up to 3 days. To reheat, place the burgers in a lightly greased skillet over medium heat until warmed through.

nutritional info (per serving)				
calories	fat	protein	carbs	fiber
443	38g	23g	4g	2g

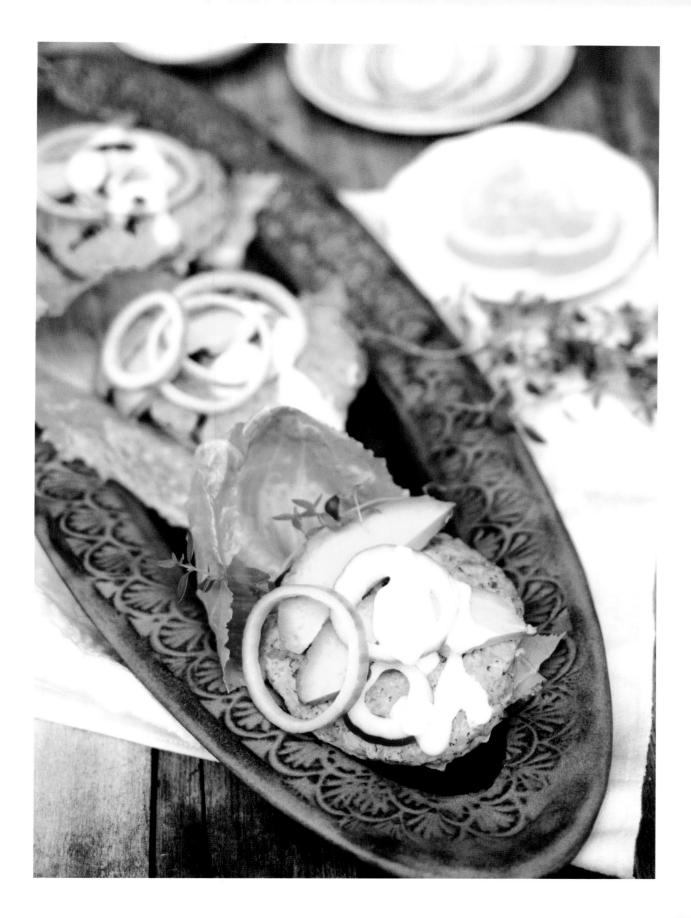

CRAB CLAWS
with Spicy Mustard Sauce

I love this recipe because crab claws are already cooked when you purchase them! All you have to do to pull this dish together is warm up the claws and make the tasty sauce while the claws are heating. A keto meal is ready in an instant!

prep time: **5 minutes**   *cook time:* **3 minutes**   *yield:* **4 servings (6 claws per serving)**

Fine sea salt

24 medium Alaskan king crab or snow crab claws, thawed

Spicy Mustard Sauce:

1 cup Baconnaise (page 34) or mayonnaise, homemade (page 34 or 35) or store-bought

¼ cup Dijon mustard

2 tablespoons prepared horseradish

2 teaspoons lime or lemon juice

2 or 3 drops hot sauce

Fine sea salt (optional)

For Garnish (optional):

Lime wedges

Fresh parsley

1. Fill a large stockpot about two-thirds full with water. Add about 2 tablespoons of salt to the water and bring to a boil. Add the crab claws and boil for 3 minutes or until warmed through.

2. Meanwhile, make the sauce: Place the baconnaise, mustard, horse-radish, lime juice, and hot sauce in a small bowl. Stir well to combine. Taste and add salt, if needed.

3. Place the crab claws on a platter and serve with a bowl of the spicy mustard sauce. Garnish the platter with lime wedges and parsley, if desired.

4. Store in an airtight container in the refrigerator for up to 4 days. Serve the leftover crab warm or chilled. To reheat, place the crab claws in boiling water until warmed through, about 3 minutes.

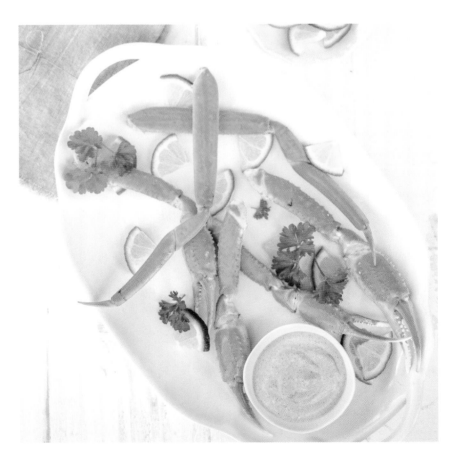

nutritional info (per serving)				
calories	fat	protein	carbs	fiber
498	40g	30g	1g	0.3g

EASY PICKLED SHRIMP
with Curry Mayo

1 pound cooked and peeled shrimp, preferably tail on (thawed if frozen)

⅓ cup coconut vinegar or white wine vinegar

⅓ cup MCT oil or extra-virgin olive oil

½ jalapeño pepper, thinly sliced

1 teaspoon fine sea salt

Curry Mayo:

⅔ cup mayonnaise, homemade (page 34 or 35) or store-bought

1 teaspoon Dijon mustard

½ teaspoon grated garlic

½ teaspoon curry powder

¼ teaspoon turmeric powder

½ teaspoon grated lime zest

1½ teaspoons lime juice

Lemon slices, for garnish (optional)

1. In large bowl, toss the shrimp with the vinegar, oil, jalapeño, and salt. Cover the bowl with a lid or plastic wrap and place in the refrigerator to chill for 20 minutes.

2. Meanwhile, in a small bowl, whisk together the ingredients for the curry mayo. Drain the shrimp and place on a platter. Garnish with lemon slices, if desired. Serve with the curry mayo for dipping.

3. Store the shrimp and curry mayo in separate airtight containers in the refrigerator for up to 3 days.

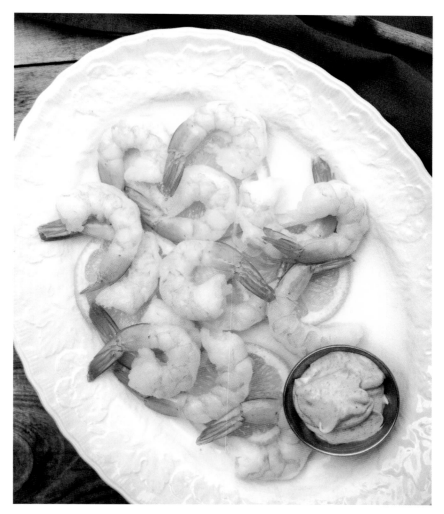

nutritional info (per serving)				
calories	fat	protein	carbs	fiber
398	31g	28g	0.3g	0.1g

BACON-WRAPPED COD

KETO   OPTION

prep time: **5 minutes** (*not including time to make tartar sauce*)
cook time: **14 minutes**   *yield:* **4 servings**

1 (1-pound) cod fillet

4 thin-cut strips bacon

1 tablespoon coconut oil or avocado oil

Lemon slices, for garnish (optional)

¼ cup Tartar Sauce (page 40), for serving (see Note)

1. Preheat the oven to 400°F.

2. Cut the cod fillet into 4 equal pieces. Starting at one end of a piece of cod, wrap a slice of bacon around it, spiraling the bacon slightly so that it overlaps at the edges and covers the whole fillet. Use a toothpick to secure the ends of the bacon. Repeat with the remaining fish and bacon.

3. Heat the oil in a cast-iron skillet over medium-high heat. Sear the bacon-wrapped cod in the hot oil for 2 minutes per side. Using an oven mitt, transfer the skillet to the oven and bake for 10 minutes or until the bacon is crisp and the fish flakes easily and is no longer translucent at the center. Garnish the fillets with lemon slices, if desired, and serve with the tartar sauce.

4. This dish is best served fresh, when the bacon is crispy; however, leftovers can be stored in an airtight container in the refrigerator for up to 3 days. To reheat, place the fish in a lightly greased skillet over medium heat until warmed through.

Note: *To make this dish egg-free, use Egg-Free Mayo (page 35) when making the tartar sauce.*

nutritional info (per serving)				
calories	fat	protein	carbs	fiber
399	36g	18g	0g	0g

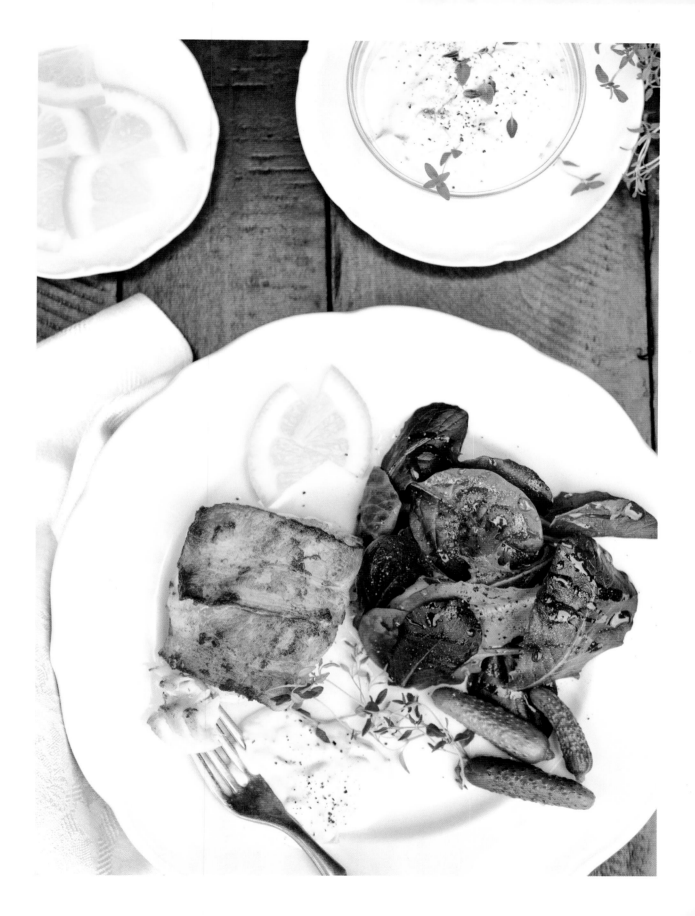

CAMARONES CUCARACHAS
(Deviled Shrimp)

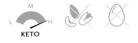

KETO

To save time, I purchase butterflied and deveined shrimp from my fishmonger. Butterflied shrimp is sometimes available in the freezer section of the grocery store, too.

prep time: **2 minutes**   *cook time:* **10 minutes**   *yield:* **4 servings**

1 tablespoon coconut oil or lard

1 pound extra-large shrimp, shell on, butterflied and deveined (thawed if frozen)

Fine sea salt and ground black pepper

1 cup tomato sauce

¼ cup medium-hot hot sauce

2 tablespoons Swerve confectioners'-style sweetener or equivalent amount of liquid or powdered sweetener (see page 29)

Chopped fresh cilantro, for garnish (optional)

For Serving (optional):

Pitted green olives

Lime wedges

1. Melt the coconut oil in a large cast-iron skillet over medium heat. Season the shrimp on all sides with salt and pepper and cook in the oil for 4 minutes or until slightly pink.

2. Add the tomato sauce, hot sauce, and sweetener. Continue to cook and stir the shrimp until they are bright pink and the sauce is bubbly, about 7 minutes. Serve garnished with cilantro, with olives and lime wedges on the side, if desired.

3. Store in an airtight container in the refrigerator for up to 3 days. To reheat, place the shrimp in a greased skillet over medium heat for a few minutes, until warmed through.

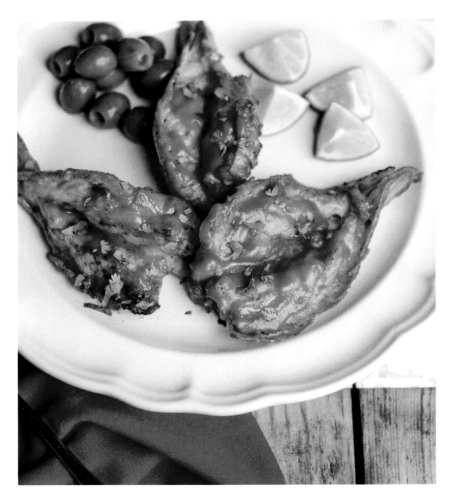

nutritional info (per serving)				
calories	fat	protein	carbs	fiber
180	6g	29g	3g	1g

SHRIMP ADOBO

prep time: **4 minutes, plus time to marinate**   cook time: **5 minutes**
yield: **4 servings**

1 pound large shrimp, peeled and deveined

¼ cup coconut vinegar

2 tablespoons lime juice

1 tablespoon wheat-free tamari, or ¼ cup coconut aminos

2 tablespoons black peppercorns

1 teaspoon fine sea salt

1 teaspoon fish sauce (or more salt)

2 cloves garlic, minced

2 tablespoons coconut oil, for the pan

For Garnish (optional):

Chopped fresh cilantro

Lime slices

1. Place the shrimp in a large bowl. Add the vinegar, lime juice, tamari, peppercorns, salt, fish sauce, and garlic and toss to coat. Cover and refrigerate for 2 hours or overnight.

2. Heat the oil in a wok or large cast-iron skillet over medium-high heat. When the oil is hot, add the shrimp along with the marinade.

3. Stir-fry for 5 minutes or until the shrimp have turned pink and are no longer translucent. Serve garnished with cilantro and lime slices, if desired.

4. Store in an airtight container in the refrigerator for up to 3 days. To reheat, place the shrimp in a lightly greased skillet over medium heat until warmed through.

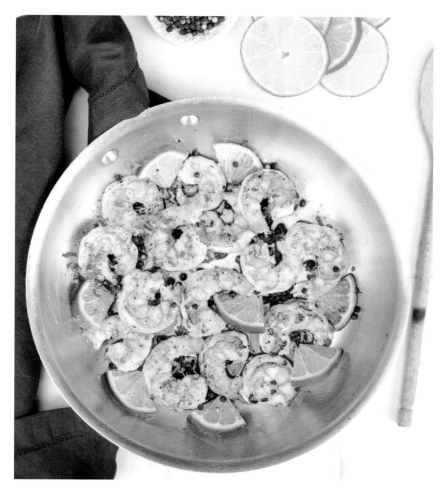

nutritional info (per serving)				
calories	fat	protein	carbs	fiber
205	9g	30g	1g	0.1g

AHI POKE

KETO · OPTION

½ pound sushi-grade ahi tuna

¾ teaspoon wheat-free tamari, or 1 tablespoon coconut aminos

¼ cup mayonnaise, homemade (page 34 or 35) or store-bought (see Notes)

2 tablespoons finely diced onions

2 tablespoons chopped scallions

Fine sea salt (optional)

2 tablespoons fish roe, preferably masago (see Notes)

For Garnish (optional):

Sliced scallions

Lemon slices

1. Cut the tuna into 1-inch pieces and place in a medium-sized bowl. Add the tamari, mayonnaise, onions, and scallions. Stir well, then season with salt to taste, if desired, keeping in mind that the roe will add saltiness.

2. Top with the fish roe and serve, garnished with sliced scallions and lemon slices, if desired.

3. This dish is best served fresh; however, leftovers can be stored in an airtight container in the refrigerator for up to 2 days.

Notes: *If using store-bought mayo, try Primal Kitchen's chipotle lime mayo. The flavors of the lime and chipotle are delicious in this recipe.*

Masago *refers to the roe (eggs) of a small fish called the capelin that is found in the northern Atlantic and Pacific oceans. Masago comes in different colors and has a fresh, sweet taste and a lovely crunchy texture. You can find it at seafood markets, specialty grocery stores, or online.*

nutritional info (per serving)				
calories	fat	protein	carbs	fiber
332	22g	31g	2g	0.4g

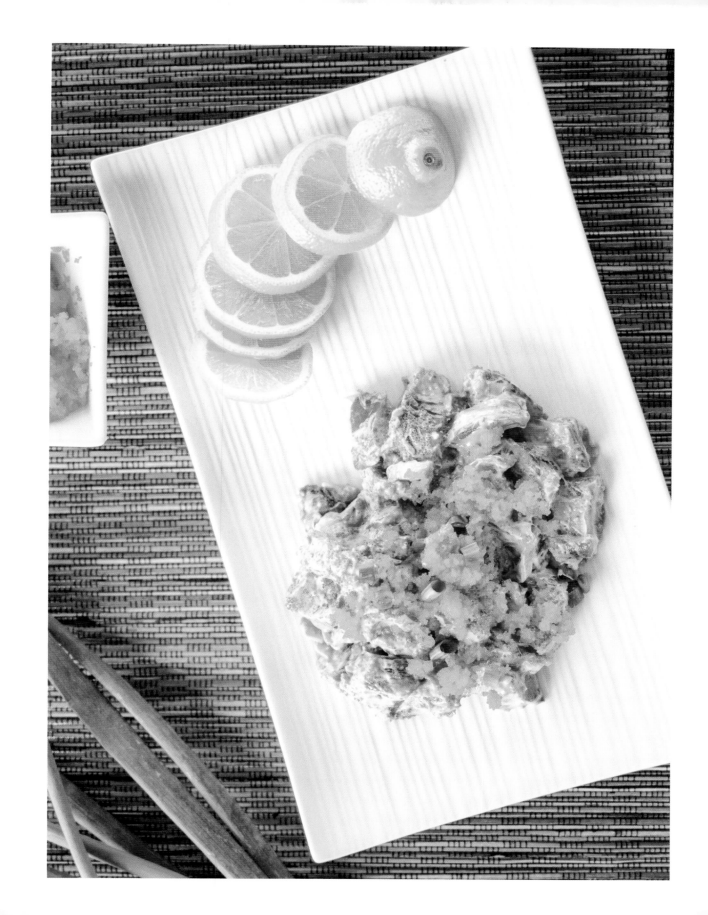

FISH IN PUTTANESCA SAUCE

prep time: **5 minutes** *cook time:* **12 minutes** *yield:* **4 servings**

2 cups marinara sauce

½ cup pitted black and green olives

2 tablespoons capers

2 tablespoons chopped fresh basil leaves

4 (4-ounce) sablefish (aka black cod or butterfish) or other white fish fillets

1 teaspoon fine sea salt

½ teaspoon ground black pepper

1 tablespoon avocado oil or melted coconut oil

1 batch Cabbage Pasta (page 152), for serving (optional)

Fresh thyme leaves, for garnish

1. Preheat the oven to 375°F.

2. Put the marinara sauce, olives, capers, and basil in a large cast-iron skillet or 13 by 9-inch baking dish; stir well. Season the fish with the salt and pepper. Place in the skillet and drizzle the fish with the oil.

3. Bake for 12 minutes or until the fish flakes easily and is no longer translucent in the center. Serve on a bed of cabbage pasta, if desired, topped with the sauce from the pan. Garnish with fresh thyme.

4. Store in an airtight container in the refrigerator for up to 3 days. To reheat, place the fish in a lightly greased skillet over medium heat until warmed through.

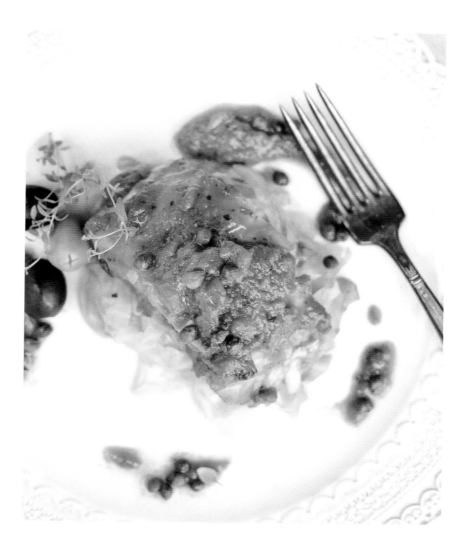

nutritional info (per serving)				
calories	fat	protein	carbs	fiber
339	26g	17g	8g	2g

GARLIC LIME BROILED SHRIMP

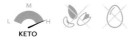

prep time: **8 minutes (not including time to make sauces)** cook time: **5 minutes**
yield: **2 servings**

2 tablespoons avocado oil or melted coconut oil

1 tablespoon lime or lemon juice

1 teaspoon fine sea salt

1 teaspoon paprika

1 clove garlic, smashed to a paste

½ pound large tail-on shrimp, peeled and deveined

Suggested Dipping Sauces:

Creamy Lime Sauce (page 38)

Satay Sauce (page 192)

Pico de Gallo (page 85) or Citrus Avocado Salsa (page 86)

Cilantro Lime Dressing (page 39)

1. Preheat the broiler to high heat. Place the oil, lime juice, salt, paprika, and garlic in a large bowl. Stir well to combine. Add the shrimp and toss to coat thoroughly in the seasonings.

2. Place the shrimp on a rimmed baking sheet and broil for 5 minutes or until the shrimp is beginning to turn pink and is no longer translucent.

3. Arrange the shrimp on a platter and serve with the dipping sauce of your choice.

4. Store in an airtight container in the refrigerator for up to 3 days. To reheat, place the shrimp in a lightly greased skillet over medium heat until warmed through.

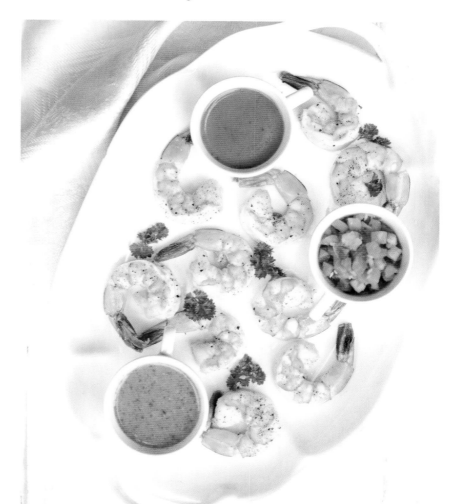

nutritional info (per serving)				
calories	fat	protein	carbs	fiber
258	16g	28g	1g	0.3g

PERSONAL SALMON EN PAPILLOTE

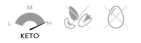

KETO

This is a super easy dinner for one. And if you have dinner guests, it's easy to make more!

prep time: **5 minutes**   *cook time:* **15 minutes**   *yield:* **1 serving**

1 (4-ounce) salmon fillet

½ teaspoon fine sea salt

1 teaspoon melted coconut oil, MCT oil, or avocado oil

1 teaspoon peeled and grated fresh ginger

1 clove garlic, minced

1 sprig fresh thyme, plus more for garnish

3 or 4 lime slices

1. Preheat the oven to 425°F.

2. Lay a 12-inch square piece of parchment paper on top of a 12-inch square piece of aluminum foil. Place the salmon in the center of the parchment. Season well on all sides with the salt. Drizzle with the oil, then sprinkle with the ginger and garlic. Place the sprig of thyme and lime slices on top of the fish.

3. To form a packet, wrap the ends of the parchment and foil tightly around the fish and fold over twice to secure. Twist the ends and fold them under the fish. Place the packet on a rimmed baking sheet.

4. Bake for 15 minutes or until the salmon is flaky and no longer translucent in the center (the exact timing will depend on the thickness of the fillet). Open and eat right out of the parchment paper for a super simple dinner. (Be careful when opening the packet, as very hot steam will escape.)

5. Store in an airtight container, without the parchment paper, for up to 3 days. To reheat, place the fish in a baking dish in a preheated 350°F oven for 5 minutes or until warmed through.

nutritional info (per serving)				
calories	fat	protein	carbs	fiber
187	9g	23g	5g	1g

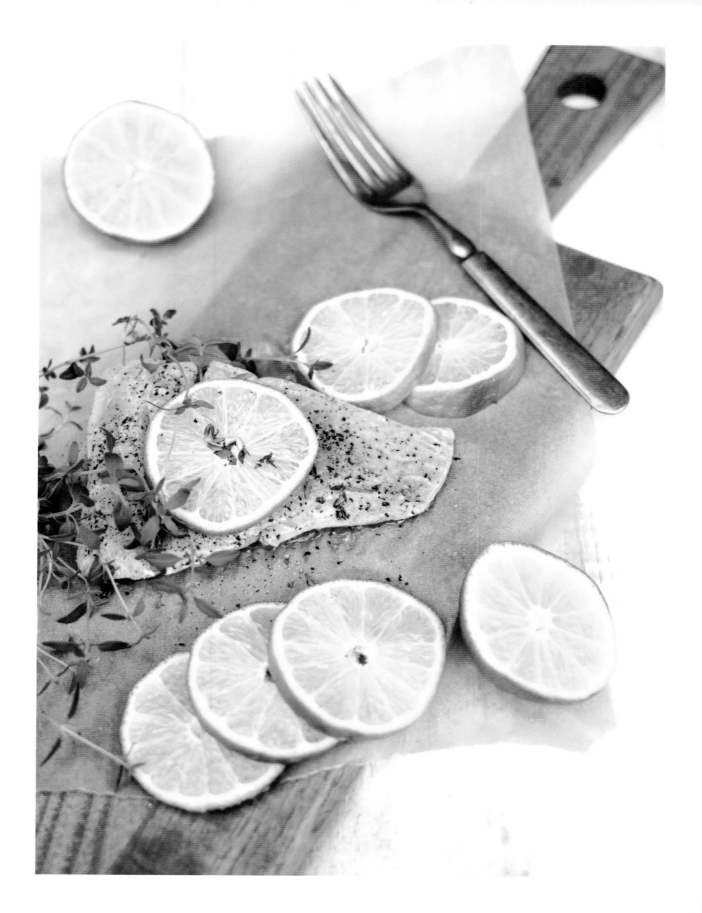

SALT-CRUSTED FISH

KETO

If you really want to impress your family or dinner guests, you must try this recipe. It will make you look like a master chef, but in reality, this method of cooking fish is very simple. And it creates tasty, tender fish!

To make this recipe even easier, I ask the fishmonger to prepare the fillet for me by removing the gills and fins.

prep time: **7 minutes (not including time to make tartar sauce)**
cook time: **25 minutes** *yield:* **4 servings**

2 tablespoons fresh herbs, such as parsley or thyme

1 lemon, thinly sliced

1 (3-pound) whole trout, gutted, gills and fins removed

4 large egg whites

2 cups coarse sea salt

¼ batch Tartar Sauce (page 40), for serving

For Garnish:

2 tablespoons diced red onions

2 tablespoons fresh dill

2 tablespoons capers

Lemon slices

1. Preheat the oven to 450°F.

2. Place the herbs and lemon slices inside the body of the fish. Set aside.

3. Place the egg whites in a mixing bowl or the bowl of a stand mixer. Whisk until soft peaks form. Gently fold the salt into the whites with a spatula.

4. Place about ¼ cup of the egg white mixture on an ovenproof platter. Spread the mixture into the size and shape of the trout. Place the trout on top of the mixture, then top the trout with the rest of the egg white mixture, covering it completely. Place the platter on a rimmed baking sheet and bake for 25 minutes or until the fish is no longer opaque and flakes easily with a fork.

5. Let the fish rest for 10 minutes. For a dramatic presentation, move the platter to the dinner table and crack the salt crust open in front of your guests. Then place pieces of fish on serving plates and garnish with diced red onions, fresh dill, capers, and lemon slices. Serve with tartar sauce.

6. Store in an airtight container in the refrigerator for up to 3 days. To reheat, place the fish in a baking dish in a preheated 350°F oven for 5 minutes or until warmed through.

nutritional info (per serving)				
calories	fat	protein	carbs	fiber
390	21g	46g	2g	1g

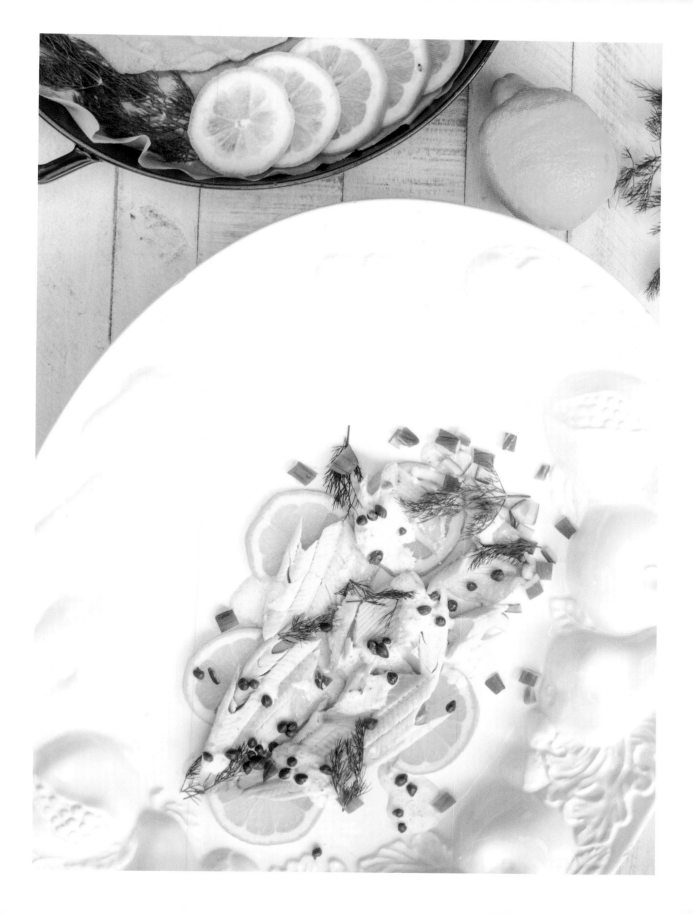

CAJUN SHRIMP

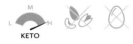

2 tablespoons avocado oil or coconut oil

¼ cup diced onions

1 clove garlic, smashed to a paste

1 pound large tail-on shrimp, peeled and deveined

1 teaspoon fine sea salt, or more to taste

½ cup tomato sauce

½ teaspoon garlic powder

½ teaspoon onion powder

½ teaspoon dried oregano leaves

⅛ teaspoon hot sauce, or more to taste

Ground black pepper (optional)

Chopped fresh parsley, for garnish (optional)

1. Heat the oil in a medium-sized saucepan over medium heat. Add the onions and sauté for 2 minutes or until soft. Add the garlic and sauté for another minute. Season the shrimp with the salt, add to the pan, and sauté for 2 minutes or until no longer translucent.

2. Add the tomato sauce, garlic powder, onion powder, oregano, and hot sauce. Bring to a boil, then remove from the heat. Taste and add more salt, hot sauce, and/or pepper, if desired. Serve garnished with parsley, if desired.

3. Store in an airtight container in the refrigerator for up to 4 days. To reheat, place the shrimp in a lightly greased skillet over medium heat until warmed through.

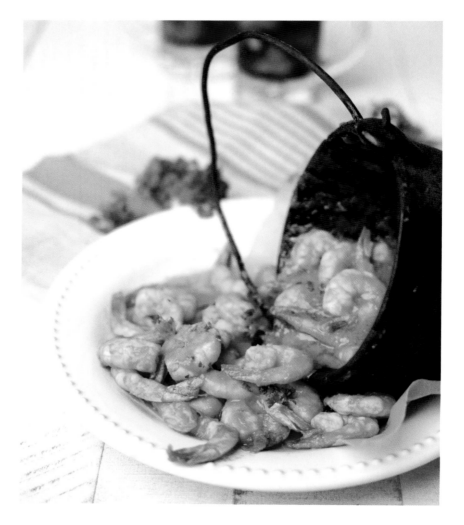

nutritional info (per serving)				
calories	fat	protein	carbs	fiber
208	9g	28g	3g	0.4g

AVOCADO SALMON CEVICHE

¼ cup plus 1 tablespoon lime juice

2 tablespoons avocado oil or extra-virgin olive oil

¼ teaspoon grated garlic

1 very fresh (6-ounce) salmon fillet (see Note), cut into ½-inch pieces

1 avocado, peeled, pitted, and cut into ½-inch pieces

1 scallion, thinly sliced

2 tablespoons diced red onions

2 tablespoons chopped cilantro leaves

1 teaspoon fine sea salt

1. Place the lime juice, oil, and garlic in a large bowl and stir to combine. Add the salmon, avocado, scallion, red onions, cilantro, and salt. Stir well to combine. Cover and refrigerate for 15 minutes before serving.

2. Store in an airtight container in the refrigerator for up to 3 days.

Note: *Let your fishmonger know that you're planning to make ceviche with the salmon and that you require ultra-fresh fish. Be sure to prepare this recipe the same day you purchase the fish.*

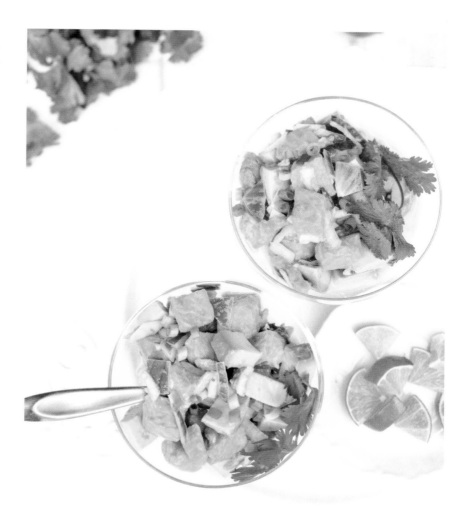

nutritional info (per serving)				
calories	fat	protein	carbs	fiber
192	15g	9g	6g	3g

ASIAN-STYLE SALMON LETTUCE CUPS

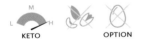

KETO   OPTION

Canned salmon is super tasty. It reminds me of canned tuna, but with less mercury and more omega-3 fatty acids! My dad makes his own canned salmon, so this recipe is in his honor.

prep. time: **6 minutes** *yield:* **2 servings**

¼ cup mayonnaise, homemade (page 34 or 35) or store-bought

1 tablespoon Swerve confectioners'-style sweetener or equivalent amount of liquid or powdered sweetener (see page 29), or more to taste (optional)

2¼ teaspoons wheat-free tamari, or 3 tablespoons coconut aminos

1 teaspoon lime juice, or more to taste (optional)

½ teaspoon peeled and grated fresh ginger, or more to taste (optional)

1 (8-ounce) can salmon, drained

Butter lettuce leaves, for serving

For Garnish:

1 tablespoon black sesame seeds or toasted sesame seeds

1 scallion, thinly sliced

Lime wedges

1. In a medium-sized bowl, mix together the mayo, sweetener (if using), tamari, lime juice (if using), and ginger. Add the salmon and stir gently to coat. Taste and adjust the seasoning to your liking, adding more ginger, lime juice, and/or sweetener, if desired.

2. Serve wrapped in lettuce leaves, garnished with sesame seeds and scallions, with lime wedges on the side.

3. Store in an airtight container in the refrigerator for up to 4 days.

Variation: *Smoked Salmon Lettuce Cups. Replace the canned salmon with 8 ounces of smoked salmon. Crumble the salmon and add it to the bowl with the mayo mixture as described above. For this recipe, be sure to use hot-smoked versus cold-smoked salmon.*

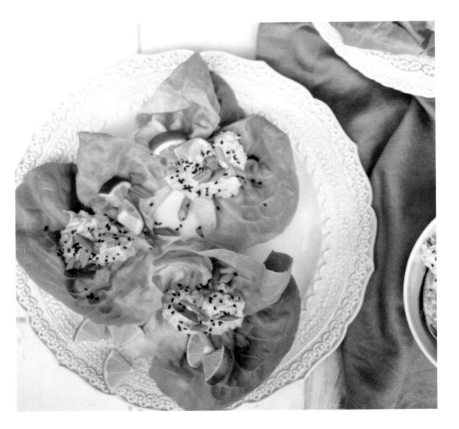

nutritional info (per serving)				
calories	fat	protein	carbs	fiber
360	28g	24g	4g	2g

YELLOW CURRY SHRIMP
over Keto Fried "Rice"

prep time: **8 minutes**   cook time: **12 minutes**   yield: **8 servings**

¼ cup coconut oil

½ cup diced onions

6 cloves garlic, minced

2 tablespoons peeled and grated fresh ginger

2 pounds medium shrimp, peeled and deveined

2 teaspoons fine sea salt

¼ cup chicken bone broth, homemade (page 106) or store-bought

3 tablespoons garam masala

2 tablespoons yellow curry paste

1 tablespoon turmeric powder

1 tablespoon lime juice

2 batches Keto Fried "Rice" (page 148), for serving

For Garnish:

Lime wedges

Fresh cilantro leaves

Sliced scallions

1. Heat the coconut oil in a large cast-iron skillet over medium-high heat. Add the onions and sauté for 3 minutes or until soft. Add the garlic and ginger and sauté for another 2 minutes.

2. Season the shrimp on all sides with the salt. Add to the skillet and cook for 2 minutes per side or until no longer translucent.

3. Add the broth, garam masala, curry paste, and turmeric powder and stir until well combined. Reduce the heat to medium and simmer for 2 minutes, then stir in the lime juice. Serve over fried "rice" and garnish with lime wedges, cilantro leaves, and sliced scallions.

4. Store in an airtight container in the refrigerator for up to 3 days. To reheat, place the shrimp in a lightly greased sauté pan over medium heat, stirring often, for 2 minutes or until warmed through.

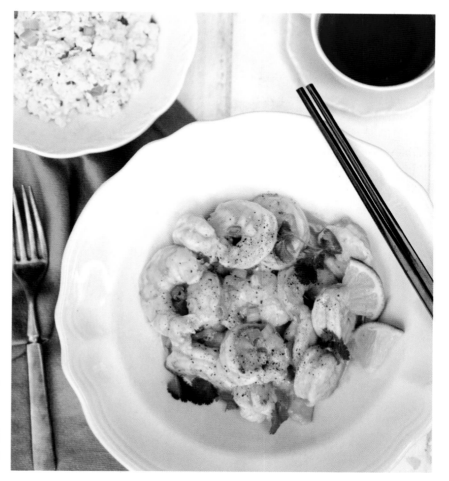

nutritional info (per serving)				
calories	fat	protein	carbs	fiber
214	10g	29g	5g	1g

SUPER FAST SHRIMP FAJITAS

KETO

prep time: **7 minutes**   *cook time:* **5 minutes**   *yield:* **4 servings**

2 tablespoons coconut oil

1 green bell pepper, thinly sliced

1 yellow or red bell pepper, thinly sliced

½ small onion, thinly sliced

1 pound precooked shrimp, peeled and deveined (see Note)

2 teaspoons chili powder

2 teaspoons paprika

1 teaspoon ground cumin

1 teaspoon fine sea salt

1 tablespoon lime juice, or more to taste

For Serving:

Boston lettuce leaves

Fresh cilantro leaves

Lime wedges

Topping Suggestions:

1 batch Guacamole (page 87)

1 cup Pico de Gallo (page 85) or Citrus Avocado Salsa (page 86)

Sliced black olives

1. Heat the coconut oil in a large cast-iron skillet over medium-high heat. Add the bell peppers and onion and sauté for 4 minutes or until crisp-tender. Add the shrimp, spices, salt, and lime juice. Stir well to coat the shrimp and veggies. Heat for 1 minute or until the shrimp is warmed through.

2. Serve wrapped in lettuce leaves with cilantro and a squirt of lime juice, along with any additional toppings of your choice.

3. Store in an airtight container in the refrigerator for up to 3 days. To reheat, place the fajitas in a lightly greased sauté pan over medium heat for 2 minutes, stirring often, or until warmed through.

Note: *You can use raw shrimp to make this recipe, but you will need to cook the shrimp until it is cooked through, about 3 minutes per side.*

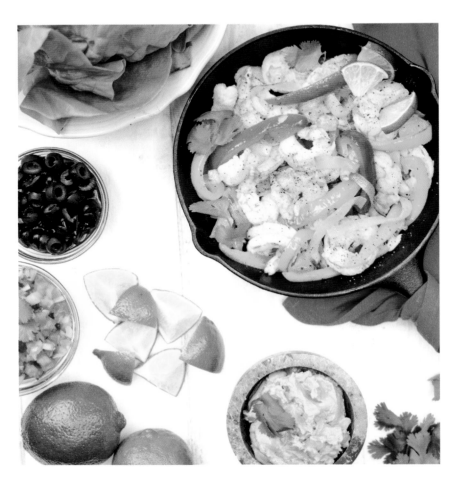

nutritional info (per serving)				
calories	fat	protein	carbs	fiber
224	9g	29g	7g	2g

SIMPLE SCALLOPS
with Garlic Sauce

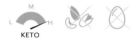

prep time: **10 minutes**   *cook time:* **8 minutes**   *yield:* **4 servings**

¼ cup butter-flavored coconut oil

1 pound large sea scallops

1 teaspoon fine sea salt

½ teaspoon ground black pepper

4 cloves garlic, minced

For Garnish (optional):

1 lemon, sliced or quartered

1 tablespoon chopped fresh parsley

1. Heat the coconut oil in a large cast-iron skillet over medium-high heat. While the oil is heating, pat the scallops dry and season on both sides with the salt and pepper. Add the garlic to the skillet and sauté for 1 minute.

2. Place the scallops in the hot skillet with the garlic and sear for 4 minutes or until golden brown, then flip and sear for another 4 minutes or until no longer translucent in the center.

3. To serve, divide the scallops among 4 plates, then drizzle with the pan juices. Garnish with lemon slices or quarters and parsley, if desired.

4. Store in an airtight container in the refrigerator for up to 3 days. To reheat, place the scallops in a lightly greased sauté pan over medium heat, stirring often, for 2 minutes or until warmed through.

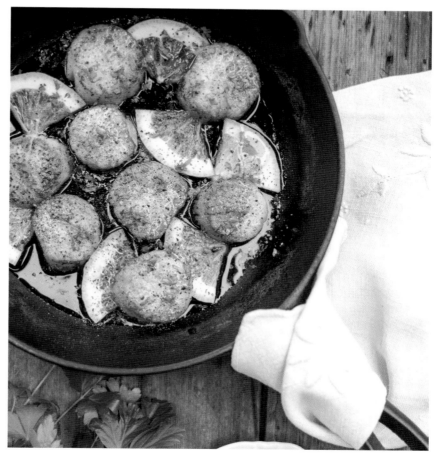

nutritional info (per serving)				
calories	fat	protein	carbs	fiber
255	15g	26g	5g	0.2g

SHRIMP FRIED "RICE"

KETO

prep time: **5 minutes**   *cook time:* **15 minutes**   *yield:* **4 servings**

8 large eggs

½ cup full-fat coconut milk

2 tablespoons beef bone broth, homemade (page 106) or store-bought

½ teaspoon wheat-free tamari, or 2 teaspoons coconut aminos

1 teaspoon fine sea salt

½ teaspoon ground black pepper

3 strips bacon, diced

¼ cup diced onions

1 clove garlic, minced

1 pound large shrimp, peeled and deveined

For Garnish (optional):

1 teaspoon crushed red pepper

Thinly sliced scallions

1. Crack the eggs into a medium-sized bowl. Add the coconut milk, broth, tamari, salt, and pepper and whisk until well combined.

2. In a large skillet over medium heat, cook the bacon until crisp, about 4 minutes. Using a slotted spoon, remove the bacon; leave the drippings in the pan. Add the onions and garlic to the skillet and sauté until the onions are translucent, about 2 minutes. Season the shrimp on all sides with salt and pepper and add to the skillet. Cook for 2 minutes on each side.

3. Make the "rice": Pour the egg mixture into the skillet and cook until the mixture thickens and small curds form, while scraping the bottom of the pan and whisking to keep large curds from forming. (A whisk works well for this task.) This will take about 7 minutes. Stir in the reserved bacon.

4. Place the "rice" on a platter. Garnish with crushed red pepper and scallions, if desired, and serve.

5. Store in an airtight container in the refrigerator for up to 3 days. To reheat, place the shrimp fried "rice" in a lightly greased sauté pan over medium heat, stirring often, for 2 minutes or until warmed through.

Note: *If the "rice" releases excess liquid, soak it up with a paper towel before serving.*

nutritional info (per serving)				
calories	fat	protein	carbs	fiber
386	21g	45g	3g	0.2g

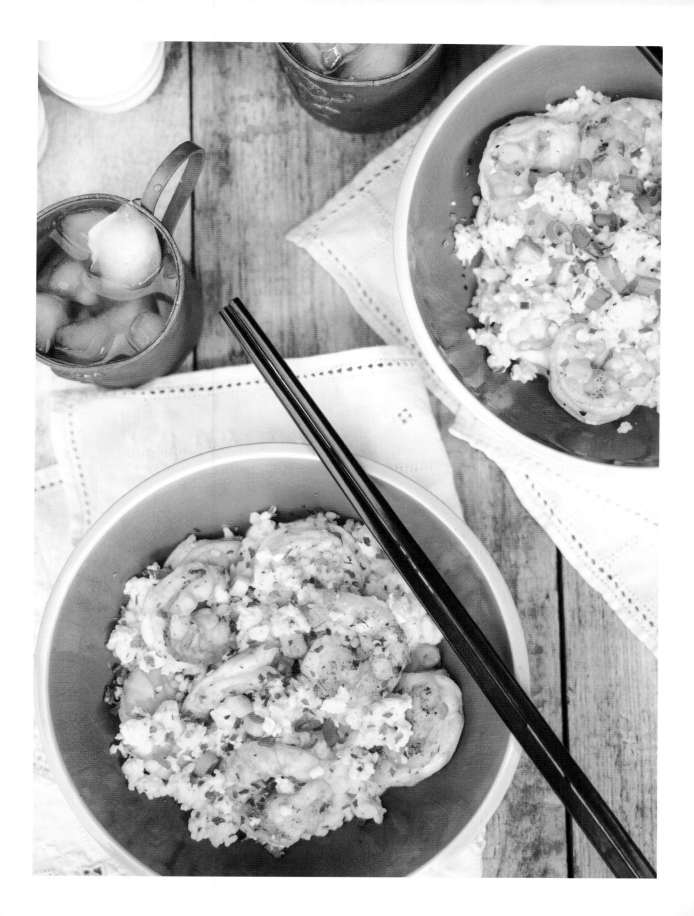

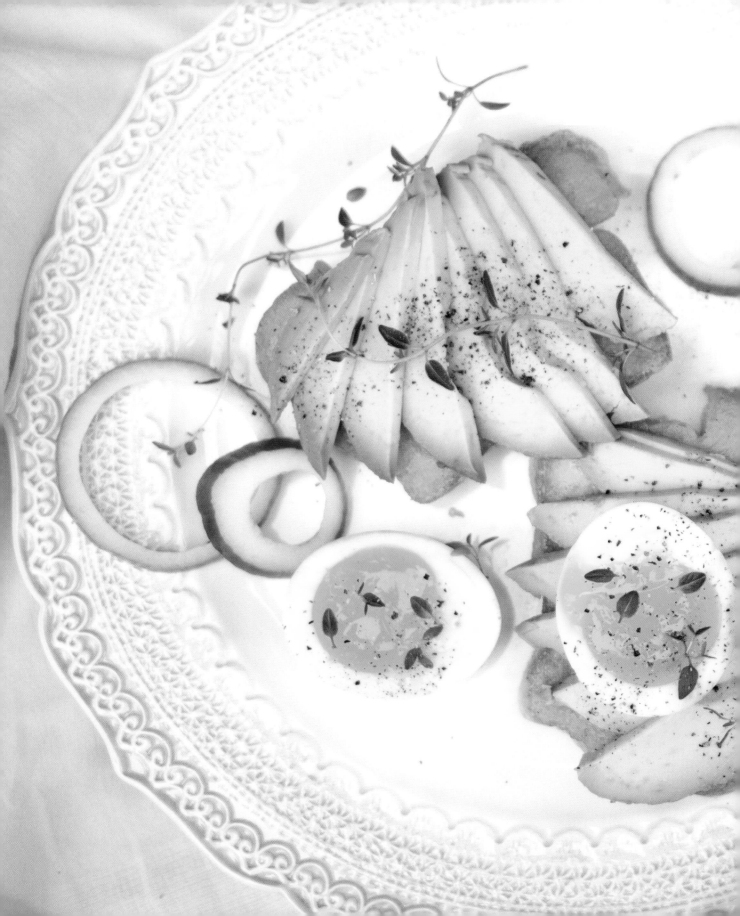

Chapter 10:
Vegetarian Dishes

SWEET 'N' SOUR CAULIFLOWER
over Vegetarian Fried "Rice"

prep time: 5 minutes   *cook time:* 15 minutes   *yield:* 6 servings

Cauliflower:

¼ cup avocado oil or coconut oil

1 head cauliflower, cut into bite-size pieces

Fine sea salt

½ cup vegetable broth

⅓ cup Swerve confectioners'-style sweetener or equivalent amount of liquid or powdered sweetener (see page 29)

¼ cup tomato sauce

1 tablespoon plus 1 teaspoon wheat-free tamari, or ⅓ cup coconut aminos

1 tablespoon coconut vinegar or apple cider vinegar

¾ teaspoon crushed red pepper

¼ teaspoon peeled and grated fresh ginger

1 clove garlic, crushed

Fried "Rice":

8 large eggs

½ cup full-fat coconut milk

2 tablespoons vegetable broth

½ teaspoon wheat-free tamari, or 2 teaspoons coconut aminos

1 teaspoon fine sea salt

½ teaspoon ground black pepper

1 teaspoon avocado oil or coconut oil

¼ cup diced onions

1 teaspoon minced garlic

For Garnish:

Scallions, sliced on the diagonal

Sesame seeds

1. Heat the oil in a wok or large cast-iron skillet over medium heat. Fry the cauliflower in the hot oil on all sides until light golden brown, about 4 minutes. Remove from the pan, sprinkle with salt, and set aside.

2. Add the remaining ingredients for the cauliflower to the wok and boil over medium heat until reduced and thickened, about 10 minutes.

3. Return the cauliflower to the pan and bring to a hard boil. Reduce the heat to medium and simmer for 5 to 10 minutes.

4. Meanwhile, make the fried "rice": Place the eggs, coconut milk, broth, tamari, salt, and pepper in a bowl and beat until well combined. Heat the oil in a large cast-iron skillet over medium-high heat. Add the onions and garlic and sauté until the onions are translucent, about 2 minutes. Add the egg mixture and cook until the mixture thickens and small curds form, while scraping the bottom of the pan and stirring to keep large curds from forming. (A whisk works well for this task.) This will take about 5 minutes. Transfer the rice to a platter.

5. Serve the cauliflower over the fried rice. (*Note:* If the rice released liquid during cooking, soak it up with a paper towel before serving.) Garnish with sliced scallions and sesame seeds.

6. Store in an airtight container in the refrigerator for up to 4 days. To reheat, place the cauliflower and rice in a lightly greased skillet, stirring occasionally, for 5 minutes or until warmed through.

nutritional info (per serving)				
calories	fat	protein	carbs	fiber
251	19g	13g	9g	3g

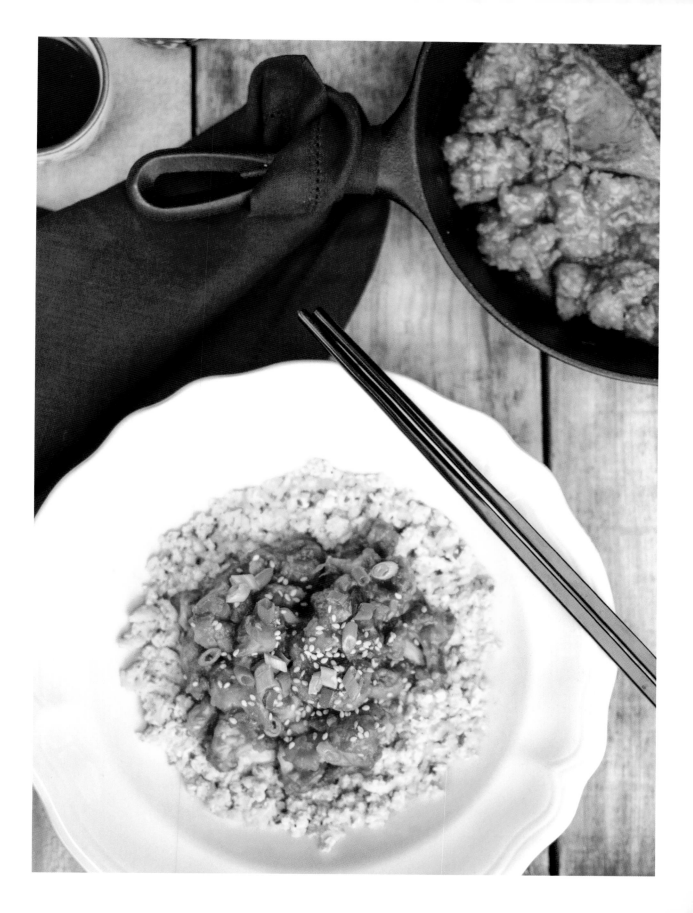

VEGETARIAN CURRY

prep time: 5 minutes (not including time to cook eggs) *cook time:* 10 minutes
yield: 6 servings

2 tablespoons coconut oil

2 teaspoons cumin seeds

¾ cup diced onions

¼ cup diced tomatoes

2 cloves garlic, smashed to a paste

1½ teaspoons red curry paste

2 teaspoons fine sea salt

1 teaspoon ground coriander

½ teaspoon turmeric powder

12 hard-boiled eggs (see page 81), whites and yolks separated

¾ cup vegetable broth

Juice of 1 lime

For Garnish:

Fresh cilantro

Scallions, sliced on the diagonal

Lime wedges

Freshly ground black pepper

Special Equipment:

Immersion blender

1. Heat the coconut oil in a cast-iron skillet over medium heat. Add the cumin seeds and cook for 1 minute, stirring often, until fragrant. (Watch the seeds closely, as they can burn quickly.) Add the onions and sauté for 3 minutes. Add the tomatoes and garlic and cook for 2 more minutes. Stir in the curry paste, salt, coriander, and turmeric.

2. Add 8 of the hard-boiled egg yolks (reserving the whites), along with the broth. Using an immersion blender, purée the mixture a bit, but leave some chunks. The yolks will thicken the curry. Cook over medium-high heat for 5 minutes, allowing the liquid to reduce a little.

3. Quarter the remaining 4 hard-boiled egg yolks and the reserved whites. Add the quartered eggs and lime juice to the pan, then stir. Serve garnished with cilantro, scallions, lime wedges, and freshly ground pepper.

4. Store in an airtight container in the refrigerator for up to 3 days. To reheat, place the curry in a saucepan over medium heat for 3 minutes or until warmed through.

nutritional info (per serving)				
calories	fat	protein	carbs	fiber
174	14g	13g	3g	1g

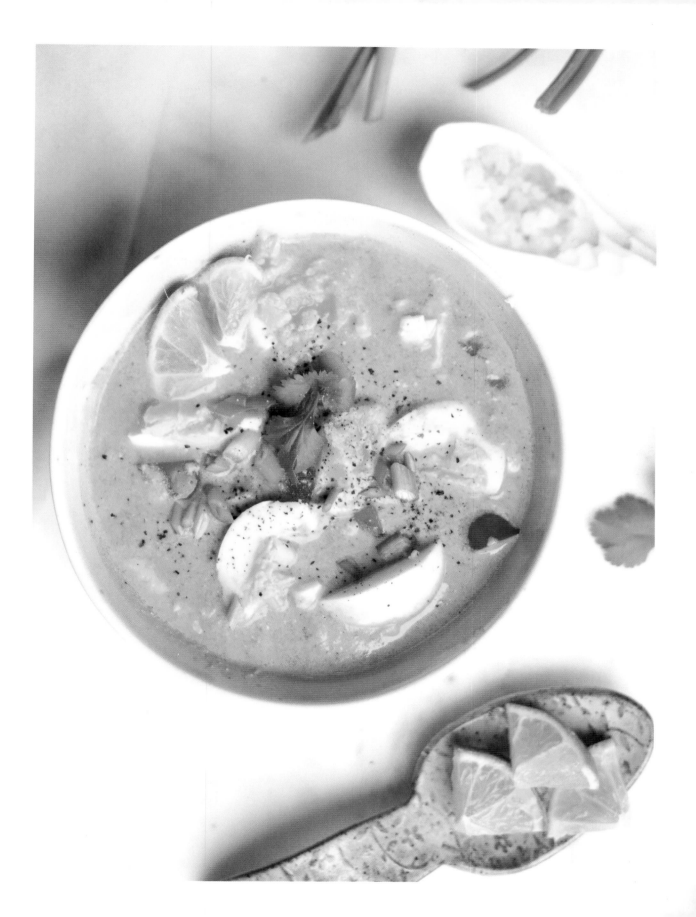

ITALIAN BAKED EGGS

KETO

prep time: **10 minutes** *cook time:* **15 minutes** *yield:* **4 servings**

4 teaspoons coconut oil or avocado oil

8 large eggs

1 teaspoon fine sea salt, divided

1 teaspoon ground black pepper, divided

8 tablespoons marinara sauce, divided

Chopped fresh parsley, for garnish

1. Preheat the oven to 350°F. Grease four 4-ounce ramekins.

2. Break 2 eggs into each ramekin. Season each with ¼ teaspoon of the salt and ¼ teaspoon of the pepper. Add 2 tablespoons of marinara sauce to each ramekin. Place the ramekins on a rimmed baking sheet.

3. Bake for 15 minutes or until the egg whites are opaque and the yolks have firm edges and are soft in the center. Garnish with parsley and serve immediately.

4. Store in an airtight container in the refrigerator for up to 4 days. Before reheating, set the chilled ramekins on the counter for 20 minutes to come to room temperature to prevent them from shattering in the oven. Then place the ramekins in a preheated 350°F oven for 5 minutes or until warmed through.

Note: Serve with toasted Keto Brioche (page 144) for a hearty meal.

nutritional info (per serving)				
calories	fat	protein	carbs	fiber
214	16g	13g	2g	0.4g

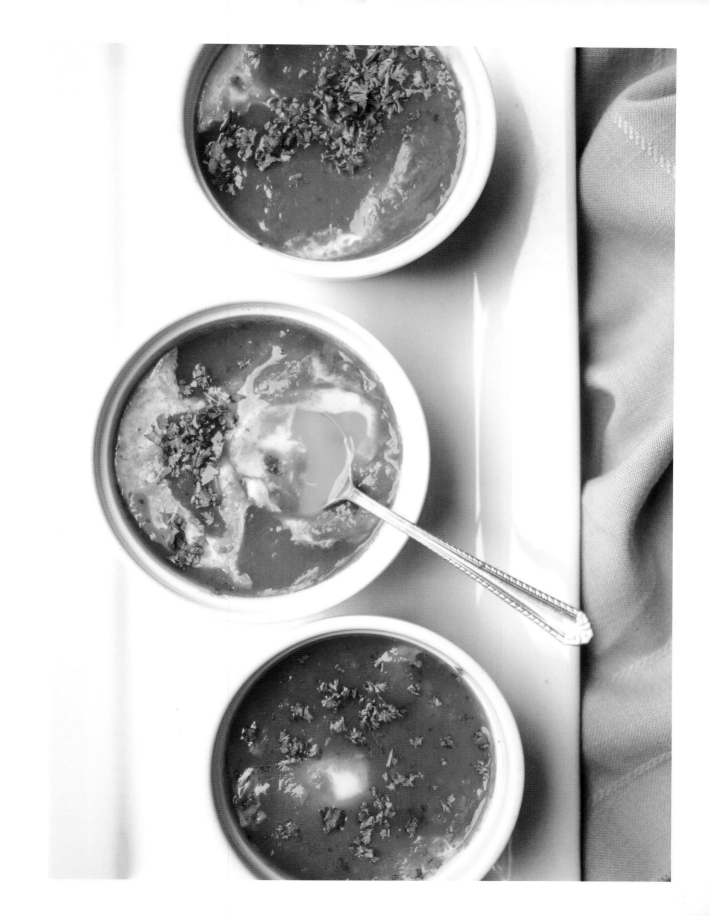

EGG ROLL IN A BOWL

KETO

I adore egg rolls. This recipe gives you the taste of the inside of an egg roll without the starchy wrapper! The mushrooms provide a meaty texture and umami taste that many vegetarians crave. You can easily double the recipe to make four servings.

prep time: 10 minutes, plus time to marinate cabbage   cook time: 8 minutes
yield: 2 servings

3 tablespoons lime juice

2 tablespoons sliced scallions, plus extra for garnish

2¼ teaspoons wheat-free tamari, or 3 tablespoons coconut aminos

1¼ teaspoons fine sea salt, divided

2 cups thinly sliced cabbage

2 tablespoons avocado oil or coconut oil

3 cloves garlic, minced

1 tablespoon peeled and grated fresh ginger

1 cup diced mushrooms

2 large eggs, beaten

⅛ teaspoon ground black pepper

1. Place the lime juice, scallions, tamari, and ¾ teaspoon of the salt in a bowl. Add the cabbage and toss to coat; set aside to marinate for up to 24 hours.

2. Heat the oil in a wok or large cast-iron skillet over medium heat. Add the garlic and ginger and cook until fragrant and softened, about 1 minute. Add the mushrooms and season with ¼ teaspoon of the salt; stir-fry for 3 minutes.

3. Add the marinated cabbage to the pan and cook until soft and wilted, about 3 minutes. Move the cabbage to the outside of the pan. Pour the beaten eggs into the center and season with the remaining ¼ teaspoon of salt and the pepper. Cook, stirring often, for 2 minutes or until cooked through. Garnish with scallions and freshly ground pepper and serve.

4. Store in an airtight container in the refrigerator for up to 4 days or in the freezer for up to a month. To reheat, place the egg roll mixture in a lightly greased skillet and stir-fry for 5 minutes or until warmed through.

nutritional info (per serving)				
calories	fat	protein	carbs	fiber
266	19g	13g	12g	3g

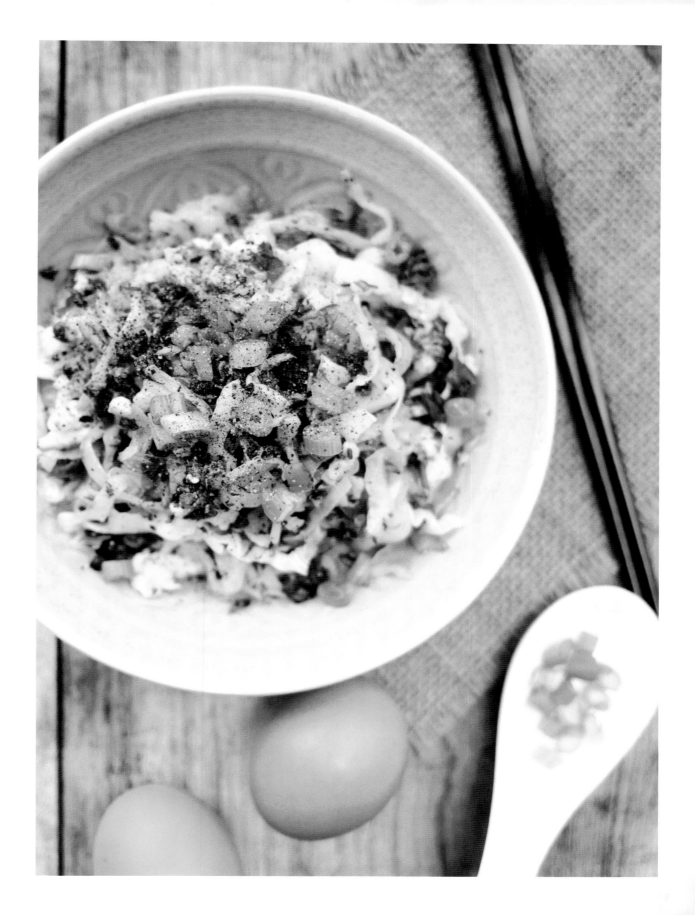

CHIPOTLE LIME EGG SALAD WRAPS

prep time: **5 minutes** (not including time to cook eggs)
yield: **4 servings**

8 hard-boiled eggs (see page 81), peeled and chopped

½ cup mayonnaise, homemade (page 34) or store-bought (see Note)

1 tablespoon lime juice

½ teaspoon fine sea salt

½ cup diced celery

8 radicchio leaves

Finely chopped fresh cilantro, for garnish

1. In a large bowl, combine the eggs, mayonnaise, lime juice, and salt. Mash well with a fork or wooden spoon. Add the celery and stir well.

2. Fill each radicchio leaf with egg salad and garnish with cilantro.

3. Store in an airtight container in the refrigerator for up to 3 days.

Note: *If using store-bought mayo, try the Primal Kitchen brand of chipotle lime mayo. The flavors of lime and chipotle are delicious in this recipe!*

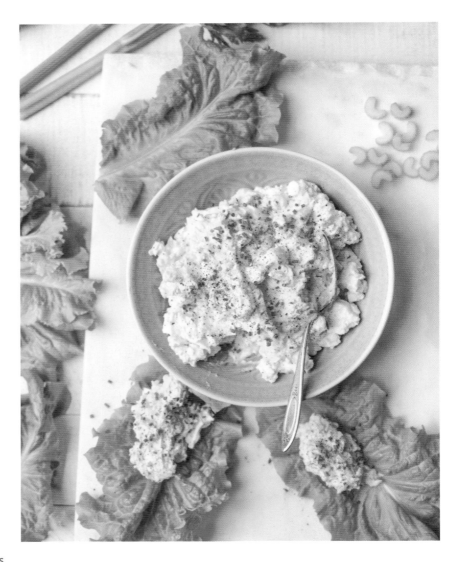

nutritional info (per serving)				
calories	fat	protein	carbs	fiber
304	29g	12g	1g	0.2g

CREAMY EGG BHURJI

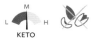

Egg bhurji is a popular dish in India and Pakistan, and once you try it, you'll see why it's so popular. There's something so comforting about a bowl of spicy eggs. It warms your belly and expands your adventurous side! Serve these eggs with toasted Keto Brioche (page 144) for a satisfying start or end to the day.

prep time: **5 minutes** *cook time:* **7 minutes** *yield:* **2 servings**

2 tablespoons avocado oil or coconut oil

¼ cup diced red onions

2 cloves garlic, smashed to a paste

¼ cup chopped tomatoes

1 tablespoon green curry paste

1 tablespoon garam masala

1 tablespoon ground coriander

1 teaspoon cayenne pepper

1 teaspoon turmeric powder

¼ teaspoon fine sea salt

4 large eggs, beaten

¼ cup full-fat coconut milk

Fresh cilantro, for garnish

Lime wedges, for serving

1. Heat the oil in a cast-iron skillet over medium-high heat. Add the onions and cook for 4 minutes or until soft, then add the garlic and sauté for another minute. Add the tomatoes, curry paste, garam masala, coriander, cayenne, turmeric, and salt and stir to combine.

2. Add the beaten eggs to the skillet and lower the heat to medium. Using a whisk, stir until the eggs are cooked through and resemble cooked rice, about 3 minutes. Serve hot, garnished with cilantro and a squirt of lime juice.

3. Store in an airtight container in the refrigerator for up to 4 days. To reheat, place the eggs in a sauté pan over medium heat for a minute or two, until warmed through.

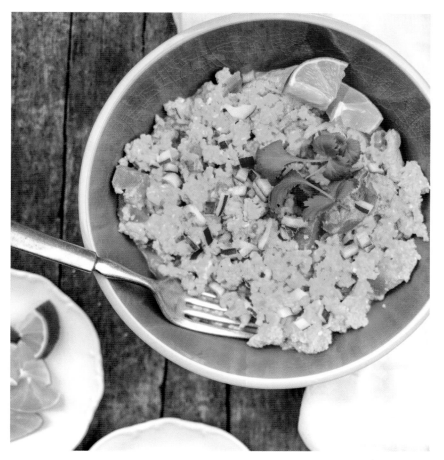

nutritional info (per serving)				
calories	fat	protein	carbs	fiber
219	18g	8g	7g	2g

VEGETARIAN DORO WATT

Doro watt is a special dish to my family. It is a staple in Ethiopia, and Craig and I ate it almost every day when we traveled there to adopt our two precious boys. Traditionally, it is made with chicken and hard-boiled eggs, but because I'm not a huge fan of poultry, I often filled my plate with the amazing sauce and plenty of eggs. You will never miss the chicken in this flavorful dish! It is also traditionally served with injera bread to scoop and soak up the yummy flavors. My Keto Tortillas (page 150) are a great substitute for injera bread.

prep time: **8 minutes** (not including time to cook eggs) *cook time:* **10 minutes**
yield: **4 servings**

Berbere Spice Mix:

(makes ⅓ heaping cup)

3 tablespoons paprika

1½ tablespoons cayenne pepper

1½ teaspoons fine sea salt

½ teaspoon garlic powder

½ teaspoon onion powder

½ teaspoon ground coriander

¼ teaspoon ginger powder

¼ teaspoon ground cardamom

¼ teaspoon ground fenugreek

¼ teaspoon ground nutmeg

⅛ teaspoon ground cloves

¼ cup coconut oil or avocado oil

1 large onion, finely chopped

1 clove garlic, minced

2 teaspoons fine sea salt

12 hard-boiled eggs (see page 81), peeled

Fresh thyme sprigs, for garnish (optional)

For Serving (optional):

1 batch Keto "Rice" (page 147)

1 batch Keto Tortillas (page 150)

1. Place the ingredients for the spice mix in a jar with a lid. Cover and shake until well combined.

2. Heat the oil in a large cast-iron skillet over medium-high heat. Add the onion, garlic, salt, and 2 tablespoons of the berbere spice. Cook, stirring occasionally, until the onions are very soft, about 10 minutes.

3. Place the onion mixture in a beautiful dish, then add the hard-boiled eggs and spoon some of the onion mixture over the eggs. Allow the eggs to warm through, if they were previously chilled. Garnish with thyme sprigs, if desired. Serve over keto "rice" and/or with a side of tortillas, if desired.

4. Store in an airtight container in the refrigerator for up to 4 days. To reheat, place in a sauté pan over medium heat for a minute or two, until warmed through.

Note: This amount of berbere spice mix is more than you'll need for this recipe, but it's good on so many things and will keep in the pantry for up to 2 months. If you crave ethnic food with a touch of spice, try this traditional Ethiopian blend on chicken, beef, or pork. If you don't want to make it yourself, you can purchase berbere spice at specialty spice stores or online.

nutritional info (per serving)				
calories	fat	protein	carbs	fiber
314	27g	18g	4g	1g

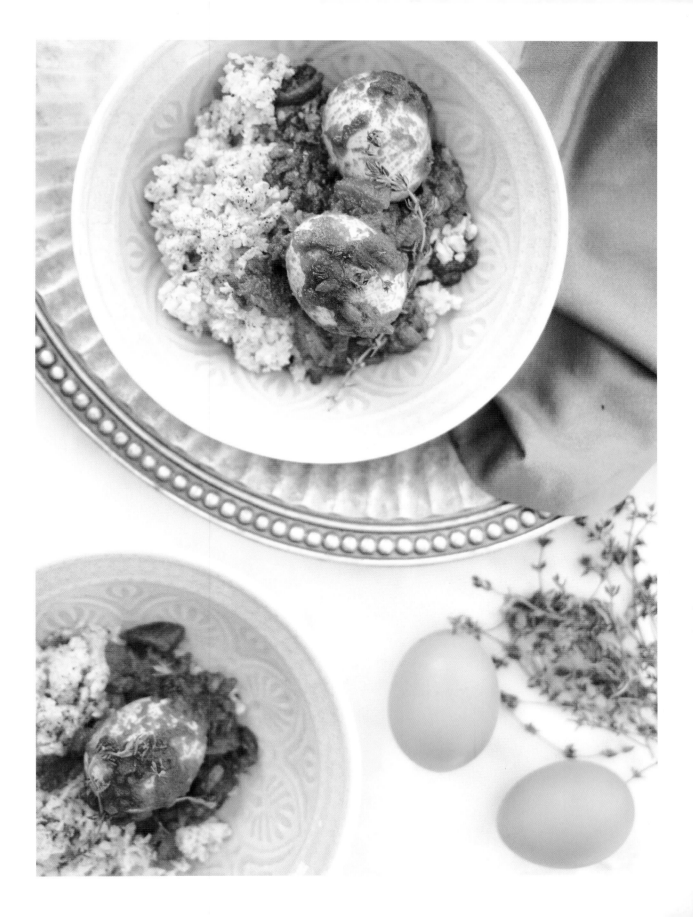

AVOCADO TOAST

KETO

prep time: 7 minutes (not including time to make brioche) cook time: 7 minutes
yield: 2 servings

4 large eggs

4 slices Keto Brioche, baked in a loaf pan (page 144)

2 tablespoons mayonnaise, homemade (page 34) or store-bought

1 small avocado

¾ teaspoon fine sea salt

½ teaspoon ground black pepper

2 teaspoons lime juice

Stone-ground mustard, for serving

Fresh herbs, such as oregano or parsley, for garnish

1. Preheat the oven to 425°F.

2. Soft-boil the eggs: Fill a medium-sized saucepan halfway with water and bring just to a simmer. Gently place the eggs in the simmering water and cook for 5 to 7 minutes, depending on how runny you prefer the yolks: 5 minutes will give you runny yolks and 7 minutes will give you yolks that are just set. Hold the water at a simmer when cooking the eggs; don't let it come to a boil.

3. Meanwhile, toast the brioche: Place the slices on a baking sheet and spread ½ tablespoon of mayonnaise on each slice. Toast in the oven for 2 to 3 minutes, until the bread is turning golden brown.

4. When the eggs are done, remove them from the water and run under cool water. Once cool, carefully peel the eggs. Slice them in half and set aside.

5. Slice the avocado in half and discard the pit. Use a sharp knife to cut ½-inch slices in the avocado while still in the peel. Use a spoon to scoop out the slices and spread like a fan on the toast. Sprinkle the avocado evenly with the salt, pepper, and lime juice. Top each avocado toast with 2 halves of a soft-boiled egg. Sprinkle the eggs lightly with salt and pepper. Serve with stone-ground mustard. Garnish with herbs. Best served fresh.

nutritional info (per serving)				
calories	fat	protein	carbs	fiber
276	24g	11g	5g	3g

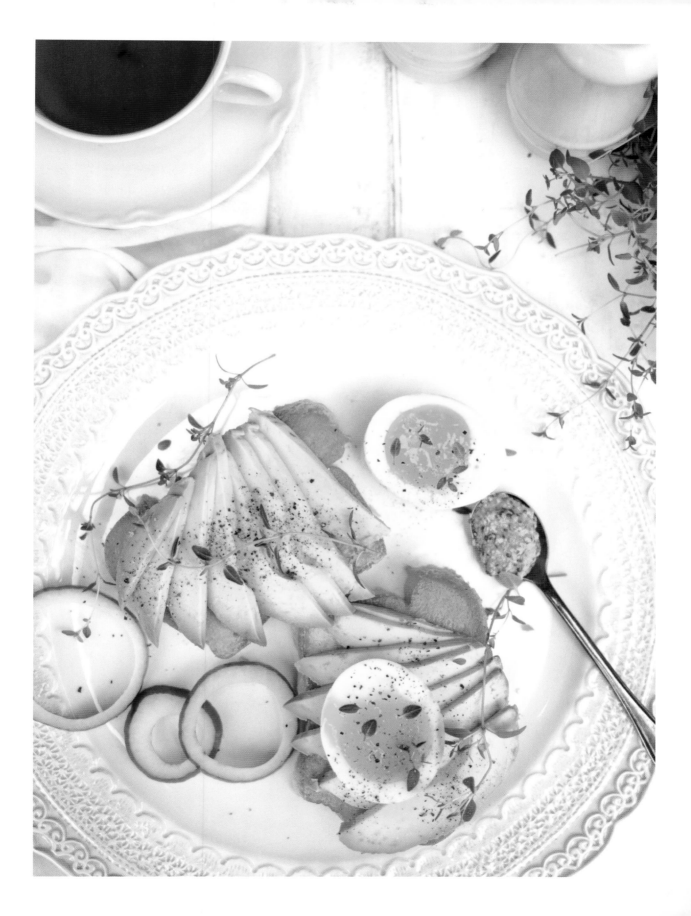

GAZPACHO

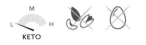

2 medium tomatoes, quartered

2 red bell peppers, seeded and coarsely chopped

1 (10-inch) cucumber, peeled, sliced in half lengthwise, and seeded

¼ cup chopped red onions

3 teaspoons minced garlic

3 cups tomato sauce

1 cup vegetable broth

¼ cup MCT oil, avocado oil, or extra-virgin olive oil, plus more for drizzling

2 tablespoons lime juice

1½ teaspoons fine sea salt

1 teaspoon ground black pepper

½ teaspoon smoked paprika

Diced avocado, for garnish

Lime wedges, for serving

1. Place the tomatoes, bell peppers, cucumber, onions, and garlic in a food processor. Pulse a few times until roughly chopped. Pour into a large bowl.

2. Add the tomato sauce, broth, oil, lime juice, salt, pepper, and paprika. Stir well to combine. Taste and adjust the seasoning to your liking.

3. Cover and place in the refrigerator to chill for at least 20 minutes before serving. Garnish with diced avocado and a drizzle of oil, and serve with lime wedges.

4. Store in an airtight container in the refrigerator for up to 4 days.

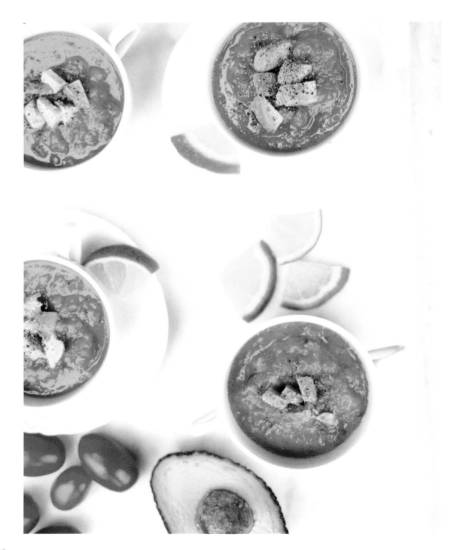

nutritional info (per serving)				
calories	fat	protein	carbs	fiber
112	8g	1g	9g	2g

EGG MASALA

prep time: 5 minutes (not including time to cook eggs) cook time: 10 minutes
yield: 2 servings

3 tablespoons coconut oil

1 cup diced onions

2 tomatoes, diced

1 cup vegetable broth

4 cloves garlic, smashed to a paste

2 teaspoons garam masala, plus more if needed

1 teaspoon turmeric powder

1½ teaspoons fine sea salt

Juice of 1 lime

6 hard-boiled eggs (see page 81)

For Garnish:

Chopped fresh cilantro

Sliced scallions

Lime wedges

1. Heat the coconut oil in a large saucepan over medium-high heat. Add the onions and sauté for 3 minutes.

2. Add the tomatoes, broth, garlic, spices, salt, and lime juice, bring to a boil, and continue to boil for 5 minutes.

3. Meanwhile, peel and quarter the eggs, then add to the sauce. Simmer for another minute. Taste and adjust the seasoning, adding more garam masala and/or salt, if desired. Garnish with chopped cilantro, sliced scallions, and lime wedges.

4. Store in an airtight container in the refrigerator for up to 4 days. To reheat, place in a saucepan, stirring occasionally, for 5 minutes or until warmed through.

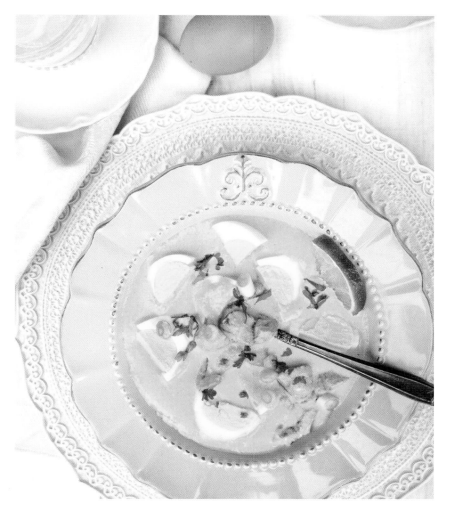

nutritional info (per serving)				
calories	fat	protein	carbs	fiber
468	38g	22g	18g	4g

VEGETARIAN FAJITAS WITH AVOCADO

KETO   OPTION

prep time: **3 minutes**   *cook time:* **16 minutes**   *yield:* **2 servings**

Tortillas:

2 large eggs

2 hard-boiled eggs (see page 81), peeled

¼ cup unsweetened cashew milk or almond milk (or hemp milk if nut-free)

¼ teaspoon fine sea salt

¼ teaspoon baking powder

2 tablespoons coconut oil, divided, for the skillet

Fillings:

1 tablespoon coconut oil

1 bell pepper (any color), thinly sliced

¼ cup thinly sliced onions

Fine sea salt

½ avocado, diced

1 small tomato, sliced

For Serving (optional):

¼ cup sugar-free salsa

2 tablespoons chopped fresh cilantro leaves

Cilantro Lime Dressing (page 39)

1. Place all the ingredients for the tortillas, except the coconut oil, in a blender and blend until very smooth.

2. Heat 1½ teaspoons of coconut oil in a nonstick skillet over medium heat. Once hot, pour one-quarter of the batter into the skillet. Cook until golden brown, about 2 minutes, then flip and cook for another 2 minutes or until cooked through. Remove from the skillet and repeat, using another 1½ teaspoons of coconut oil for each tortilla.

3. Prepare the fillings: Heat 1 tablespoon of coconut oil in a sauté pan over medium-high heat. Add the sliced bell pepper and onions and sauté for 5 minutes or until soft. Season to taste with couple pinches of salt.

4. To assemble the fajitas, divide the diced avocado, tomato slices, and sautéed peppers and onions evenly among the tortillas. Wrap up and serve with the salsa, cilantro, and/or dressing, if desired.

5. Store leftover tortillas and fillings in separate airtight containers in the refrigerator for up to 4 days. Reheat the tortillas in a lightly greased skillet over medium heat for 2 minutes or until warmed through. Reheat the sautéed bell peppers and onions in a small skillet over medium heat for 3 minutes or until warmed through.

nutritional info (per serving)				
calories	fat	protein	carbs	fiber
354	29g	25g	1g	0g

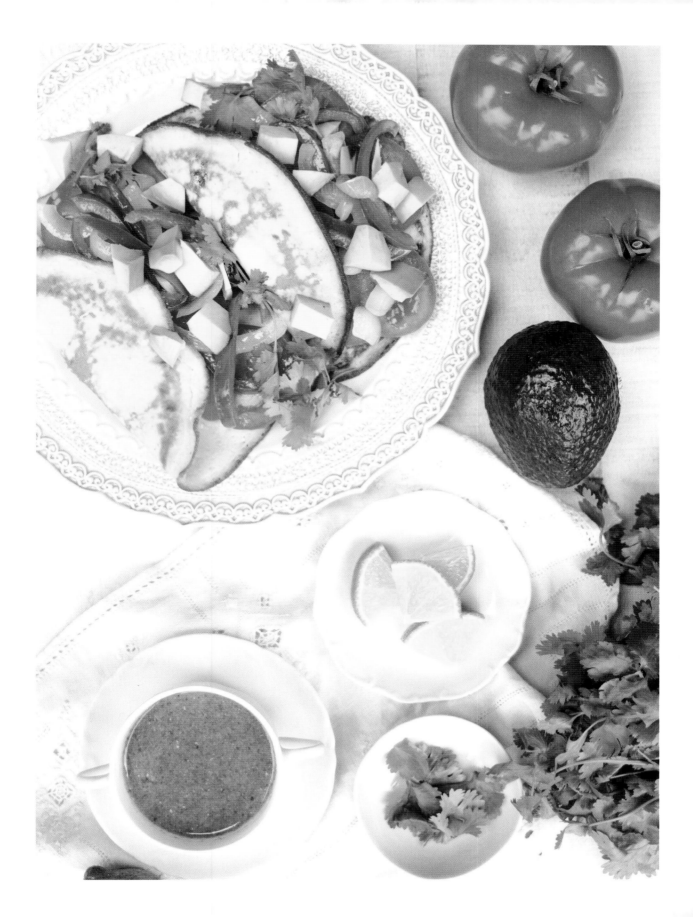

VEGETARIAN FAJITA STEW

KETO

prep time: **5 minutes** *cook time:* **15 minutes** *yield:* **2 servings**

2 tablespoons avocado oil or coconut oil

1 cup diced onions

1 green bell pepper, thinly sliced

3 cups vegetable broth

½ cup sugar-free salsa

¼ cup diced pickled jalapeños

2½ teaspoons fine sea salt

2 teaspoons chili powder

1 teaspoon paprika

1 teaspoon ground cumin

½ teaspoon ground black pepper

4 large eggs

2 limes, halved

For Garnish (optional):

Chopped fresh cilantro

Avocado slices

Lime wedges

Drizzle of MCT oil, avocado oil, or extra-virgin olive oil

1. Heat the oil in a saucepan over medium-high heat. Add the onions and bell pepper and sauté for 4 minutes. Add the broth, salsa, pickled jalapeños, salt, and spices and reduce the heat to medium. Simmer for 10 minutes.

2. Meanwhile, soft-boil the eggs: Fill a medium-sized saucepan halfway with water and bring just to a simmer. Gently slide the eggs into the simmering water and cook for 5 to 7 minutes, depending on how you like the yolks: 5 minutes will give you runny yolks and 7 minutes will give you yolks that are just set. Hold the water at a simmer while cooking the eggs; don't let it come to a boil.

3. When the eggs are done, remove them from the water and run under cool water. Once cool, carefully peel the eggs, slice them in half, and set aside.

4. Stir the stew well and squeeze in the lime juice. Stir once more, then taste and add more salt, if desired. Garnish with chopped cilantro, avocado slices, lime wedges, and/or a drizzle of oil, if desired.

5. Store in an airtight container in the refrigerator for up to 5 days. To reheat, place the stew in a pot over medium heat for 3 minutes or until warmed through.

nutritional info (per serving)				
calories	fat	protein	carbs	fiber
372	25g	15g	26g	6g

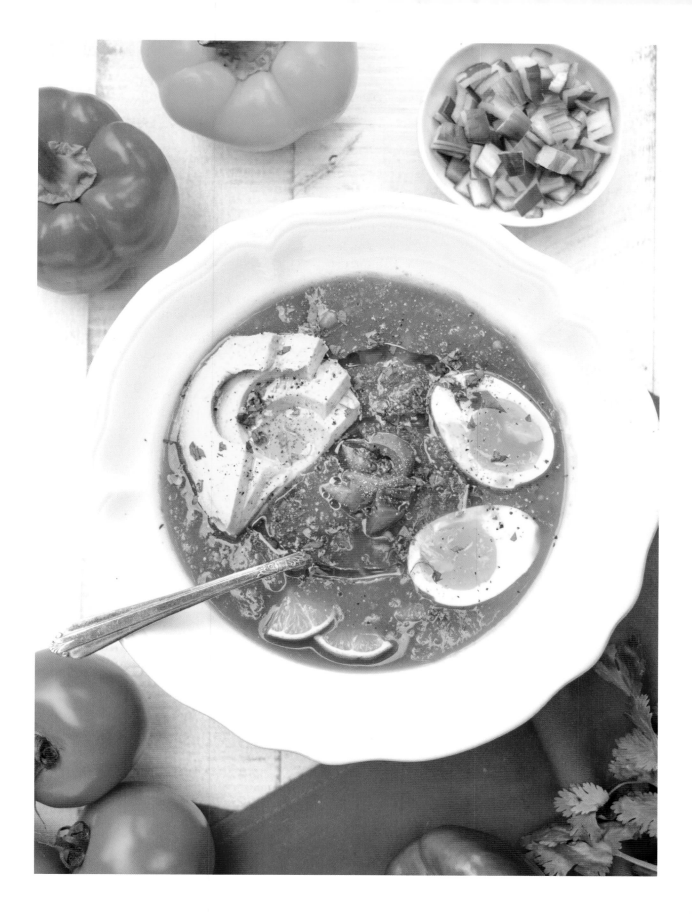

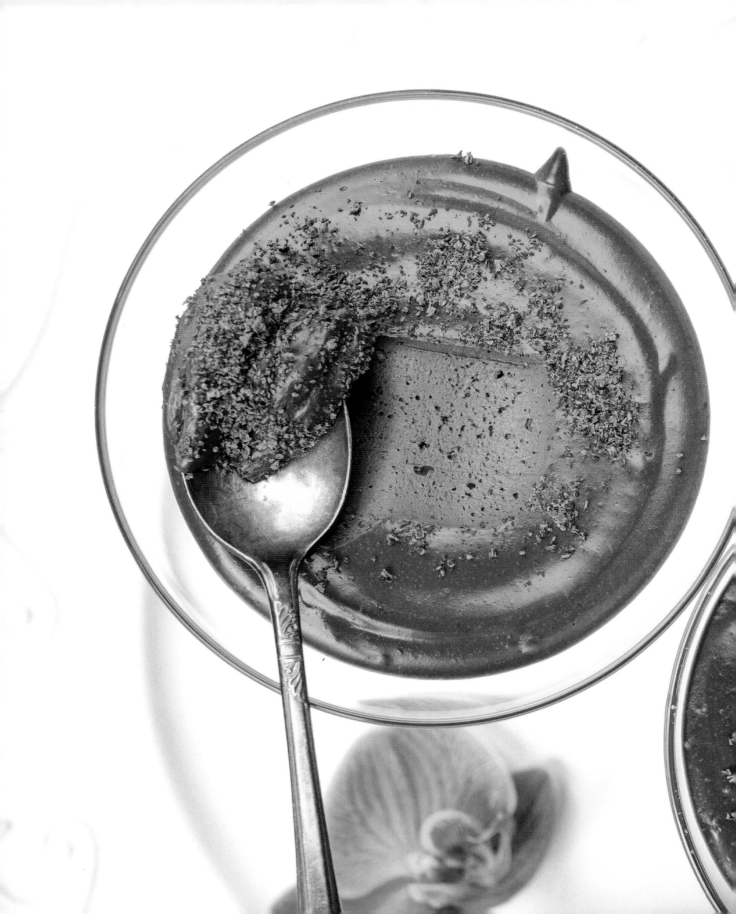

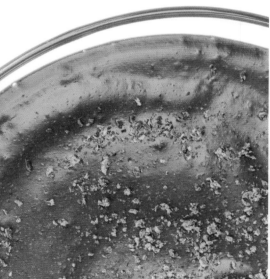

Chapter 11:
Sweet Endings

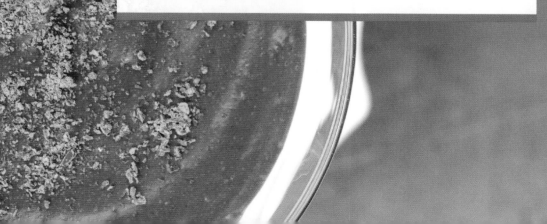

GRAND MARNIER CHOCOLATE CANDIES

prep time: **5 minutes, plus time to set** *yield:* **24 candies (4 per serving)**

½ cup coconut oil (preferably butter-flavored), softened

2 tablespoons unsweetened cocoa powder

2 teaspoons orange extract, or 8 drops orange oil

¼ teaspoon orange-flavored liquid stevia, or ¼ cup Swerve confectioners'-style sweetener or equivalent amount of liquid or powdered sweetener (see page 29)

Special Equipment:

24 (½-ounce-capacity) candy molds (optional)

1. Mix all of the ingredients in a medium-sized bowl until well combined.

2. Divide the mixture evenly among 24 candy molds. Or use a 24-well mini muffin pan, filling each well with about ¼ inch of the mixture.

3. Freeze until set, about 15 minutes. Serve chilled.

4. Store in an airtight container in the refrigerator for up to a week or in the freezer for up to a month.

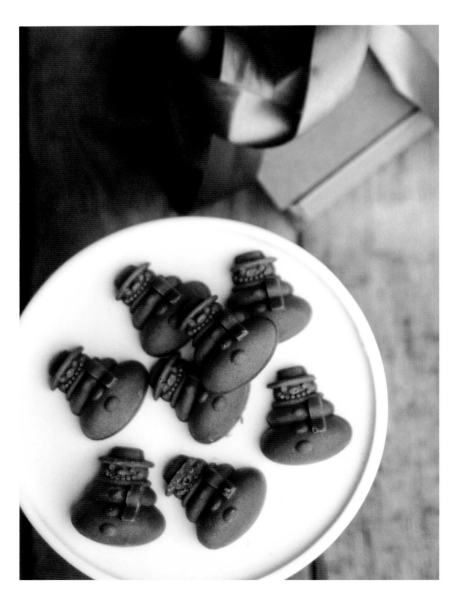

nutritional info (per serving)				
calories	fat	protein	carbs	fiber
168	20g	0.3g	1g	0.3g

SOUR PATCH CANDY

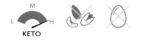

2 tablespoons unflavored gelatin

1 hibiscus tea bag

1 teaspoon citric acid, plus more for dusting

½ teaspoon watermelon-flavored liquid stevia or other fruit-flavored liquid stevia of choice, plus more if desired

2 tablespoons Swerve confectioners'-style sweetener or equivalent amount of liquid or powdered sweetener (see page 29)

Special Equipment:

20 (¼-ounce) candy molds

1. Place 1 cup of water in a microwave-safe cup. Whisk in the gelatin and stir until dissolved. Add the tea bag and heat in the microwave until boiling. Stir well. Squeeze out the liquid from the tea bag and discard the bag.

2. Add the citric acid to the cup and stir to combine, then add the liquid stevia and Swerve and stir. Taste and add more sweetener, if desired.

3. Pour into candy molds and place in the refrigerator until set, about 2 hours. *Note:* The longer gelatin sits, the chewier the candy will be.

4. Dust the candy with citric acid for more sour taste, if desired.

5. Store in an airtight container in the refrigerator for up to 5 days.

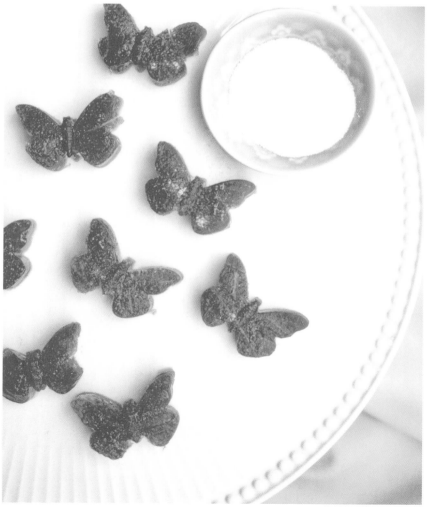

nutritional info (per serving)				
calories	fat	protein	carbs	fiber
25	0g	6g	0g	0g

SNICKERDOODLE BITES

1 cup coconut oil, soft but not liquid

½ cup strong-brewed cinnamon tea or chai tea, chilled

¾ cup Swerve confectioners'-style sweetener or equivalent amount of powdered sweetener (see page 29)

1 teaspoon ground cinnamon

For Sprinkling (optional):

Ground cinnamon

Swerve confectioners'-style sweetener or equivalent amount of powdered sweetener (see page 29)

1. Line an 8 by 4-inch loaf pan with parchment paper.

2. Place the coconut oil, tea, sweetener, and cinnamon in a blender or food processor and combine until smooth. Immediately pour into the prepared loaf pan. (*Note:* If the mixture sits out at room temperature after being blended, it will separate; if that happens, puree again until smooth.)

3. Place in the freezer or refrigerator until set, 10 to 20 minutes. Remove from the pan and cut into 1-inch squares. If sprinkling the bites with cinnamon and sweetener, mix equal parts of both in a small bowl, then sprinkle the bites with the mixture. Serve chilled.

4. Store in the refrigerator for up to a week or in the freezer for up to a month.

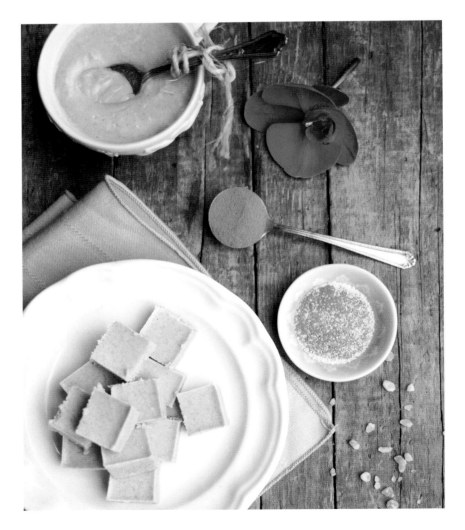

nutritional info (per serving)				
calories	fat	protein	carbs	fiber
235	28g	0g	0.2g	0.2g

BERRY ICE POPS

prep time: 5 minutes, plus time to freeze   *yield:* 8 ice pops (1 per serving)

2 cups water or berry-flavored sparkling water or seltzer water (see Notes)

¼ cup lime or lemon juice

A few drops of berry-flavored liquid stevia, or more to taste

½ teaspoon citric acid (optional, for sourness)

Special Equipment:

8 (3.4-ounce) ice pop molds (see Notes)

1. Place all of the ingredients in a large pitcher and stir well to combine. Taste and adjust the sweetness to your liking.

2. Pour the mixture into 8 ice pop molds and place in the freezer to set, about 3 hours.

3. Store in the freezer for up to a month.

Notes: *If using a berry-flavored sparkling water or seltzer water, look for a clean, naturally flavored water with no added sugars. I use LaCroix brand strawberry-kiwi–flavored sparkling water for these ice pops.*

To make these ice pops, I used silicone molds from FoodWorks. You can use any type of ice pop mold you like; just be sure to use molds with a similar capacity.

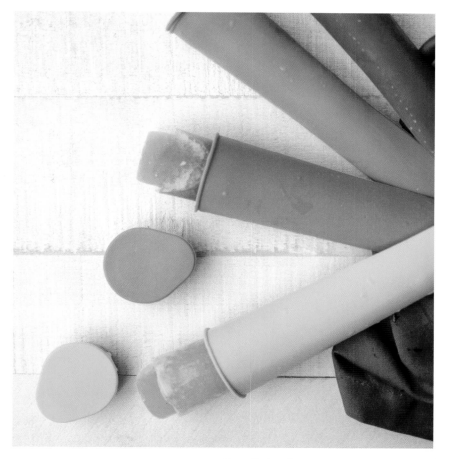

nutritional info (per serving)				
calories	fat	protein	carbs	fiber
2	0g	0.1g	1g	0.2g

PERSONAL FLOURLESS CHOCOLATE TORTES

KETO

I like my tortes a touch underbaked for a gooey center. They taste great with dairy-free ice cream on top!

prep time: **7 minutes**   *cook time:* **10 minutes**   *yield:* **8 small tortes (1 per serving)**

7 ounces unsweetened baking chocolate, finely chopped

¾ cup plus 2 tablespoons butter-flavored coconut oil

1¼ cups Swerve confectioners'-style sweetener or equivalent amount of liquid or powdered sweetener (see page 29)

5 large eggs

1 tablespoon coconut flour

Pinch of fine sea salt

1. Preheat the oven to 325°F. Grease eight 4-ounce ramekins and set on a rimmed baking sheet or in a large baking dish.

2. Place the chocolate and coconut oil in a heavy saucepan or in a double boiler over medium heat and stir until the chocolate is completely melted. Remove the pan from the heat, then add the rest of the ingredients to the melted chocolate and stir until smooth. If you're not concerned about consuming raw eggs, taste and adjust the sweetness to your liking.

3. Pour the batter into the prepared ramekins and bake for 8 to 10 minutes, until the tortes are set. (For tortes with a gooey center, remove after 8 minutes; for tortes with centers that are just set, bake for the full 10 minutes.) Serve warm or chilled.

4. Store in an airtight container in the refrigerator for up to 5 days or in the freezer for up to a month.

Note: *If using these cakes to make Dirt Cake (page 327), bake them for 15 minutes or until totally baked through with no gooey center.*

nutritional info (per serving)				
calories	fat	protein	carbs	fiber
414	40g	8g	8g	6g

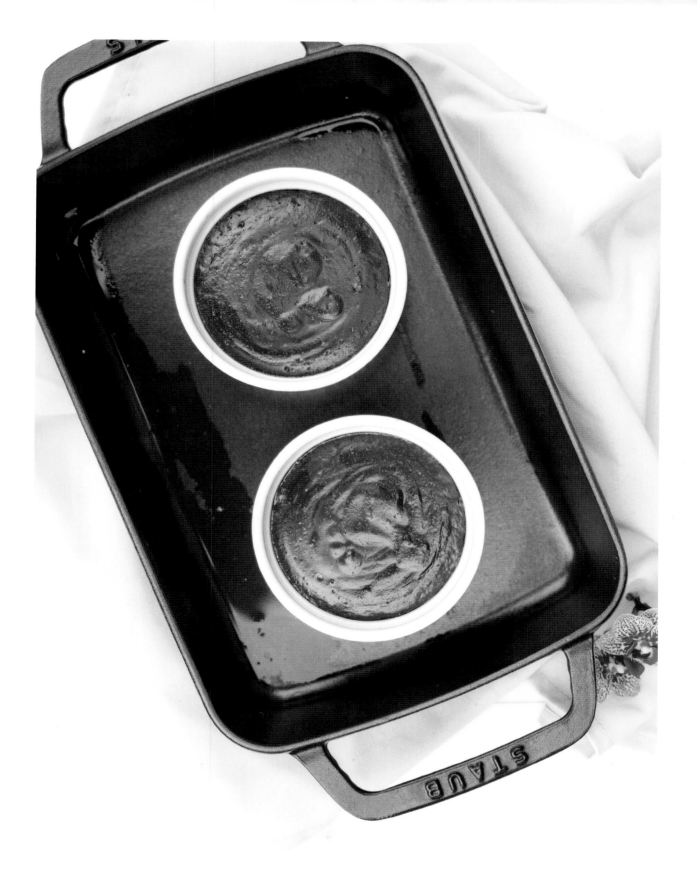

MINT CHOCOLATE CHUNK GELATO

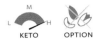

KETO   OPTION

This gelato recipe uses raw eggs. If you are not comfortable consuming raw eggs, feel free to purchase pasteurized eggs for this recipe.

If you enjoy the flavor of mint pure and simple, omit the chocolate.

prep time: 10 minutes, plus time to set chocolate and churn gelato
yield: 6 cups (1 cup per serving)

Chocolate Chunks:

1 cup melted coconut oil

1 cup unsweetened cocoa powder

¾ cup Swerve confectioners'-style sweetener or equivalent amount of liquid or powdered sweetener (see page 29)

1 teaspoon vanilla extract

¼ teaspoon fine sea salt

Gelato Base:

¾ cup plus 2 tablespoons coconut oil

½ cup unsweetened cashew milk (or hemp milk for nut-free)

¼ cup MCT oil

4 large eggs

4 large egg yolks

¼ cup Swerve confectioners'-style sweetener or equivalent amount of liquid or powdered sweetener (see page 29)

¼ cup fresh mint leaves, or 2 teaspoons mint extract

½ teaspoon fine sea salt

Fresh mint sprigs, for garnish (optional)

Special Equipment:

Ice cream maker

1. Line the bottom of a 9-inch pie pan with a round piece of parchment paper.

2. Place the ingredients for the chocolate chunks in a blender and pulse until smooth. Taste and adjust the sweetness to your liking. Pour the mixture into the lined pie pan and place in the freezer or refrigerator until the chocolate is fully set and hard, 10 to 15 minutes.

3. Transfer the chocolate to a cutting board and cut in half. Coarsely chop half of the chocolate and set aside. Use the remaining half of chocolate for other recipes; it will keep in an airtight container in the refrigerator for up to a week or in the freezer for up to a month.

4. Make the gelato base: Place the ingredients for the base in a blender and puree until the mint leaves are completely broken down. Taste and add more sweetener, if desired.

5. Pour the gelato base into an ice cream maker and churn, according to the manufacturer's directions, until set. About three-quarters of the way through churning, add the chopped chocolate.

6. Serve the gelato garnished with fresh mint, if desired.

7. Store in an airtight container in the freezer for up to a month.

nutritional info (per serving)				
calories	fat	protein	carbs	fiber
447	48g	6g	1g	0.3g

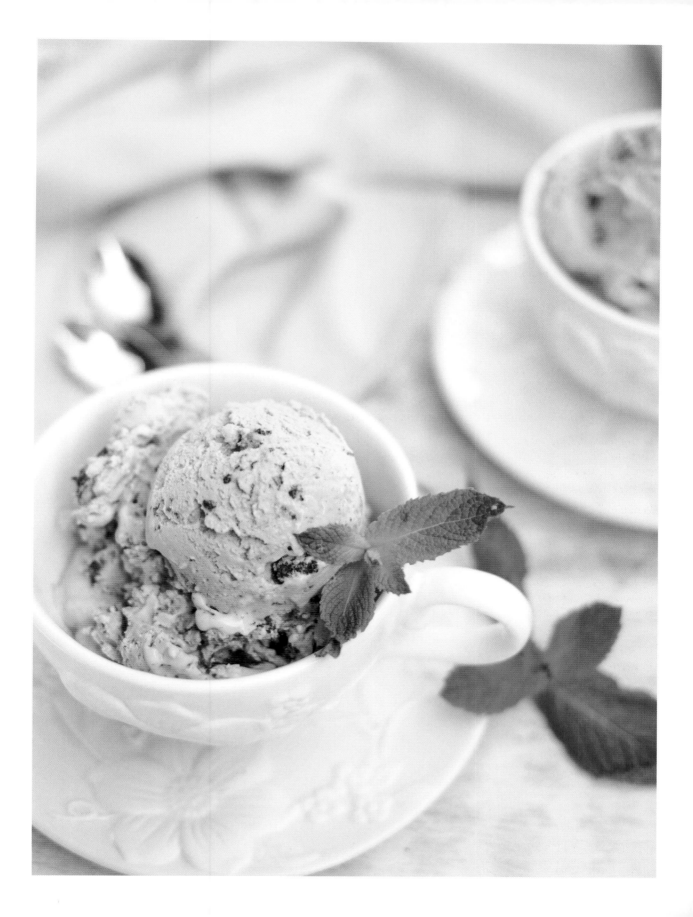

MOCHA FUDGE MUG CAKES

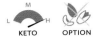

KETO   OPTION

You can make these as individual cakes in the oven or as a single layer cake in a slow cooker (see the variation below). They are great either way!

prep time: **10 minutes**   *cook time:* **10 minutes in the oven or 2 hours in a slow cooker**
yield: **12 servings**

¼ cup coconut oil (preferably butter-flavored)

3 ounces unsweetened chocolate, finely chopped

1½ cups Swerve confectioners'-style sweetener or equivalent amount of liquid or powdered sweetener (see page 29)

3 large eggs (6 eggs if using coconut flour)

¾ cup Kite Hill brand cream cheese style spread

1½ cups blanched almond flour (or ¾ cup coconut flour for nut-free)

1½ teaspoons baking soda

¾ cup hot decaf espresso or strong-brewed decaf coffee

1½ teaspoons vanilla or chocolate extract

½ teaspoon fine sea salt

1. Preheat the oven to 350°F. Grease twelve 4-ounce ramekins or oven-safe mugs or cups and set on a rimmed baking sheet.

2. Heat the coconut oil in a large saucepan over medium-high heat, stirring often. Once hot, remove the pan from the heat and add the chocolate. Let sit for a minute or two to melt, then stir well to combine.

3. Add the sweetener and mix thoroughly. Beat in the eggs, then the cream cheese spread.

4. Sift the flour and baking soda into another bowl, then add to the chocolate mixture. Beat in the coffee, vanilla extract, and salt.

5. Pour the batter into the ramekins or mugs, filling each about two-thirds full. Bake for about 10 minutes, until a toothpick inserted in the center of a cake comes out clean.

6. Store in an airtight container in the refrigerator for up to 4 days or in the freezer for up to a month. Allow frozen cake(s) to thaw to room temperature before serving.

Variation: *Slow Cooker Mocha Fudge Cake. Line the bottom of a 6-quart slow cooker with parchment paper, then grease the parchment well. Complete Steps 2 through 4 above, then pour the batter into the slow cooker. Cover and cook on low until the cake is fully baked on the edges but still gooey in the center, 2 to 3 hours. To serve, scoop into twelve 4-ounce ramekins, mugs, or cups.*

nutritional info (per serving)				
calories	fat	protein	carbs	fiber
164	14g	5g	4g	2g

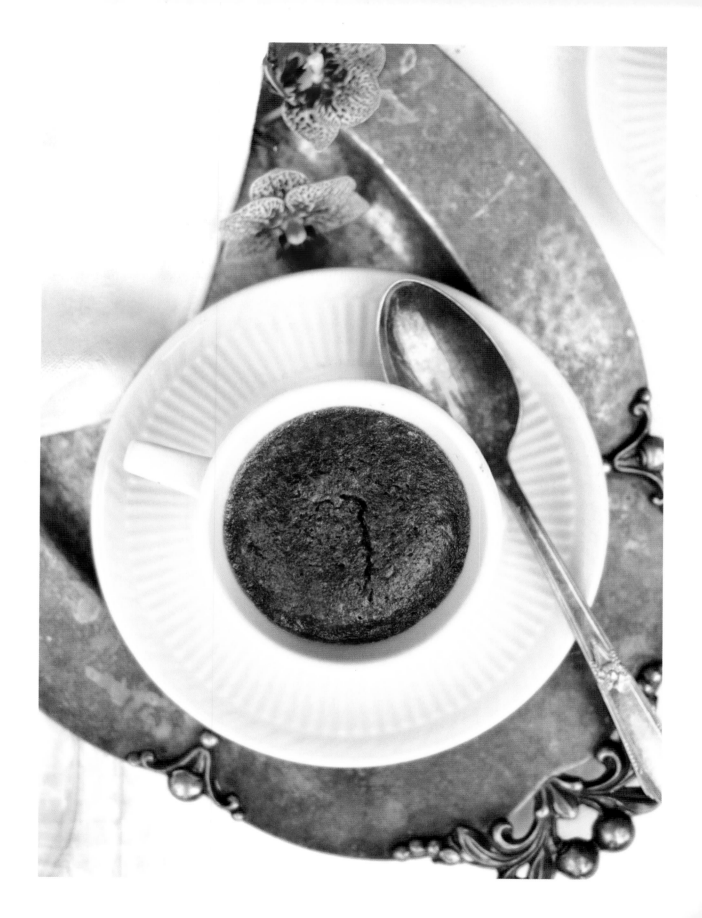

CLASSIC SHERBET

You can take this basic sherbet recipe and change up the flavor in multiple ways by playing around with different flavors of extract, oil, liquid stevia, and even sparkling water—it's so easy!

prep time: **3 minutes, plus time to churn** *yield:* **2 cups (½ cup per serving)**

1 cup full-fat coconut milk

1 cup flavored sparkling water or seltzer water, such as coconut, lime, or strawberry (see Note)

½ cup strong-brewed hibiscus tea, chilled (optional, for added pink color; if using, reduce the amount of sparkling water by half)

1 teaspoon orange extract, or a few drops of orange oil (or other fruit-flavored extract/oil, such as strawberry)

¼ teaspoon fruit-flavored liquid stevia (such as orange or strawberry)

3 tablespoons Swerve confectioners'-style sweetener or equivalent amount of liquid or powdered sweetener (see page 29)

½ teaspoon fine sea salt

Special Equipment:

Ice cream maker

1. Place all of the ingredients in a blender and combine until smooth. Taste and adjust the intensity of the fruit flavor and sweetness to your liking.

2. Pour into an ice cream maker and churn, following the manufacturer's directions, until set.

3. Store in an airtight container in the freezer for up to a month.

Note: *When choosing a flavored sparkling water or seltzer water, look for a clean, naturally flavored water with no added sugars. I use the LaCroix brand of sparkling water.*

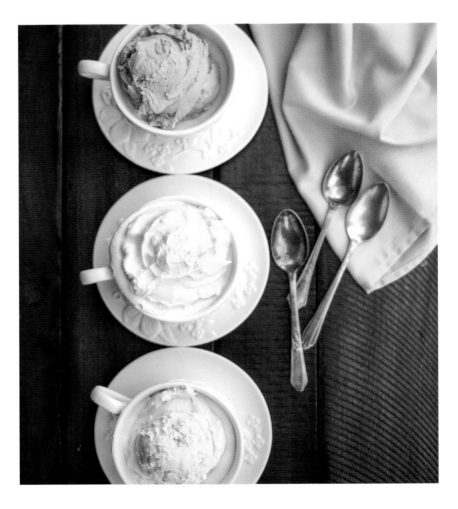

nutritional info (per serving)				
calories	fat	protein	carbs	fiber
92	9g	1g	1g	0g

DIRT CAKE

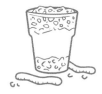

When I was about ten years old, my mom made me a dirt cake for my birthday. It was made with crushed Oreos, layered with Cool Whip, and filled with gummy worms. I decided to re-create dirt cake for my boys using keto ingredients. I thought they'd get a kick out of this cake, and they sure did! They had never seen a gummy worm before, so when I offered them my "healthified" version, they didn't know what to think. They didn't realize that you can eat such a crazy-looking "food," but once they popped them into their mouths, they couldn't get enough!

It is crazy how much we eat with our eyes, and kids are no exception. They love bright-colored food. That's why I use hibiscus tea to make bright-colored gummy worms!

prep time: **10 minutes** *(not including time to make tortes or gummy worms)*
cook time: **10 minutes** *yield:* **12 servings**

Cream Filling:

1 cup coconut cream or Kite Hill brand cream cheese style spread, softened

¼ cup Swerve confectioners'-style sweetener or equivalent amount of liquid or powdered sweetener (see page 29)

1 teaspoon vanilla extract

Pinch of fine sea salt

"Dirt":

1 batch Personal Flourless Chocolate Tortes (page 320), crumbled

"Worms":

1 batch Gummy Worms (page 328)

1. Place the ingredients for the cream filling in a small bowl. Mix until well combined.

2. To assemble the cake, place 2 tablespoons of "dirt" in a small serving cup. Top with 1 to 2 tablespoons of the cream filling, then another 2 tablespoons of "dirt." Garnish with gummy worms and serve.

3. Store in an airtight container in the refrigerator for up to 5 days.

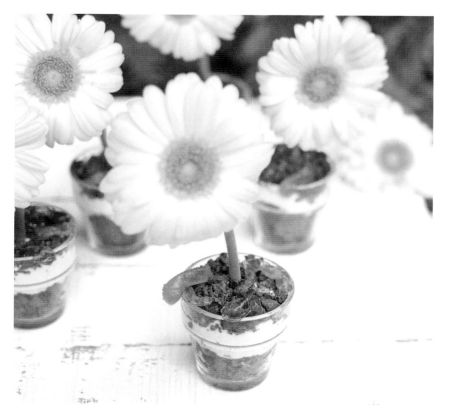

nutritional info (per serving)				
calories	fat	protein	carbs	fiber
327	32g	6g	5g	4g

GUMMY WORMS

One of my favorite products is Everly drink mix. The mix is sweetened with stevia and does not contain food dyes. If you do not have hibiscus tea, you can use 2 tablespoons of any flavor of Everly mixed into ½ cup of water. This will sweeten your gummy worms and give them a natural color.

prep time: **4 minutes, plus time to set** *yield:* **1 cup (¼ cup per serving)**

½ cup strong-brewed hibiscus tea, or 2 tablespoons Everly mixed into ½ cup water

¼ cup Swerve confectioners'-style sweetener or equivalent amount of liquid or powdered sweetener (see page 29) (omit if using Everly)

3 tablespoons unflavored gelatin

1 teaspoon citric acid (optional, for sourness)

Special Equipment:

3 (20-cavity) gummy worm molds

1. Place the tea and sweetener in a microwave-safe cup. Add the gelatin and stir until dissolved. Microwave on high for 40 seconds or until boiling.

2. Add the citric acid, if using, and stir well. Pour into the gummy worm molds. Place in the refrigerator until set, about 2 hours or overnight. The longer they sit, the more they will firm up.

3. Store in an airtight container in the refrigerator for up to 5 days.

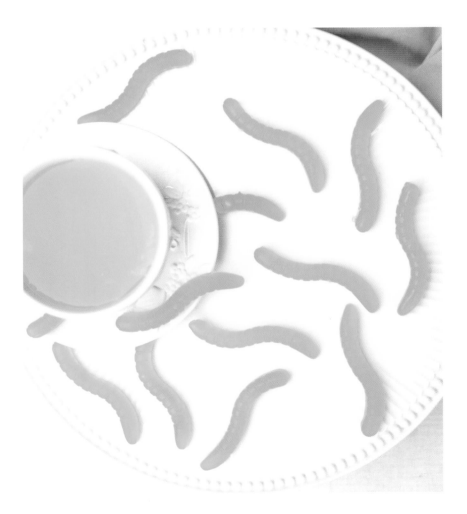

nutritional info (per serving)				
calories	fat	protein	carbs	fiber
19	0g	5g	0g	0g

MEXICAN CHOCOLATE MOUSSE

2 ounces unsweetened chocolate, finely chopped

¼ cup Swerve confectioners'-style sweetener or equivalent amount of liquid or powdered sweetener (see page 29)

1½ tablespoons unsweetened cocoa powder

1 teaspoon ground cinnamon

⅛ teaspoon fine sea salt

2 large eggs

½ cup unsweetened cashew milk or almond milk (or hemp milk for nut-free)

½ cup full-fat coconut milk

¼ cup butter-flavored coconut oil

Seeds scraped from 1 vanilla bean (about 8 inches long), or 1 teaspoon vanilla extract

Shaved unsweetened chocolate or homemade sweetened chocolate (use Chocolate Chunks, page 322), for garnish

1. Place the chocolate, sweetener, cocoa powder, cinnamon, and salt in a blender. Pulse for a few seconds or until the mixture is very fine. Add the eggs and pulse until well combined.

2. Place the cashew milk, coconut milk, and coconut oil in a saucepan and bring to a boil over medium-high heat. Remove from the heat and, with the blender running on low speed, slowly pour the hot milk mixture into the blender jar. Add the vanilla and puree until light and fluffy, about 1 minute. Taste and add more sweetener, if desired.

3. Pour the mixture into 4 decorative glasses, cover, and refrigerate until ready to serve. Serve chilled, and garnish with chocolate shavings just before serving.

4. Store in an airtight container in the refrigerator for up to 5 days.

Note: *A touch of cinnamon gives this mousse a Mexican flair!*

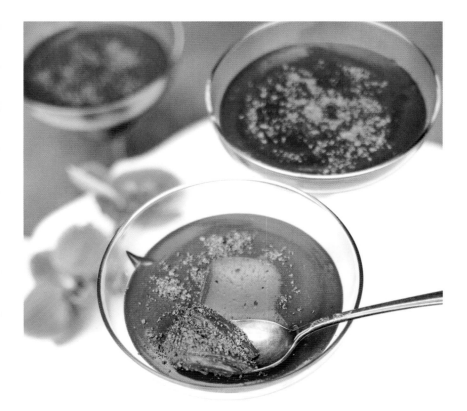

nutritional info (per serving)				
calories	fat	protein	carbs	fiber
304	29g	6g	6g	4g

BANANA BREAD

prep time: 5 minutes (not including time to cook eggs)
cook time: 20 minutes for mini loaves or 45 minutes for large loaf
yield: 8 mini loaves or 1 large loaf (12 servings)

8 large eggs

8 hard-boiled eggs (see page 81), peeled

½ cup Swerve confectioners'-style sweetener or equivalent amount of liquid or powdered sweetener (see page 29)

½ cup vanilla-flavored egg white or beef protein powder

3 tablespoons ground cinnamon

1½ teaspoons baking powder

½ teaspoon fine sea salt

½ cup coconut oil, melted

1 tablespoon plus 1 teaspoon banana extract

Cinnamon Glaze (optional):

¼ cup coconut oil, melted

2 tablespoons Swerve confectioners'-style sweetener or equivalent amount of liquid or powdered sweetener (see page 29)

1 teaspoon ground cinnamon

1. Preheat the oven to 325°F. Grease an 8-well mini loaf pan or an 8½ by 4½-inch loaf pan.

2. Place the raw eggs, hard-boiled eggs, sweetener, protein powder, cinnamon, baking powder, and salt in a blender or food processor and pulse until smooth and thick. Add the melted coconut oil and banana extract and pulse to combine well.

3. Pour into the greased mini loaf pan, filling each well about three-quarters full, or pour into the loaf pan.

4. Bake for 15 to 20 minutes for mini loaves or 40 to 45 minutes for a large loaf. A toothpick should come out clean when inserted into the center.

5. Meanwhile, make the glaze, if using: Place the ingredients for the glaze in a bowl and stir well. Taste and adjust the sweetness to your liking.

6. When the bread is done, remove it from the oven and allow to cool in the pan for 10 minutes. To serve, cut the large loaf into 12 slices or serve two-thirds of each mini loaf per person. Drizzle the bread with the glaze, if desired.

7. Store in an airtight container in the refrigerator for up to 5 days or in the freezer for up to a month.

nutritional info (per serving)				
calories	fat	protein	carbs	fiber
182	16g	11g	1g	0.3g

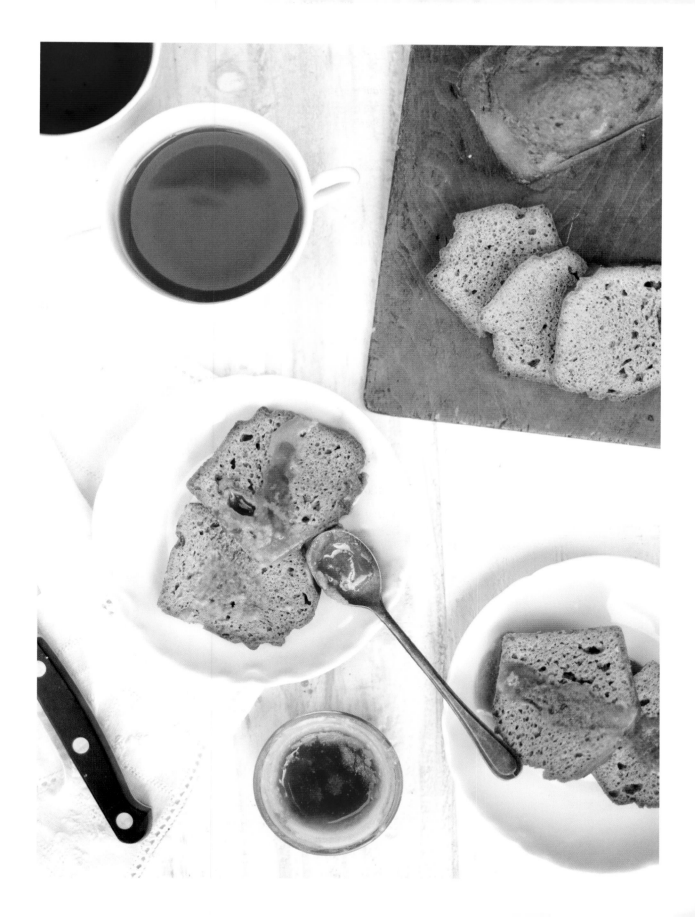

MALTED MILK PUSH POPS

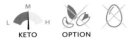

When I was a child, I adored malts. There was something special about that malt flavor. But to my dismay, malted milk powder is filled with gluten and sugar. I searched for a way to replicate that malt flavor for about seven years, and I finally found it—maca powder! It not only has great healing benefits, but it also adds that malt flavor I was looking for. Yahoo!

prep time: **6 minutes, plus time to set** *yield:* **8 pops (1 per serving)**

1 cup full-fat coconut milk

¼ cup Swerve confectioners'-style sweetener or equivalent amount of liquid or powdered sweetener (see page 29), or more to taste

2 tablespoons maca powder, or more to taste

Seeds scraped from 1 vanilla bean (about 8 inches long), or 1 teaspoon vanilla extract

1 cup unsweetened cashew milk (or hemp milk for nut-free)

Special Equipment:

8 push pop or ice pop molds

1. Place the coconut milk, sweetener, maca powder, and vanilla in a blender and pulse on high for about 1 minute to whip some air into the mixture.

2. Add the cashew milk and blend until well combined and pourable. Taste and adjust the sweetness and malt flavor to your liking.

3. Pour the mixture into the molds and place in the freezer until set, about 4 hours.

4. Store in an airtight container in the freezer for up to a month.

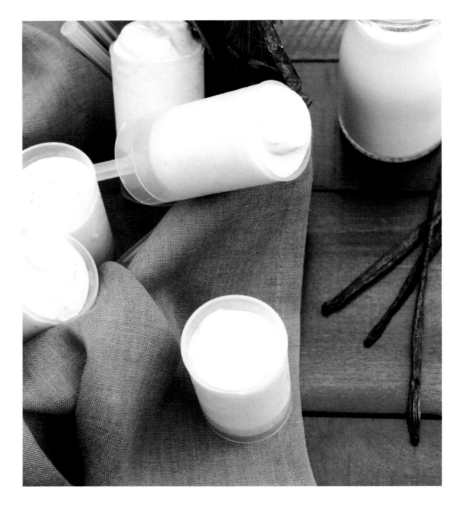

nutritional info (per serving)				
calories	fat	protein	carbs	fiber
228	23g	2g	7g	2g

CHOCOLATE PUDDING POPS

4 hard-boiled eggs (see page 81), peeled (see Note)

1 (13½-ounce) can full-fat coconut milk

½ cup Swerve confectioners'-style sweetener or equivalent amount of liquid or powdered sweetener (see page 29)

1 teaspoon stevia glycerite, or more to taste

¼ cup unsweetened cocoa powder, or more to taste

Seeds scraped from 2 vanilla beans (about 8 inches long), or 2 teaspoons vanilla extract

1 teaspoon ground cinnamon

⅛ teaspoon fine sea salt

Special Equipment:

12 ice pop molds

1. Place all of the ingredients in a blender and puree until very smooth. Taste and add up to an additional teaspoon of stevia glycerite and/or more cocoa powder, if desired.

2. Pour the mixture into the ice pop molds and place in the freezer until set, about 4 hours.

3. Store in an airtight container in the freezer for up to a month.

Note: *If you're making these pudding pops for a child under the age of one, use only the egg yolks.*

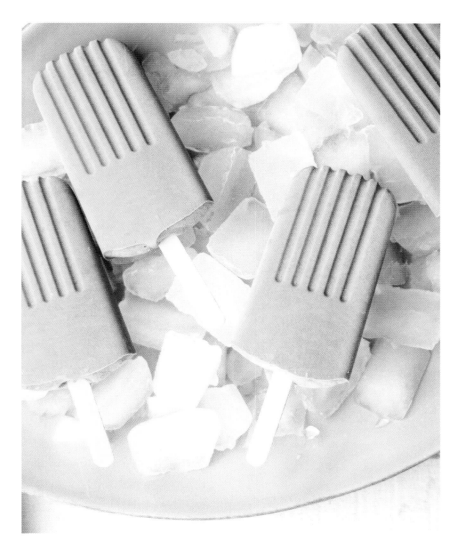

nutritional info (per serving)				
calories	fat	protein	carbs	fiber
76	7g	3g	1g	1g

HIBISCUS STRAWBERRY ICE LOLLIES

2 cups strong-brewed hibiscus tea, chilled

¼ cup Swerve confectioners'-style sweetener or equivalent amount of liquid or powdered sweetener (see page 29)

2 teaspoons strawberry extract

⅛ teaspoon fine sea salt

Special Equipment:

8 ice pop molds

1. Place all of the ingredients in a blender and blend until smooth. Pour into the ice pop molds and place in the freezer until set, at least 2 hours.

2. Store in an airtight container in the freezer for up to a month.

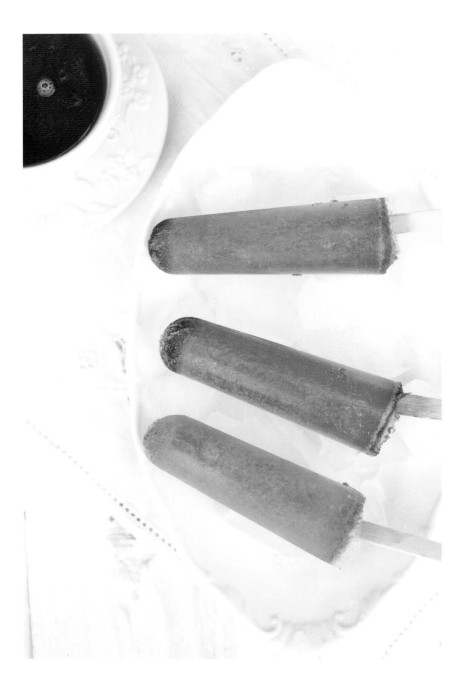

nutritional info (per serving)				
calories	fat	protein	carbs	fiber
0	0g	0g	0g	0g

TAPIOCA PUDDING

prep time: **2 minutes**   cook time: **5 minutes**   yield: **1 serving**

2 large eggs

⅓ cup full-fat coconut milk

2 tablespoons Swerve confectioners'-style sweetener or equivalent amount of liquid or powdered sweetener (see page 29)

1 teaspoon vanilla extract

¼ teaspoon fine sea salt

2 tablespoons coconut oil

Ground cinnamon, for garnish

1. In a small bowl, whisk together the eggs, coconut milk, sweetener, vanilla extract, and salt.

2. Melt the coconut oil in a medium-sized saucepan over medium heat. Add the egg mixture and cook, scraping the bottom of the pan with a whisk, until the mixture thickens and starts to curdle, about 4 minutes. Use the whisk to separate the curds.

3. Remove from the heat and transfer to a serving bowl. Sprinkle with cinnamon and allow the flavors to meld for 2 minutes before serving.

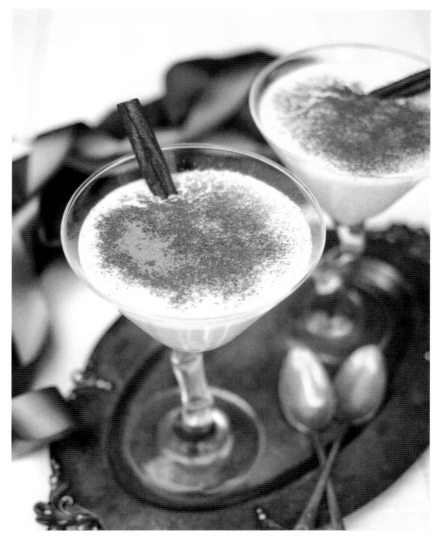

nutritional info (per serving)				
calories	fat	protein	carbs	fiber
395	36g	14g	2g	0g

KETO PINK SQUIRRELS

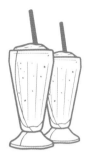

When I was a little girl, my parents would take my brother and me to eat at the local fish and steak restaurant called the High View every Friday night. It was perfectly situated on a small lake, where my brother and I would fish until our dinner was ready. Now, as a parent myself, I realize how awesome it must have been for my parents to have the opportunity to talk on their own while the restaurant cooks prepared our meal.

We always concluded our meal with nonalcoholic Pink Squirrels, a tasty after-dinner ice cream drink with almond and chocolate undertones. If you have never had one, you must try this recipe! Traditionally, the pink color comes from crème de Noyaux (which also provides the almond flavor) and the chocolate flavor comes from white crème de cacao, but since I don't recommend consuming alcohol, I switched it up a little to make it almond and cherry flavored. As a kid, I always associated the drink's pretty pink color with cherry. Sometimes the memory of something creates something even better than the original!

The first step in making a Pink Squirrel is to make the almond- and cherry-flavored ice cream as the base. The MCT oil is needed to create a smooth ice cream. And don't skip the salt. It does more than add flavor; it also helps keep the ice cream soft.

prep. time: 10 minutes, plus time to churn ice cream
yield: 3 cups ice cream (½ cup per serving), or 6 drinks

Pink Squirrel Ice Cream:

(makes enough for 6 drinks)

¾ cup plus 2 tablespoons coconut oil (preferably butter-flavored)

½ cup unsweetened almond milk

¼ cup Swerve confectioners'-style sweetener or equivalent amount of liquid or powdered sweetener (see page 29)

4 large eggs

4 large egg yolks

¼ cup MCT oil

¼ teaspoon almond extract

¼ teaspoon cherry extract

¼ teaspoon fine sea salt

Pink Squirrels:

(makes 1 drink)

½ cup Pink Squirrel Ice Cream

¼ cup unsweetened almond milk, chilled

¼ teaspoon almond extract

¼ teaspoon cherry extract

Special Equipment:

Ice cream maker

1. Place the ice cream ingredients in a blender and puree until smooth. Pour into an ice cream maker and churn, following the manufacturer's instructions, until set. Use immediately to make Pink Squirrels or enjoy as is. The ice cream can be stored in an airtight container in the freezer for up to a month.

2. To make a Pink Squirrel, place the drink ingredients in a blender and blend until smooth.

nutritional info (per serving for ice cream)				
calories	fat	protein	carbs	fiber
242	26g	3g	0.4g	0g

nutritional info (per serving for drink)				
calories	fat	protein	carbs	fiber
502	57g	6g	0.8g	0g

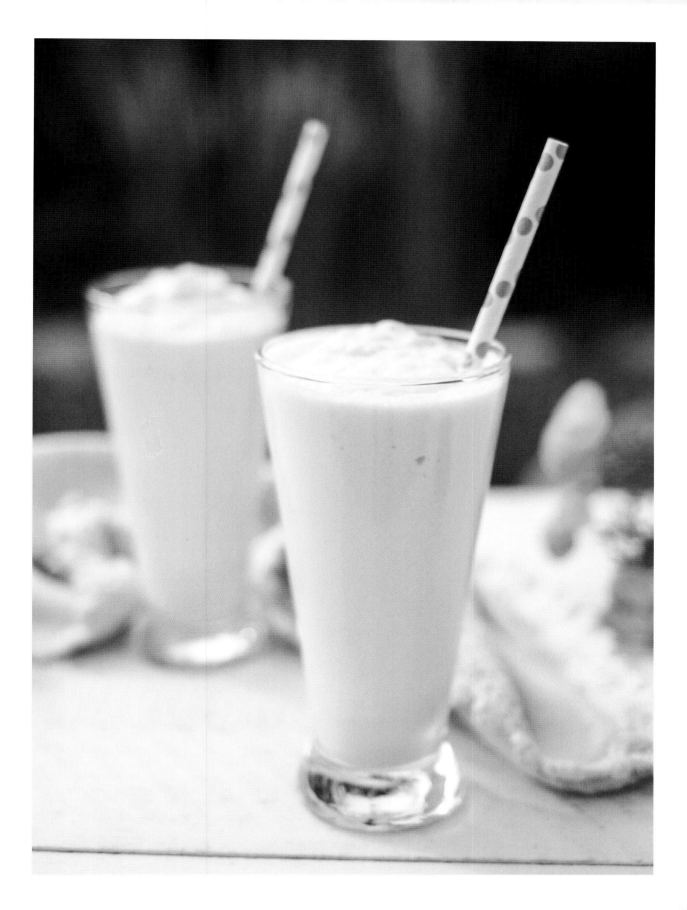

STRAWBERRY HIBISCUS SORBET

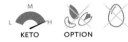

prep time: 5 minutes, plus time to churn   *yield:* 3 cups (¾ cup per serving)

1 cup unsweetened almond milk (or hemp milk if nut-free)

1 cup strong-brewed hibiscus tea, chilled

1 teaspoon strawberry extract, or more to taste

3 tablespoons Swerve confectioners'-style sweetener or equivalent amount of liquid or powdered sweetener (see page 29), or more to taste

¼ teaspoon fine sea salt

Special Equipment:

Ice cream maker

1. Place all of the ingredients in a blender and blend until smooth. Taste and add more strawberry extract and/or sweetener, if desired.

2. Pour into an ice cream maker and churn according to the manufacturer's instructions.

3. Store in an airtight container in the freezer for up to a month.

Note: *To change things up, you can use different flavors of fruit extract. Banana extract is nice, for example.*

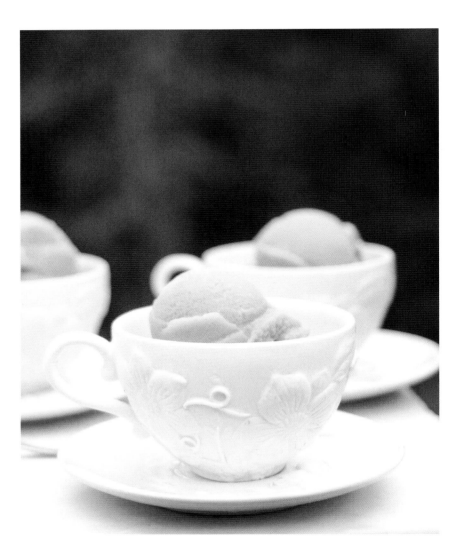

nutritional info (per serving)				
calories	fat	protein	carbs	fiber
103	10g	2g	1g	0g

KETO CUSTARD

KETO   OPTION

prep time: **5 minutes**   *cook time:* **10 minutes**   *yield:* **4 servings**

4 large eggs

2 cups unsweetened cashew milk or almond milk (or hemp milk if nut-free)

½ cup Swerve confectioners'-style sweetener or equivalent amount of liquid or powdered sweetener (see page 29), or more to taste

1 teaspoon vanilla extract

½ teaspoon ground nutmeg

⅛ teaspoon fine sea salt

1. Preheat the oven to 325°F.

2. Place all of the ingredients in a medium-sized bowl and whisk until smooth. Taste and adjust the sweetness to your liking. Pour into four 4-ounce ramekins and bake for 8 to 10 minutes, until the custard is set. Enjoy warm or chill before serving.

3. Store in an airtight container in the refrigerator for up to 4 days.

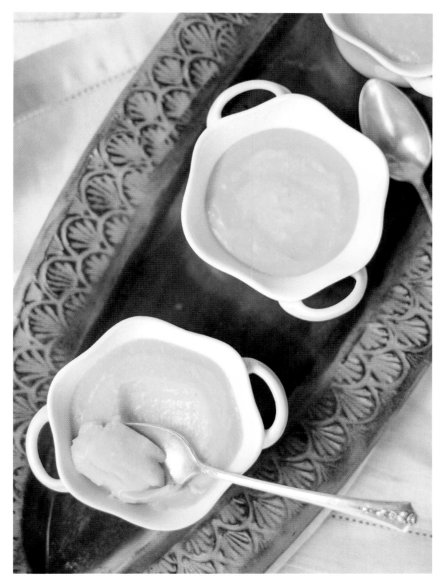

nutritional info (per serving)				
calories	fat	protein	carbs	fiber
93	6g	7g	1g	0.1g

STRAWBERRIES AND CREAM PANNA COTTA

prep time: **6 minutes, plus time to set**   *cook time:* **3 minutes**
yield: **6 servings**

1 (13½-ounce) can full-fat coconut milk

1 cup strong-brewed hibiscus tea

⅓ cup Swerve confectioners'-style sweetener or equivalent amount of liquid or powdered sweetener (see page 29)

⅛ teaspoon fine sea salt

2 teaspoons strawberry extract (see Notes)

1 tablespoon unflavored gelatin (see Notes)

Fresh mint leaves, for garnish (optional)

1. In a small saucepan, warm the coconut milk and tea over medium heat. Add the sweetener, salt, and extract and stir to combine. Simmer for 3 minutes, stirring often, then remove from the heat.

2. Place the gelatin in a small bowl and add 2 tablespoons of water; stir and allow the gelatin to soften for a minute. Pour the gelatin into the coconut milk mixture and stir well.

3. Pour the panna cotta mixture into six 4-ounce ramekins and refrigerate until set. Serve garnished with mint leaves, if desired.

4. Store in an airtight container in the refrigerator for up to 5 days.

Notes: *If you don't have strawberry extract on hand, you can substitute the same amount of vanilla extract to make a vanilla-flavored panna cotta.*

Food made with gelatin can easily become rubbery if it sits in the refrigerator overnight. If you plan on making the panna cotta ahead of time and not serving it the same day it is made, I suggest using ¼ teaspoon less gelatin than called for. This will create the perfect creamy texture after a day of resting in the fridge.

nutritional info (per serving)				
calories	fat	protein	carbs	fiber
103	10g	2g	1g	0g

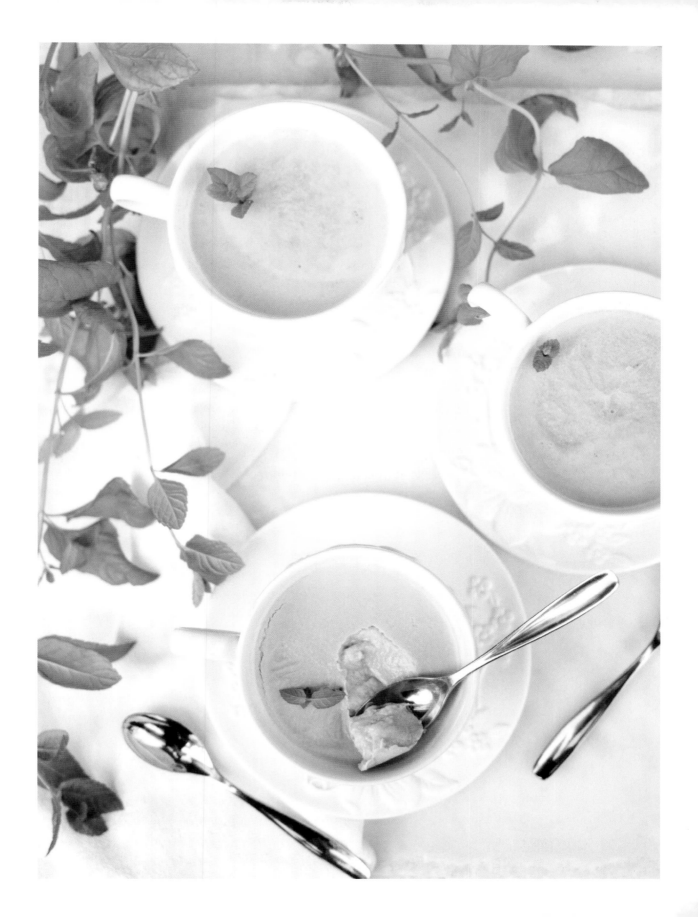

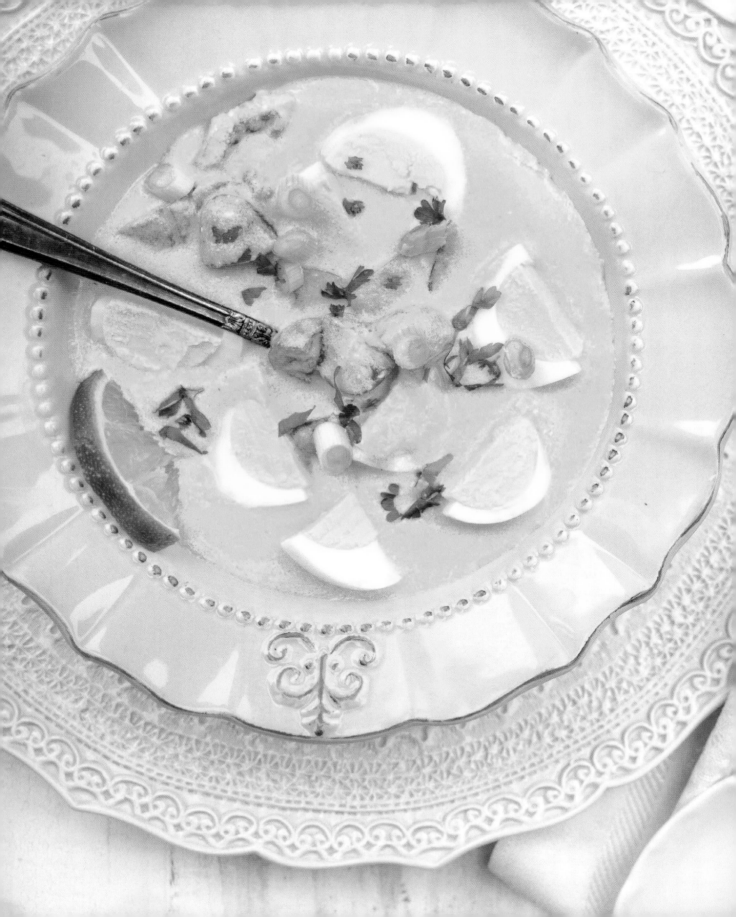

Chapter 12:
Meal Plans

Note: These meal plans are designed to serve one person, but in most cases the recipes make plenty of food for two or more. The yield for each recipe is listed in parentheses in the meal plans; you can double or triple a recipe if needed to feed a larger group.

28-Day Basic Meal Plan

	BREAKFAST	DINNER	SIDE DISH	NUTRITION INFO (per serving)	
DAY 1	Cherry Almond Breakfast Shake (2) — 54	T-Bone Steaks with Romanesco Sauce (4) — 206	Manhattan Clam Chowder (4) — 120	calories (kcal)	1100
				fat	75 g
				carbohydrate	22 g
				protein	85 g
DAY 2	Snickerdoodle Mini Muffins (6) — 72	Chicken Shawarma (4) — 158	Dry-Rubbed Baked Wings (8) — 94	calories (kcal)	1097
				fat	89 g
				carbohydrate	7 g
				protein	71 g
DAY 3	Lemon Poppyseed Waffles (4) — 67	T-Bone Steaks with Romanesco Sauce — LEFTOVER	Manhattan Clam Chowder — LEFTOVER	calories (kcal)	1165
				fat	81 g
				carbohydrate	17 g
				protein	91 g
DAY 4	Loaded Scrambled Eggs (2) — 64	Chicken Shawarma — LEFTOVER	Dry-Rubbed Baked Wings — LEFTOVER	calories (kcal)	1030
				fat	77 g
				carbohydrate	7 g
				protein	79 g
DAY 5	Snickerdoodle Mini Muffins — LEFTOVER	Pan-Fried Fish with Tartar Sauce (4) — 266	Dry-Rubbed Baked Wings — LEFTOVER	calories (kcal)	1141
				fat	94 g
				carbohydrate	2 g
				protein	72 g
DAY 6	Lemon Poppyseed Waffles — LEFTOVER	Hawaiian Luau Pork (4) — 254	Dry-Rubbed Baked Wings — LEFTOVER	calories (kcal)	1226
				fat	95 g
				carbohydrate	8 g
				protein	87 g
DAY 7	Spicy Fried Eggs with Chorizo (2) — 66	Pan-Fried Fish with Tartar Sauce — LEFTOVER	Steak Fajita Soup (4) — 121	calories (kcal)	1267
				fat	94 g
				carbohydrate	15 g
				protein	85 g

Week 1 Grocery List

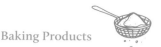

Baking Products
Baking powder, 1¾ teaspoons

Broth
Beef bone broth, 6 cups
Chicken bone broth, 4½ cups

Canned and Jarred Pantry Items
Baby clams, 2 (10-ounce) cans
Dill pickles, ¼ cup
Greek olives, 1 handful
Roasted red peppers, 1 (12-ounce) jar

Condiments and Sauces
Almond butter, ¼ cup
Clam juice, 1 (8-ounce) bottle
Dill pickle juice, ¼ cup
Lemon juice, 2 tablespoons
Liquid smoke, 1½ tablespoons
Mayonnaise, 1 cup
Sugar-free salsa, 1 cup
Tomato paste, 2 tablespoons
Wheat-free tamari, 1 tablespoon

Dairy-Free Subs
Kite Hill brand cream cheese style spread, ½ cup

Dried Herbs, Spices, and Extracts
Almond extract, ½ teaspoon
Bay leaves, 2
Cherry extract, 1 teaspoon
Chili powder, 1 tablespoon
Crushed red pepper, ⅛ teaspoon
Fine sea salt, ¼ cup
Garlic powder, ½ teaspoon

Ground black pepper, 1 tablespoon + 1 teaspoon
Ground cinnamon, 2 tablespoons + 1¼ teaspoons
Ground cumin, 2 teaspoons
Italian seasoning, 1 tablespoon
Lemon extract, 2 teaspoons
Onion powder, ½ teaspoon
Paprika, 1 tablespoon + ½ teaspoon
Poppy seeds, 2 tablespoons
Thyme leaves, ½ teaspoon
Turmeric powder, ½ teaspoon
Vanilla extract, 1 tablespoon + 1 teaspoon

Eggs
Eggs, 16 large
Hard-boiled eggs, 8

Fats and Oils
Avocado oil, ¼ cup
Butter-flavored coconut oil, 1 tablespoon
Coconut oil, 1¼ cups + 2 tablespoons

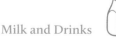

Fresh Herbs
Basil, 2 tablespoons chopped
Cilantro, for garnish
Flat-leaf parsley, for garnish

Milk and Drinks
Cherry tea, 1 cup brewed
Unsweetened cashew milk, 1 cup

Other Recipes
Greek Vinaigrette (page 46)
Keto Tortillas (page 150), 1 batch
Lemon Syrup (page 67), ¼ cup

Produce
Celery, 1 stalk
Garlic, 10 cloves
Grape tomatoes, 1 handful
Green bell peppers, 2
Jalapeño peppers, 2
Lemons, 3
Limes, 4
Mushrooms, ¼ cup sliced
Onions, 1 cup diced
Red bell peppers, ½ cup diced
Red onions, ¼ cup sliced
Scallions, for garnish
Tomato, 1 large
Zucchini, 1 small

Protein Powder
Vanilla-flavored egg white or beef protein powder, ¼ cup + 2 tablespoons

Proteins
Bacon, 4 strips
Boneless beef roast, 1 pound
Boneless pork shoulder, 2 pounds
Boneless, skinless chicken thighs, 1 pound
Chicken wings or drumettes, 30
Halibut, 4 (5-ounce) skin-on fillets
Ham, ¼ cup diced
Mexican-style fresh (raw) chorizo, 4 ounces
T-bone steaks, 2 (1 pound each)

Sweeteners
Swerve confectioners, 1¾ cups

28-Day Basic Meal Plan

	BREAKFAST	DINNER	SIDE DISH	NUTRITION INFO (per serving)	
DAY 8	Irish Breakfast (4) — 74	Easy BBQ Brisket (8) — 208	French Onion Meatball Soup (8) — 126	calories (kcal)	1233
				fat	97 g
				carbohydrate	11 g
				protein	77 g
DAY 9	Soft-Boiled Eggs with Bacon-Wrapped Asparagus Dunkers (2) — 76	Grilled Jerk Chicken Thighs (6) — 168	Slow Cooker Thai Soup (4) — 129	calories (kcal)	1105
				fat	76 g
				carbohydrate	16 g
				protein	86 g
DAY 10	Irish Breakfast — LEFTOVER	Easy BBQ Brisket — LEFTOVER	French Onion Meatball Soup — LEFTOVER	calories (kcal)	1233
				fat	97 g
				carbohydrate	11 g
				protein	77 g
DAY 11	Reuben Eggs Benedict (2) — 78	Grilled Jerk Chicken Thighs — LEFTOVER	Crab Louie Salad (4) — 140	calories (kcal)	1356
				fat	98 g
				carbohydrate	15 g
				protein	100 g
DAY 12	French Toast Pudding (4) — 80	Grilled Jerk Chicken Thighs — LEFTOVER	Slow Cooker Thai Soup — LEFTOVER	calories (kcal)	1174
				fat	85 g
				carbohydrate	17 g
				protein	86 g
DAY 13	Super Keto Pancakes (2) — 79	Easy BBQ Brisket — LEFTOVER	French Onion Meatball Soup — LEFTOVER	calories (kcal)	1114
				fat	85 g
				carbohydrate	12 g
				protein	73 g
DAY 14	French Toast Pudding — LEFTOVER	Halibut Smothered in Tomato Basil Cream (4) — 267	Crab Louie Salad — LEFTOVER	calories (kcal)	935
				fat	69 g
				carbohydrate	14 g
				protein	62 g

Week 2 Grocery List

Baking Products
Baking powder, ¼ teaspoon

Broth
Beef bone broth, 5½ cups +
  2 tablespoons
Chicken bone broth, 3 cups
Fish bone broth, ¼ cup

Canned and Jarred Pantry Items
Black olives, ½ cup sliced
Canned crabmeat, 8 ounces
Dill pickles, 1 tablespoon chopped

Condiments and Sauces
Coconut vinegar, ½ cup
Fermented sauerkraut, ¼ cup
Lime juice, 3 tablespoons
Liquid smoke, 2 teaspoons
Mayonnaise, 3 tablespoons
Red curry paste, 2 tablespoons
Tomato sauce, 2¼ cups +
  1 tablespoon
Wheat-free tamari, ¾ cup

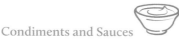

Dried Herbs, Spices, and Extracts
Dry mustard, 1 tablespoon
Fine sea salt, 3 tablespoons
Garlic powder, 1 tablespoon
Ground allspice, ½ teaspoon
Ground black pepper, 1 tablespoon
  + ¼ teaspoon
Ground cinnamon, 1 tablespoon
Ground cloves, ½ teaspoon
Ground nutmeg, ½ teaspoon

Ground thyme, garnish
Lemongrass, 1 teaspoon
Maple extract, 2½ teaspoons
Onion powder, 1 tablespoon
Thyme leaves, 2 teaspoons
Vanilla extract, 1 teaspoon

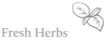

Eggs
Eggs, 12 large
Hard-boiled eggs, 16

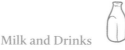

Fats and Oils
Avocado oil, ½ cup
Bacon fat, 2 teaspoons (or more
  coconut oil)
Coconut oil, 1½ teaspoons
Lard, ¼ cup

Fresh Herbs
Basil leaves, 1 tablespoon chopped
Cilantro, ⅓ cup chopped
Thyme, 1 tablespoon chopped +
  garnish

Milk and Drinks
Coconut milk, 2 (13½-ounce) cans
  + ¼ cup

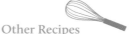

Other Recipes
Cinnamon Syrup (page 47), ¼ cup
Crab Louie Dressing (page 44),
  ¾ cup
Keto Brioche (page 144), 2

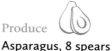

Produce
Asparagus, 8 spears
Button mushrooms, 1 cup sliced
Cherry tomatoes, for garnish
Garlic, 2 cloves
Ginger root, 1 tablespoon grated
Jalapeño pepper, 1
Mushrooms, 4 cups sliced
Onions, 3 medium
Red bell peppers, ½ cup sliced
Red onions, ¼ cup diced
Romaine lettuce, 1 head
Scallions, 10
Tomatoes, 2

Proteins
Bacon, 12 strips
Bone-in, skin-on chicken thighs,
  1½ pounds
Boneless, skinless chicken thighs,
  1½ pounds
Breakfast sausage, 4 links
Brisket, 4 pounds
Corned beef, 8 slices
Ground beef, 2 pounds
Halibut, 4 (4-ounce) skinless
  fillets

Sweeteners
Stevia glycerite, 2 teaspoons
Swerve confectioners, 1¼ cups

	BREAKFAST	DINNER	SIDE DISH	NUTRITION INFO (per serving)	
DAY 15	Silky Egg Breakfast Soup (2) — 70	Crab Claws with Spicy Mustard Sauce (4) — 270	Chef's Salad (4) — 142	calories (kcal)	1392
				fat	99 g
				carbohydrate	11 g
				protein	109 g
DAY 16	Loaded Scrambled Eggs (2) — 64	Cilantro Lime Slow Cooker Ribs (8) — 256	Salad Kabobs (4) — 141	calories (kcal)	1465
				fat	119 g
				carbohydrate	9 g
				protein	87 g
DAY 17	Cherry Almond Breakfast Shake (2) — 54	Crab Claws with Spicy Mustard Sauce — LEFTOVER	Salad Kabobs — LEFTOVER	calories (kcal)	1262
				fat	102 g
				carbohydrate	13 g
				protein	76 g
DAY 18	Baked Eggs and Ham (2) — 57	Cilantro Lime Slow Cooker Ribs — LEFTOVER	Chef's Salad — LEFTOVER	calories (kcal)	1281
				fat	103 g
				carbohydrate	8 g
				protein	75 g
DAY 19	Breakfast Asparagus (2) — 65	Cilantro Lime Slow Cooker Ribs — LEFTOVER	Chicken and "Rice" Soup (8) — 130	calories (kcal)	1181
				fat	91 g
				carbohydrate	11 g
				protein	76 g
DAY 20	Silky Egg Breakfast Soup (2) — 70	Salmon Burgers with Dill Sauce (6) — 268	Grilled Avocado (4) — 143	calories (kcal)	1147
				fat	83 g
				carbohydrate	18 g
				protein	85 g
DAY 21	Reuben Eggs Benedict (2) — 78	Salmon Burgers with Dill Sauce — LEFTOVER	Chicken and "Rice" Soup — LEFTOVER	calories (kcal)	1212
				fat	92 g
				carbohydrate	10 g
				protein	88 g

Week 3 Grocery List

Broth
Chicken bone broth, 14 cups

Canned and Jarred Pantry Items
Black olives, 1 cup pitted
Dill pickles, 3 spears
Fermented sauerkraut, ¼ cup
Pink salmon, 1 (14-ounce) can
Roasted red peppers, ¼ cup

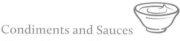

Condiments and Sauces
Almond butter, ¼ cup
Dijon mustard, ¼ cup
Fish sauce, ¼ cup + 1 tablespoon
Hot sauce, 2 or 3 drops
Lemon juice, 2 tablespoons +
   1 teaspoon
Lime juice, ¾ cup + 2 teaspoons
Mayonnaise, 3 tablespoons
Prepared horseradish,
   2 tablespoons
Ranch dressing, ½ cup
Tomato sauce, ½ cup +
   1 tablespoon

Dried Herbs, Spices, and Extracts
Almond extract, ½ teaspoon
Bay leaf, 1
Cherry extract, 1 teaspoon
Fine sea salt, 1½ teaspoons
Ground black pepper, 1 teaspoon

Eggs
Eggs, 31 large
Hard-boiled eggs, 12

Fats and Oils
Butter-flavored coconut oil,
   1 tablespoon
Coconut oil, 1½ tablespoons
Lard, 2 tablespoons
MCT oil, 1 tablespoon

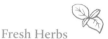

Fresh Herbs
Chives, 3 tablespoons chopped
Cilantro, ¼ cup chopped
Dill, 2 tablespoons chopped
Flat-leaf parsley, for garnish
Ginger root, 2 tablespoons grated
Thyme, 2 sprigs

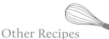

Milk and Drinks
Cherry tea, 1 cup brewed
Unsweetened cashew milk, 1 cup

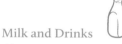

Other Recipes
Baconnaise (page 34), 3¼ cups +
   2 tablespoons
Keto Brioche (page 144), 1

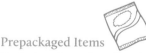

Prepackaged Items
Pork dust (powdered pork rinds),
   ⅓ cup

Produce
Asparagus, 6 spears
Avocados, 4
Celery, 1 cup diced
Cherry tomatoes, 1 cup
Chives, 2½ tablespoons chopped
Garlic, 2 cloves
Iceberg lettuce, ½ head
Jalapeño pepper, 1
Limes, 3
Mushrooms, ¼ cup sliced
Onion, 1 medium
Red bell peppers, ¼ cup diced
Red onion, ½
Romaine lettuce, 1 head + 6 leaves
Scallions, 2

Proteins
Alaskan king or snow crab claws,
   24 medium
Bacon, 2 strips
Boneless, skinless chicken breast
   halves, 4 (about 2 pounds)
Boneless, skinless chicken thighs, 4
Corned beef, 8 slices
Ham, 1 pound + ¼ cup chopped
Ham, deli-style, 4 slices
Pork ribs, 4 pounds
Roast beef, thinly sliced, ½ pound
Smoked salmon, 2 ounces

Sweeteners
Swerve confectioners, ¼ cup +
   2 tablespoons

28-Day Basic Meal Plan

	BREAKFAST	DINNER	SIDE DISH	NUTRITION INFO (per serving)	
DAY 22	Breakfast Sausage Soup with Soft-Boiled Eggs (6) — 68	Simple Spaghetti (8) — 213	Slow Cooker Thai Soup (4) — 129	calories (kcal)	1192
				fat	88 g
				carbohydrate	20 g
				protein	78 g
DAY 23	Deviled Green Eggs and Ham (6) — 96	Saucy BBQ Wraps (4) — 214	Coconut Ginger Chicken Soup (8) — 110	calories (kcal)	1252
				fat	88 g
				carbohydrate	16 g
				protein	94 g
DAY 24	Breakfast Sausage Soup with Soft-Boiled Eggs — LEFTOVER	Simple Spaghetti — LEFTOVER	Slow Cooker Thai Soup — LEFTOVER	calories (kcal)	1192
				fat	88 g
				carbohydrate	20 g
				protein	78 g
DAY 25	Breakfast Sausage Soup with Soft-Boiled Eggs — LEFTOVER	Simple Spaghetti — LEFTOVER	Coconut Ginger Chicken Soup — LEFTOVER	calories (kcal)	1167
				fat	83 g
				carbohydrate	20 g
				protein	80 g
DAY 26	Deviled Green Eggs and Ham — LEFTOVER	Saucy BBQ Wraps — LEFTOVER	Coconut Ginger Chicken Soup — LEFTOVER	calories (kcal)	1252
				fat	88 g
				carbohydrate	16 g
				protein	94 g
DAY 27	Reuben Eggs Benedict (2) — 78	Hungarian Goulash (4) — 216	Cute Kitty Deviled Eggs (12) — 98	calories (kcal)	1131
				fat	83 g
				carbohydrate	19 g
				protein	77 g
DAY 28	Deviled Green Eggs and Ham — LEFTOVER	Hungarian Goulash — LEFTOVER	Cute Kitty Deviled Eggs — LEFTOVER	calories (kcal)	1074
				fat	81 g
				carbohydrate	19 g
				protein	66 g

Week 4 Grocery List

Broth

Beef bone broth, 1½ cups
Chicken bone broth, 6 cups

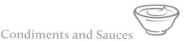

Canned and Jarred Pantry Items

Baby dill pickles, ½ cup
Capers, 24
Crushed tomatoes, 2 cups
Dill pickles, 1 tablespoon chopped
Fermented sauerkraut, ¼ cup

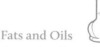

Condiments and Sauces

Coconut vinegar, 1 teaspoon
Distilled white vinegar,
    1 teaspoon
Fish sauce, 3 tablespoons
Lime juice, 3 tablespoons
Liquid smoke, 2 teaspoons
Mayonnaise, 1¼ cups +
    3 tablespoons
Prepared yellow mustard, ¼ cup
    + 1 teaspoon
Red curry paste, 2 tablespoons
Tomato paste, 1 (7-ounce) jar
Tomato sauce, 3½ cups +
    1 tablespoon

Dried Herbs, Spices, and Extracts

Black peppercorns, 48
Chives, for garnish
Fine sea salt, 2½ tablespoons
Garlic powder, 2 teaspoons
Ground black pepper, 2 teaspoons
Ground white pepper, 1 teaspoon
Italian seasoning, 2 tablespoons
Lemongrass, 1 teaspoon
Onion powder, 2 teaspoons
Smoked paprika, ¼ cup +
    2 tablespoons

Eggs

Eggs, 12 large
Hard-boiled eggs, 24

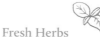

Fats and Oils

Avocado oil, 2 tablespoons
Coconut oil, 1½ teaspoons

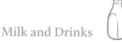

Fresh Herbs

Chives, 1 bunch
Cilantro, ⅓ cup chopped
Ginger root, ¼ cup + 1 tablespoon
    grated
Lemongrass, 4 stalks
Rosemary, 2 sprigs
Sage, 1 teaspoon minced
Thyme, 4 sprigs + garnish

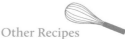

Milk and Drinks

Coconut milk, 1 (13½-ounce) can
    + 4 cups

Other Recipes

Keto Brioche (page 144), 1
Simple BBQ Sauce (page 43),
    ¼ cup

Produce

Avocado, ½ small
Boston lettuce, 1 head
Cauliflower, 4 cups florets
Garlic, 2 large + 5 medium cloves
Limes, 3
Mushrooms, 6 cups sliced
Onions, 1½ cups diced
Red bell peppers, ½ cup sliced
Red onions, ⅓ cup sliced
Scallions, 4
Serrano chile peppers, 5
Shallots, 5
Zucchini, 2 medium

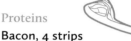

Proteins

Bacon, 4 strips
Boneless, skinless chicken breast
    halves, 4 (about 2 pounds)
Boneless, skinless chicken thighs,
    1½ pounds
Bulk breakfast sausage, 1 pound
Cold-smoked salmon, 2 ounces
Corned beef, 8 slices
Ground beef, 4 pounds
Ham, deli-style, 24 very thin
    slices

Sweeteners

Swerve confectioners,
    2 tablespoons

28-Day Egg-Free Meal Plan

	BREAKFAST	DINNER	SIDE DISH	NUTRITION INFO (per serving)	
DAY 1	Cherry Almond Breakfast Shake (2) 54	30-Minute Porchetta (4) 249	Slow Cooker Thai Soup (4) 129	calories (kcal)	1010
				fat	74 g
				carbohydrate	15 g
				protein	76 g
DAY 2	French Toast Cereal (1) 58	Ginger Lime Pork Lettuce Cups (4) 240	Steak Fajita Soup (4) 121	calories (kcal)	1265
				fat	101 g
				carbohydrate	21 g
				protein	75 g
DAY 3	Texas BBQ Brisket Soup (8) 114	Tender Coconut Chicken (4) 174	Salmon Soup (4) 133	calories (kcal)	1424
				fat	103 g
				carbohydrate	21 g
				protein	99 g
DAY 4	Cherry Almond Breakfast Shake (2) 54	30-Minute Porchetta LEFTOVER	Slow Cooker Thai Soup LEFTOVER	calories (kcal)	1010
				fat	74 g
				carbohydrate	15 g
				protein	76 g
DAY 5	Texas BBQ Brisket Soup LEFTOVER	Ginger Lime Pork Lettuce Cups LEFTOVER	Steak Fajita Soup LEFTOVER	calories (kcal)	1238
				fat	89 g
				carbohydrate	28 g
				protein	83 g
DAY 6	Texas BBQ Brisket Soup LEFTOVER	Tender Coconut Chicken LEFTOVER	Salmon Soup LEFTOVER	calories (kcal)	1424
				fat	103 g
				carbohydrate	21 g
				protein	99 g
DAY 7	French Toast Cereal (1) 58	Easy Pickled Shrimp with Curry Mayo (4) 271	Steak Fajita Soup LEFTOVER	calories (kcal)	1310
				fat	105 g
				carbohydrate	13 g
				protein	80 g

Week 1 Grocery List

Broth

Beef bone broth, 12 cups
Chicken bone broth, 3¼ cups
Fish bone broth, 4 cups

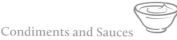

Condiments and Sauces

Almond butter, ½ cup
Asian chile sauce, 1 teaspoon
Coconut vinegar, ⅓ cup +
    1 tablespoon
Dijon mustard, 1 teaspoon
Fish sauce, 3½ tablespoons
Lime juice, ¾ cup +
    1½ tablespoons
Liquid smoke, 1 teaspoon
Mayonnaise, ⅔ cup
Red curry paste, 2 tablespoons
Sugar-free salsa, 1 cup
Tomato sauce, ¾ cup
Wheat-free tamari, ¾ teaspoon

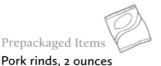

Dried Herbs, Spices, and Extracts

Almond extract, 1 teaspoon
Cherry extract, 2 teaspoons
Chili powder, 2 tablespoons
Curry powder, ½ teaspoon
Fine sea salt, 2 tablespoons +
    1 teaspoon
Ground black pepper, 2 teaspoons
Ground cinnamon, 2 teaspoons
Ground cumin, 1 teaspoon
Lemongrass, 1 teaspoon
Maple extract, 1 teaspoon
Paprika, 1 teaspoon
Smoked paprika, 3 tablespoons
Turmeric powder, ¼ teaspoon

Fats and Oils

Avocado oil, 3½ tablespoons
Coconut oil, ¾ cup
MCT oil, ⅓ cup
Toasted (dark) sesame oil,
    2 teaspoons

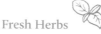

Fresh Herbs

Basil, ½ bunch
Cilantro, 3 bunches
Dill, 3 tablespoons chopped
Ginger root, ¼ cup grated
Mint, ½ bunch
Rosemary, 1½ tablespoons finely
    chopped

Milk and Drinks

Cherry tea, 2 cups brewed
Coconut milk, 1 (13½-ounce) can
    + 1 cup
Unsweetened cashew milk, 4 cups

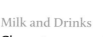

Prepackaged Items

Pork rinds, 2 ounces

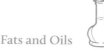

Produce

Butter lettuce, 1 head
Fennel bulb, 1 tablespoon finely
    diced
Garlic, 22 cloves
Green bell peppers, 2
Jalapeño peppers, 3
Limes, 4
Mushrooms, 4 cups sliced
Onions, 2½ cups diced
Red bell peppers, ½ cup sliced
Red onions, ¼ cup thinly sliced
Scallions, 4
Tomatoes, 1 large + 3 medium
Yellow onions, 1½ cups
Zucchini, 1 medium

Proteins

Bacon, 6 thin-cut strips
Bone-in, skin-on chicken thighs, 8
Boneless beef roast, 1 pound
Boneless, skinless chicken thighs,
    1½ pounds
Brisket, 1½ pounds
Ground pork, 1 pound
Pork tenderloin, 1 pound
Salmon fillets, skinned, 1 pound
Shrimp, 1 pound

Sweeteners

Swerve confectioners, 1¼ cups +
    1 tablespoon

28-Day Egg-Free Meal Plan

	BREAKFAST	DINNER	SIDE DISH	NUTRITION INFO (per serving)	
DAY 8	French Toast Cereal (1) 58	Spanish Spiced Lamb Chops (6) 202	Shrimp Adobo (4) 275	calories (kcal)	1160
				fat	95 g
				carbohydrate	4 g
				protein	76 g
DAY 9	Pork Chops with Dijon Gravy (4) 242	Saucy BBQ Wraps (4) 214	Easy Pickled Shrimp with Curry Mayo (4) 271	calories (kcal)	1025
				fat	73 g
				carbohydrate	8 g
				protein	74 g
DAY 10	Bacon-Wrapped Cod (4) 272	Spanish Spiced Lamb Chops LEFTOVER	Shrimp Adobo LEFTOVER	calories (kcal)	1133
				fat	89 g
				carbohydrate	2 g
				protein	79 g
DAY 11	Pork Chops with Dijon Gravy LEFTOVER	Spanish Spiced Lamb Chops LEFTOVER	Easy Pickled Shrimp with Curry Mayo LEFTOVER	calories (kcal)	1232
				fat	94 g
				carbohydrate	2 g
				protein	84 g
DAY 12	French Toast Cereal (1) 58	Saucy BBQ Wraps LEFTOVER	Manhattan Clam Chowder (4) 120	calories (kcal)	1054
				fat	79 g
				carbohydrate	22 g
				protein	68 g
DAY 13	Bacon-Wrapped Cod LEFTOVER	30-Minute Porchetta (4) 249	Bacon-Wrapped Portobello Fries with ranch dressing (2) 154	calories (kcal)	970
				fat	78 g
				carbohydrate	4 g
				protein	63 g
DAY 14	Bacon-Wrapped Scallops with Avocado Cream (4) 260	30-Minute Porchetta LEFTOVER	Manhattan Clam Chowder LEFTOVER	calories (kcal)	1108
				fat	82 g
				carbohydrate	20 g
				protein	76 g

Week 2 Grocery List

Broth

Chicken bone broth, 5 cups

Canned and Jarred Pantry Items

Baby clams, 2 (10-ounce) cans
Baby dill pickles, ½ cup

Condiments and Sauces

Clam juice, 1 (8-ounce) bottle
Coconut vinegar, ½ cup +
    3 tablespoons
Dijon mustard, ¼ cup +
    2 tablespoons + 1 teaspoon
Fish sauce, 1 teaspoon
Lemon juice, 3 tablespoons
Lime juice, ¼ cup + 1½ teaspoons
Liquid smoke, 2 teaspoons
Mayonnaise, ⅔ cup
Prepared yellow mustard, ¼ cup
Ranch dressing, ¼ cup
Tomato paste, 2 tablespoons
Tomato sauce, ½ cup
Wheat-free tamari, 1 tablespoon

Dried Herbs, Spices, and Extracts

Bay leaves, 2
Black peppercorns, 2 tablespoons
Cayenne pepper, ¼ teaspoon
Curry powder, ½ teaspoon
Fine sea salt, 2 tablespoons +
    2 teaspoons
Garlic powder, 2 teaspoons
Ground allspice, ½ teaspoon
Ground black pepper,
    2½ teaspoons
Ground cinnamon, 2½ teaspoons
Ground coriander, 1 teaspoon

Ground cumin, 1½ teaspoons
Maple extract, 1 teaspoon
Onion powder, 2 teaspoons
Oregano leaves, ¼ teaspoon
Paprika, 1½ teaspoons
Smoked paprika, 2 tablespoons
Thyme leaves, ½ teaspoon
Turmeric powder, ¼ teaspoon

Fats and Oils

Avocado oil, 1 cup
Coconut oil, ½ cup
MCT oil, ⅓ cup

Fresh Herbs

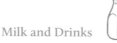

Chives, ⅓ cup chopped + garnish
Cilantro, ¼ cup
Flat-leaf parsley, for garnish
Oregano, 1 tablespoon +
    1 teaspoon
Rosemary, 1½ tablespoons finely
    chopped
Thyme, for garnish

Milk and Drinks

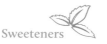

Unsweetened cashew milk, 2 cups

Other Recipes

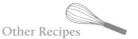

Creamy Lime Sauce (page 38),
    ¼ cup
Simple BBQ Sauce (page 43),
    ¼ cup
Tartar Sauce (page 40), ¼ cup

Prepackaged Items

Pork rinds, 2 ounces

Produce

Avocado, 1
Boston lettuce, 1 head
Celery, 1 stalk
Fennel bulb, 1 tablespoon finely
    diced
Garlic, 13 cloves
Green bell pepper, 1
Jalapeño pepper, 1
Limes, 3
Onions, ½ cup diced
Portobello mushrooms, 2 large
Red onions, ⅓ cup sliced
Tomato, 1 large
Zucchini, 1 small

Proteins

Bacon, 1 package thin-cut +
    1 package regular
Bone-in pork chops, 4 (¾ inch
    thick)
Cod, 1 (1-pound) fillet
Ground beef, 1 pound
Lamb loin chops, 6 (5 ounces
    each)
Pork tenderloin, 1 pound
Sea scallops, ½ pound
Shrimp, 2 pounds

Sweeteners

Swerve confectioners, ¼ cup

	BREAKFAST	DINNER	SIDE DISH	NUTRITION INFO (per serving)	
DAY 15	Camarones Cucarachas (Deviled Shrimp) (4) 274	Lamb Chops with Gyro Salad (8) 228	Smoky Spicy Chicken Stew (12) 122	calories (kcal)	1054
				fat	75 g
				carbohydrate	14 g
				protein	82 g
DAY 16	Personal Salmon en Papillote (2) 280	Cilantro Lime Slow Cooker Ribs (8) 256	Thai Red Curry Shrimp Soup (4) 132	calories (kcal)	1145
				fat	85 g
				carbohydrate	16 g
				protein	82 g
DAY 17	Camarones Cucarachas (Deviled Shrimp) LEFTOVER	Lamb Chops with Gyro Salad LEFTOVER	Bacon-Wrapped Portobello Fries with ranch dressing (2) 154	calories (kcal)	1054
				fat	75 g
				carbohydrate	14 g
				protein	82 g
DAY 18	Bacon-Wrapped Scallops with Avocado Cream (4) 260	Cilantro Lime Slow Cooker Ribs LEFTOVER	Smoky Spicy Chicken Stew LEFTOVER	calories (kcal)	1362
				fat	113 g
				carbohydrate	14 g
				protein	71 g
DAY 19	Simple Scallops with Garlic Sauce (4) 289	Lamb Chops with Gyro Salad LEFTOVER	Thai Red Curry Shrimp Soup LEFTOVER	calories (kcal)	1240
				fat	91 g
				carbohydrate	13 g
				protein	89 g
DAY 20	Bacon-Wrapped Scallops with Avocado Cream LEFTOVER	Cilantro Lime Slow Cooker Ribs LEFTOVER	Smoky Spicy Chicken Stew LEFTOVER	calories (kcal)	1390
				fat	111 g
				carbohydrate	21 g
				protein	77 g
DAY 21	Simple Scallops with Garlic Sauce LEFTOVER	Lamb Chops with Gyro Salad LEFTOVER	Manhattan Clam Chowder (4) 120	calories (kcal)	1108
				fat	86 g
				carbohydrate	10 g
				protein	72 g

Week 3 Grocery List

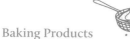

Baking Products

Unsweetened baking chocolate,
1 ounce

Broth

Chicken bone broth, 9¾ cups

Canned and Jarred Pantry Items

Baby clams, 2 (10-ounce) cans
Diced tomatoes, 1 (28-ounce) can
Greek olives, 2 cups pitted

Condiments and Sauces

Clam juice, 1 (8-ounce) bottle
Dijon mustard, 2 teaspoons
Hot sauce, ¼ cup
Lemon juice, 3 tablespoons
Lime juice, ¾ cup
Ranch dressing, ¼ cup
Red curry paste, 1½ tablespoons
Red wine vinegar, ¼ cup +
    1 tablespoon
Tomato paste, 2 tablespoons
Tomato sauce, 1 cup

Dried Herbs, Spices, and Extracts

Bay leaves, 2
Cayenne pepper, 1 teaspoon
Fine sea salt, 3 tablespoons
Ground black pepper, 2 teaspoons
Ground cumin, 1 tablespoon +
    ½ teaspoon
Ground oregano, 1 tablespoon +
    1 teaspoon
Paprika, ½ teaspoon
Smoked paprika, 2 tablespoons
Thyme leaves, ½ teaspoon

Fats and Oils

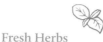

Avocado oil, ¼ cup + 1 tablespoon
Butter-flavored coconut oil, ¼ cup
Coconut oil, 1 tablespoon + 1
    teaspoon
Lard, 1 tablespoon

Fresh Herbs

Basil leaves, ½ teaspoon
Chives, 2 tablespoons chopped +
    garnish
Cilantro, 1 cup
Flat-leaf parsley, 1 tablespoon
    chopped + garnish
Ginger root, 2 tablespoons +
    1 teaspoon grated
Oregano, 4 sprigs
Thyme, 2 sprigs

Milk and Drinks

Coconut milk, 1 (14-ounce) can
Lime-flavored sparkling water,
    1 (12-ounce) can

Other Recipes

Baconnaise (page 34), 1 cup
Greek Vinaigrette (page 46),
    1 batch

Produce

Avocado, 1
Celery, 1 stalk
Cucumber, 1 medium
Garlic, 2 heads
Green bell pepper, 1
Jalapeño peppers, 2
Limes, 6
Onion, 1 medium
Portobello mushrooms, 2 large
Red onions, ¼ cup diced
Scallions, ¼ cup sliced
Shallots, 3
Tomatoes, 1 medium + 1 large
Zucchini, 1 small

Proteins

Bacon, 26 strips
Boneless, skinless chicken
    thighs, 2
Ground chicken, 2 pounds
Lamb loin chops, 8 (1¼ inches
    thick)
Pork ribs, 4 pounds
Salmon fillet, 1 (4 ounces)
Sea scallops, 1½ pounds
Shrimp, 1 pound medium +
    1 pound extra-large

Sweeteners

Swerve confectioners,
    2 tablespoons

28-Day Egg-Free Meal Plan

	BREAKFAST	DINNER	SIDE DISH	NUTRITION INFO (per serving)	
DAY 22	Cherry Almond Breakfast Shake (2) — 54	Cowboy Steak for Two (2) — 225	Bacon-Wrapped Portobello Fries with ranch dressing (2) — 154	calories (kcal)	1256
				fat	100 g
				carbohydrate	11 g
				protein	85 g
DAY 23	Chicken with Sausage and Greens (4) — 172	Juicy Pork Tenderloin (12) — 246	Bacon Chips with Dips (6) — 91	calories (kcal)	1157
				fat	83 g
				carbohydrate	23 g
				protein	79 g
DAY 24	Lemon Pepper Chicken Tenders and asparagus (4) — 176	Saucy BBQ Wraps (4) — 214	Bacon Chips with Dips — LEFTOVER	calories (kcal)	1156
				fat	82 g
				carbohydrate	30 g
				protein	76 g
DAY 25	Chicken with Sausage and Greens — LEFTOVER	Juicy Pork Tenderloin — LEFTOVER	Bacon-Wrapped Portobello Fries with ranch dressing — LEFTOVER	calories (kcal)	985
				fat	67 g
				carbohydrate	8 g
				protein	83 g
DAY 26	Simple Scallops with Garlic Sauce (4) — 289	Saucy BBQ Wraps — LEFTOVER	Slow Cooker Thai Soup (4) — 129	calories (kcal)	1043
				fat	70 g
				carbohydrate	19 g
				protein	84 g
DAY 27	Simple Scallops with Garlic Sauce — LEFTOVER	Juicy Pork Tenderloin — LEFTOVER	Slow Cooker Thai Soup — LEFTOVER	calories (kcal)	937
				fat	55 g
				carbohydrate	13 g
				protein	95 g
DAY 28	Lemon Pepper Chicken Tenders and asparagus — LEFTOVER	South of the Border Steak (8) — 200	Bacon-Wrapped Portobello Fries with ranch dressing (2) — 154	calories (kcal)	991
				fat	66 g
				carbohydrate	14 g
				protein	84 g

Week 4 Grocery List

Broth

Chicken bone broth, 3 cups

Canned and Jarred Pantry Items

Baby dill pickles, ½ cup

Condiments and Sauces

Almond butter, ¼ cup
Lime juice, ½ cup + 1 tablespoon
Liquid smoke, 2 teaspoons
Prepared yellow mustard, ¼ cup
Ranch dressing, ½ cup
Red curry paste, 2 tablespoons
Tomato sauce, ½ cup
Wheat-free tamari, 3 tablespoons

Dried Herbs, Spices, and Extracts

Almond extract, ½ teaspoon
Black peppercorns, 1 teaspoon
Cherry extract, 1 teaspoon
Chili powder, 1 tablespoon
Cumin, 1 tablespoon
Fine sea salt, ¼ cup
Garlic powder, 2 teaspoons
Ground black pepper,
    2½ teaspoons
Ground cumin, 1 tablespoon +
    1 teaspoon
Lemongrass, 1 teaspoon
Lemon pepper seasoning,
    2 tablespoons
Onion powder, 2 teaspoons
Orange oil, 10 drops
Smoked paprika, 2 tablespoons

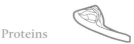

Fats and Oils

Avocado oil, ¾ cup
Butter-flavored coconut oil,
    ¼ cup

Fresh Herbs

Chives, ⅓ cup chopped
Cilantro, ⅓ cup chopped + garnish
Flat-leaf parsley, 1 tablespoon
    chopped + garnish

Milk and Drinks

Cherry tea, 1 cup brewed
Coconut milk, 1 (13½-ounce) can
Unsweetened cashew milk, 1 cup

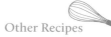

Other Recipes

Citrus Avocado Salsa (page 86),
    1 batch
Guacamole (page 87), 1 batch
Simple BBQ Sauce (page 43),
    ¼ cup
Steak Sauce (page 36), ½ cup

Produce

Asparagus, 8 ounces
Avocado, 1
Boston lettuce, 1 head
Broccoli slaw, ¼ cup
Garlic, 21 cloves
Ginger root, 2 tablespoons grated
Kale, 1 cup chopped
Lemons, 3

Limes, 2
Mushrooms, 4 cups sliced
Onions, ¼ cup diced
Portobello mushrooms, 4 large
Radicchio, 1 cup chopped
Red bell peppers, ½ cup sliced
Red onions, ⅓ cup sliced
Scallions, 4 + garnish

Proteins

Bacon, 24 strips
Bone-in rib-eye steak, 1
    (1½ pounds; about 1½ inches
    thick)
Bone-in, skin-on chicken thighs, 4
Boneless, skinless chicken breast
    halves, 4 (about 2 pounds)
Boneless, skinless chicken thighs,
    1½ pounds
Flank steak or skirt steak,
    2 pounds
Ground beef, 1 pound
Italian sausage, 1 pound
Pork tenderloins, 2 (2 pounds
    each)
Sea scallops, 1 pound large

Sweeteners

Swerve confectioners, ¾ cup

7-Day Nightshade-Free Meal Plan

	BREAKFAST	DINNER	SIDE DISH	NUTRITION INFO (per serving)	
DAY 1	Easy Breakfast Sandwich (1) (omit tomato) 73	Baked Sole with Zucchini (4) 264	French Onion Meatball Soup (8) 126	calories (kcal)	979
				fat	80 g
				carbohydrate	15 g
				protein	54 g
DAY 2	Baked Eggs and Ham (2) 57	30-Minute Porchetta (4) 249	Mexican Lime Chicken Soup (6) 111	calories (kcal)	833
				fat	56 g
				carbohydrate	5 g
				protein	76 g
DAY 3	Silky Egg Breakfast Soup (2) 70	Baked Sole with Zucchini LEFTOVER	French Onion Meatball Soup LEFTOVER	calories (kcal)	1045
				fat	73 g
				carbohydrate	15 g
				protein	83 g
DAY 4	French Toast Cereal (1) 58	Chicken with Sausage and Greens (4) 172	Mexican Lime Chicken Soup LEFTOVER	calories (kcal)	1172
				fat	96 g
				carbohydrate	9 g
				protein	72 g
DAY 5	French Toast Pudding (4) 80	Simple Lamb Chops with Lemon Mustard Gravy (4) 220	French Onion Meatball Soup LEFTOVER	calories (kcal)	1415
				fat	114 g
				carbohydrate	9 g
				protein	86 g
DAY 6	Smoked Salmon, Egg, and Avocado (1) with Greek Vinaigrette 62	Chicken with Sausage and Greens LEFTOVER	Turkey and "Orzo" Soup (6) 119	calories (kcal)	1133
				fat	87 g
				carbohydrate	16 g
				protein	72 g
DAY 7	Breakfast Asparagus (1) 65	Simple Lamb Chops with Lemon Mustard Gravy LEFTOVER	Turkey and "Orzo" Soup LEFTOVER	calories (kcal)	1244
				fat	91 g
				carbohydrate	10 g
				protein	91 g

Grocery List

Broth

Beef bone broth, 4½ cups +
2 tablespoons
Chicken bone broth, 14 cups

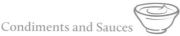

Condiments and Sauces

Dijon mustard, 2 tablespoons
Distilled white vinegar,
1 tablespoon
Fish sauce, 2½ tablespoons
Lemon juice, 1 tablespoon
Lime juice, 2 tablespoons
Red wine vinegar, ¼ cup +
1 tablespoon
Stone-ground mustard,
2 tablespoons

Dried Herbs, Spices, and Extracts

Chives, 2 tablespoons
Fine sea salt, 3 tablespoons
Ground black pepper,
2½ teaspoons
Ground cinnamon, 1 tablespoon
Ground cumin, 1 teaspoon
Maple extract, 1 tablespoon
Thyme leaves, 2 teaspoons

Eggs

Eggs, 15 large
Hard-boiled eggs, 10

Fats and Oils

Avocado oil, ¾ cup +
1½ teaspoons
Coconut oil, 3 tablespoons +
1 teaspoon
Lard, 1 tablespoon

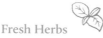

Fresh Herbs

Chives, 1½ teaspoons chopped
Cilantro, 2¼ cups chopped
Dill, 3 tablespoons chopped +
sprigs for garnish
Rosemary, 1½ tablespoons finely
chopped
Thyme, 4 sprigs + 1 teaspoon
leaves

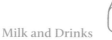

Milk and Drinks

Coconut milk, 1 (13½-ounce) can
Unsweetened cashew milk, 1 cup

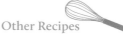

Other Recipes

Greek Vinaigrette (page 46),
1 tablespoon

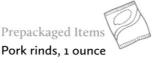

Prepackaged Items

Pork rinds, 1 ounce

Produce

Asparagus, 6 spears
Avocado, ½ medium
Broccoli slaw, ¼ cup
Cauliflower, 2 cups coarsely
chopped florets
Fennel bulb, 1 tablespoon finely
diced
Garlic, 10 cloves
Kale, 1 cup chopped
Leafy lettuce, 1 cup torn
Lemons, 2
Limes, 2
Onions, 2 medium
Radicchio, 1 cup chopped
Red onion, 1 slice
Scallions, 4 + garnish
Zucchini, 1 medium

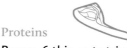

Proteins

Bacon, 6 thin-cut strips +
2 regular strips
Bone-in, skin-on chicken thighs, 4
Boneless, skinless chicken breast
halves, 2 (about 1 pound, for 2
cups chopped cooked chicken)
Boneless, skinless chicken thighs,
1¼ pounds
Ground beef, 2 pounds
Ham, deli-style, 8 slices
Italian sausage, 1 pound
Lamb chops, 8 (½ inch thick)
Pork tenderloin, 1 pound
Smoked salmon, 2 ounces
Sole, 4 (4-ounce) fillets
Turkey, roasted, 1½ cups diced

Sweeteners

Stevia glycerite, 1 to 2 teaspoons
Swerve confectioners, ½ cup +
3 tablespoons

7-Day Vegetarian Meal Plan

	BREAKFAST	DINNER	SIDE DISH	DESSERT	NUTRITION INFO (per serving)	
DAY 1	Italian Baked Eggs (4) — 298	Chipotle Lime Egg Salad Wraps (4) — 302	Vegetarian Fajita Stew (2) — 312	Personal Flourless Chocolate Tortes (8) — 320	calories	1304
					fat	110 g
					carbs	37 g
					protein	48 g
DAY 2	Lemon Poppyseed Waffles (4) — 67	Vegetarian Fajitas with Avocado (2) — 310	Vegetarian Doro Watt (4) — 304	Banana Bread (12) — 330	calories	1176
					fat	94 g
					carbs	30 g
					protein	66 g
DAY 3	Snickerdoodle Mini Muffins (6) — 72	Chipotle Lime Egg Salad Wraps — LEFTOVER	Sweet 'n' Sour Cauliflower (6) — 294	Personal Flourless Chocolate Tortes — LEFTOVER	calories	1317
					fat	122 g
					carbs	20 g
					protein	44 g
DAY 4	Italian Baked Eggs — LEFTOVER	Creamy Egg Bhurji (2) — 303	Vegetarian Doro Watt — LEFTOVER	Personal Flourless Chocolate Tortes — LEFTOVER	calories	1347
					fat	113 g
					carbs	37 g
					protein	56 g
DAY 5	Super Keto Pancakes (2) — 79	Vegetarian Fajitas with Avocado — LEFTOVER	Vegetarian Doro Watt (4) — 304	Personal Flourless Chocolate Tortes — LEFTOVER	calories	1268
					fat	110 g
					carbs	16 g
					protein	63 g
DAY 6	Lemon Poppyseed Waffles — LEFTOVER	Egg Masala (2) — 309	Sweet 'n' Sour Cauliflower — LEFTOVER	Banana Bread — LEFTOVER	calories	983
					fat	85 g
					carbs	14 g
					protein	52 g
DAY 7	Snickerdoodle Mini Muffins — LEFTOVER	Vegetarian Fajitas with Avocado (2) — 310	Vegetarian Doro Watt — LEFTOVER	Banana Bread — LEFTOVER	calories	1135
					fat	98 g
					carbs	13 g
					protein	60 g

Grocery List

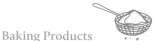

Baking Products

Baking powder, 1 tablespoon +
1 teaspoon
Coconut flour, 1 tablespoon
Unsweetened baking chocolate,
7 ounces

Broth

Vegetable broth, 4½ cups +
2 tablespoons

Canned and Jarred Pantry Items

Pickled jalapeños, ¼ cup diced

Condiments and Sauces

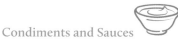

Coconut vinegar, 1 tablespoon
Green curry paste, 1 tablespoon
Lemon juice, 2 tablespoons
Lime juice, 1 tablespoon
Marinara sauce, ½ cup
Mayonnaise, ½ cup
Sugar-free salsa, ½ cup
Tomato sauce, ¼ cup
Wheat-free tamari, 1 tablespoon
+ 1½ teaspoons

Dried Herbs, Spices, and Extracts

Banana extract, 1 tablespoon +
1 teaspoon
Cayenne pepper, 1 tablespoon +
2½ teaspoons
Chili powder, 2 teaspoons
Crushed red pepper, ¾ teaspoon
Fine sea salt, ½ cup
Garam masala, 1 tablespoon +
2 teaspoons

Garlic powder, ½ teaspoon
Ginger powder, ¼ teaspoon
Ground black pepper, 2 teaspoons
Ground cardamom, ¼ teaspoon
Ground cinnamon, ¼ cup +
2 tablespoons
Ground cloves, ⅛ teaspoon
Ground coriander, 1 tablespoon +
½ teaspoon
Ground cumin, 1 teaspoon
Ground fenugreek, ¼ teaspoon
Ground nutmeg, ¼ teaspoon
Lemon extract, 2 teaspoons
Onion powder, ½ teaspoon
Paprika, 3 tablespoons +
1 teaspoon
Poppy seeds, 2 tablespoons
Sesame seeds, for garnish
Turmeric powder, 2 teaspoons
Vanilla extract, 1 tablespoon +
2 teaspoons

Eggs

Eggs, 51 large
Hard-boiled eggs, 60

Fats and Oils

Avocado oil, ½ cup + 1 teaspoon
Butter-flavored coconut oil,
¾ cup + 2 tablespoons
Coconut oil, 3 cups

Fresh Herbs

Cilantro, ¼ cup chopped + garnish
Flat-leaf parsley, for garnish
Ginger root, ¼ teaspoon grated
Thyme sprigs, for garnish

Milk and Drinks

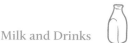

Coconut milk, ¾ cup
Unsweetened cashew milk, ½ cup

Other Recipes

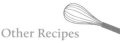

Cinnamon Syrup (page 47), ¼ cup
Keto Fried "Rice" (page 148),
2 batches
Keto Tortillas (page 150), 2 batches
Lemon Syrup (page 48), ¼ cup

Produce

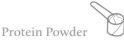

Avocado, 1 + garnish
Bell peppers (any color), 2
Cauliflower, 1 head
Celery, ½ cup diced
Garlic, 10 cloves
Green bell pepper, 1
Limes, 5
Onions, 2 large + 2¼ cups diced +
½ cup thinly sliced
Radicchio, 8 leaves
Red onions, ¼ cup diced
Scallions, for garnish
Tomatoes, 2 medium + 3 small

Protein Powder

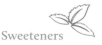

Unflavored egg white protein
powder, 2 tablespoons
Vanilla-flavored egg white protein
powder, ¾ cup

Sweeteners

Swerve confectioners, 3½ cups +
2 tablespoons

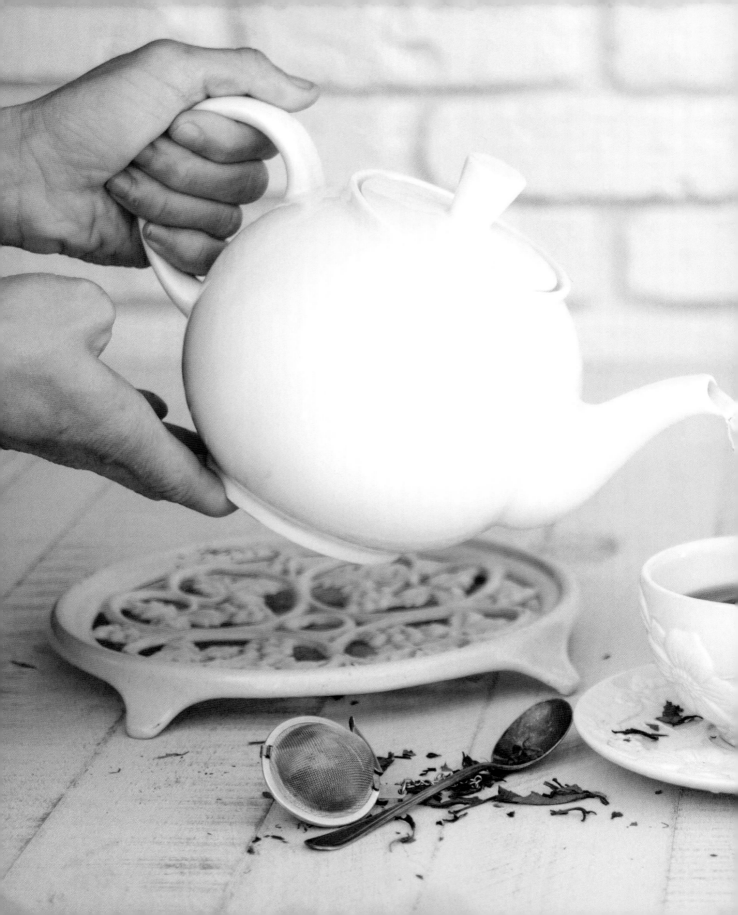

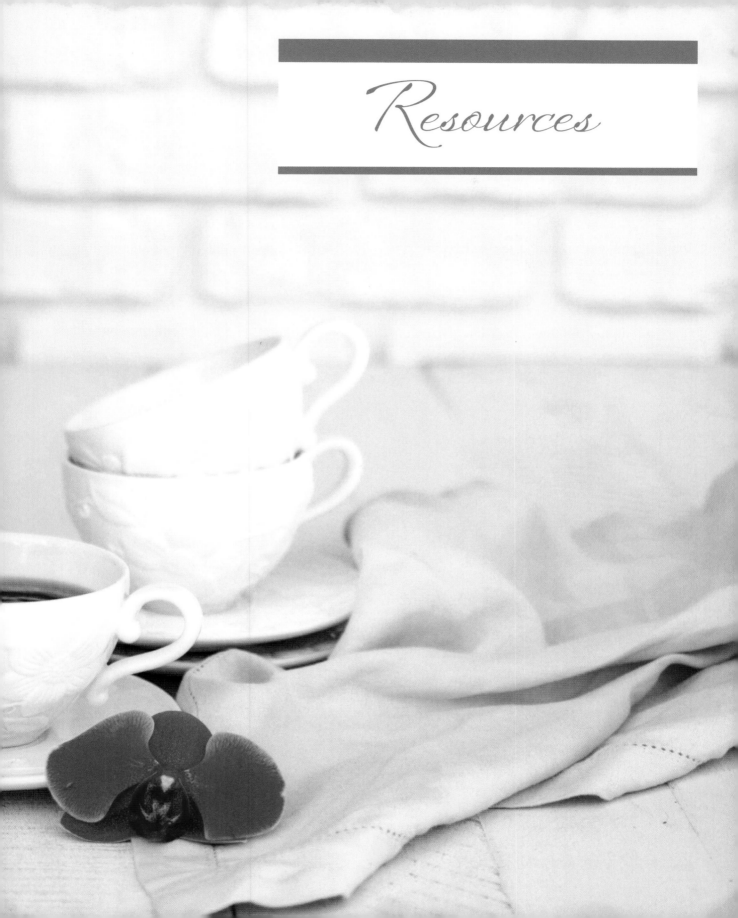

Resources

Quick Reference

H ⌣ KETO   M ⌣ KETO   L ⌣ KETO   ● Omits Ingredient   ○ Optional Ingredient

RECIPES	PAGE	L̂ H	🌿	🥚
Mayonnaise	34	H	O	
Egg-Free Mayo	35	H	●	●
Steak Sauce	36	L	●	●
Comeback Sauce	37	H	●	O
Creamy Lime Sauce	38	H	●	O
Cilantro Lime Dressing	39	L	●	●
Tartar Sauce	40	H	●	O
Béarnaise Sauce	41	H	●	
Romanesco Sauce	42	M	●	●
Simple BBQ Sauce	43	L	●	●
Crab Louie Dressing	44	H	●	O
Creamy Ranch Dressing	45	H	●	O
Greek Vinaigrette	46	H	●	●
Cinnamon Syrup	47	H	●	●
Lemon Syrup	48	H	●	●
Iced Green Tea Latte	52	L	O	●
Cherry Almond Breakfast Shake	54	M		●
Amazing Protein Shake	56	H	O	
Baked Eggs and Ham	57	H	●	
French Toast Cereal	58	H	O	●
Breakfast Bacon Fat Bombs	59	H	●	
Lemon Minute Muffins	60	M	●	
Smoked Salmon, Egg, and Avocado	62	H	●	
Loaded Scrambled Eggs	64	H	●	
Breakfast Asparagus	65	H	●	
Spicy Fried Eggs with Chorizo	66	H	●	
Lemon Poppyseed Waffles	67	H	●	
Breakfast Sausage Soup with Soft-Boiled Eggs	68	H	●	O
Silky Egg Breakfast Soup	70	H	●	
Snickerdoodle Mini Muffins	72	H	●	
Easy Breakfast Sandwich	73	H	●	
Irish Breakfast	74	H	●	
Soft-Boiled Eggs with Bacon-Wrapped Asparagus Dunkers	76	H	●	
Reuben Eggs Benedict	78	H	●	
Super Keto Pancakes	79	H	●	
French Toast Pudding	80	H	●	
Perfect Hard-Boiled Eggs	81	H	●	
Shrimp Cocktail	84	H	●	●
Pico de Gallo	85	L	●	●
Citrus Avocado Salsa	86	L	●	●
Guacamole	87	H	●	●
Jicama Crostini—Two Ways	88	M	●	O
Almost Deviled Eggs	90	H	●	
Bacon Chips with Dips	91	L	●	●
Amazing Marinated Olives	92	H	●	●
Simple Shrimp Parfait	93	H	●	●
Dry-Rubbed Baked Wings	94	H	●	O
Devilish Deviled Eggs	95	H	●	
Deviled Green Eggs and Ham	96	H	●	
Cute Kitty Deviled Eggs	98	H	●	
Moroccan Deviled Eggs	99	H	●	
Homemade Ginger Ale	100	L	●	●
Naked Gimlet	102	L	●	●

RECIPES	PAGE	L—M—H	🌿	🥚
Virgin Strawberry Margarita	103	M	●	●
Super Fast Bone Broth	106	H	●	●
Chinese Beef and Broccoli Soup	108	M	●	●
Coconut Ginger Chicken Soup	110	H	●	●
Mexican Lime Chicken Soup	111	H	●	●
Caldo de Costilla (Colombian Beef Rib Broth)	112	H	●	●
Texas BBQ Brisket Soup	114	H	●	●
Pizza Soup	115	L	●	●
Cilantro Lime Meatball Soup	116	H	●	
Chilled Tomato and Ham Soup	118	H	●	O
Turkey and "Orzo" Soup	119	H	●	●
Manhattan Clam Chowder	120	L	●	●
Steak Fajita Soup	121	M	●	●
Smoky Spicy Chicken Stew	122	H	●	●
Tuscan Sausage and "Rice" Stew	124	H	●	
French Onion Meatball Soup	126	H	●	
Ham and Fauxtato Soup	128	M	●	●
Slow Cooker Thai Soup	129	H	●	●
Chicken and "Rice" Soup	130	H	●	
Italian "Orzo" Soup	131	M	●	
Thai Red Curry Shrimp Soup	132	H	●	●
Salmon Soup	133	H	●	●
Creamy Smoked Salmon Soup	134	H	●	
Asparagus Cobb Salad with Ranch Dressing	138	H	●	O
BLT Grilled Romaine	139	H	●	●
Crab Louie Salad	140	H	●	O
Salad Kabobs	141	H	●	
Chef's Salad	142	H	●	
Grilled Avocado	143	M	●	●
Keto Brioche	144	H	●	
Brioche Croutons	146	H	●	
Keto "Rice"	147	H	●	
Keto Fried "Rice"	148	H	●	
Cauliflower Rice	149	M	●	●
Keto Tortillas	150	H	●	
Cabbage Pasta	152	M	●	●
Chow Chow	153	L	●	●
Bacon-Wrapped Portobello Fries	154	H	●	O
Asian Coleslaw	155	M	●	●
Chicken Shawarma	158	H	●	O
BLT Chicken Kabobs	160	H	●	O
Chicken Tinga with Keto Tortillas	162	M	●	O
Guacamole Lovers' Stuffed Chicken	164	H	●	●
Chicken and Asparagus Curry	166	M	●	●
Curry Braised Chicken Legs	167	H	●	●
Grilled Jerk Chicken Thighs	168	H	●	●
Easy Asian Chicken Legs	169	H	●	●
Chicken and Mushroom Kabobs	170	H	●	O
Chicken with Sausage and Greens	172	H	●	●
Tender Coconut Chicken	174	H	●	O
Lemon Pepper Chicken Tenders	176	H	●	●
Bundt Pan Chicken	178	H	●	●
Sheet Pan BBQ Chicken Breasts with Bacon-Wrapped Avocado Fries	180	H	●	●
Bacon-Wrapped Chicken Fingers	181	H	●	●
Simple Sesame Chicken	182	H	●	O
Paella	184	H	●	●

RECIPES	PAGE	L $\widehat{M}$ H	🌿	🥚
Greek Chicken Thighs	186	H	●	●
Tender Chicken Livers	188	H	●	O
Dijon Chicken	189	H	●	●
Curry Chicken Meatballs	190	H	●	O
Grilled Chicken and Avocado	191	H	●	●
Chicken Satay with Dipping Sauce	192	H	●	●
Easy Chicken and Asparagus Stir-Fry	194	H	●	●
Mole Chicken Legs	195	H	●	●
Devil Chicken	196	H	●	●
South of the Border Steak	200	H	●	●
Spanish Spiced Lamb Chops	202	H	●	●
Slow Cooker Philly Steak Sandwiches	204	H	●	
T-Bone Steaks with Romanesco Sauce	206	H	●	●
Easy BBQ Brisket	208	H	●	●
Herby Broth Fondue	210	H	●	O
Curry Short Ribs	212	H	●	●
Simple Spaghetti	213	H	●	●
Saucy BBQ Wraps	214	H	●	●
Hungarian Goulash	216	L	●	●
Jamaican Jerk Pot Roast	217	H	●	●
Fajita Kabobs	218	H	●	●
Simple Lamb Chops with Lemon Mustard Gravy	220	H	●	●
Kung Pao Meatballs in Lettuce Cups	222	H	●	
Chinese Five-Spice Roast Beef	224	H	●	●
Cowboy Steak for Two	225	H	●	●
Shan Beef Stir-Fry	226	H	●	
Lamb Chops with Gyro Salad	228	H	●	●
Italian Beef Tips	230	H	●	●
Citrus Pork Shoulder with Spicy Cilantro-Ginger Sauce	234	H	●	O
Spring Ham Bake with Dijon Sauce	236	H	●	
Easy Barbecue Ribs	238	H	●	●
Saucy Barbecue Pork Chops	239	H	●	●
Ginger Lime Pork Lettuce Cups	240	H	●	●
Pork Chops with Dijon Gravy	242	H	●	●
Sausage Zucchini Ravioli	244	H	●	●
Juicy Pork Tenderloin	246	H	●	●
Thai Pulled Pork with Keto Fried "Rice"	248	H	●	O
30-Minute Porchetta	249	H	●	●
Sweet 'n' Sour Pork Meatballs	250	H	●	
Deviled Ham	252	H	●	O
Mustard-Glazed Ham	253	H	●	●
Hawaiian Luau Pork	254	H	●	O
Cilantro Lime Slow Cooker Ribs	256	H	●	
Bacon-Wrapped Scallops with Avocado Cream	260	H	●	●
Halibut Confit	262	H	●	●
Baked Sole with Zucchini	264	H	●	●
Pan-Fried Fish with Tartar Sauce	266	H	●	●
Halibut Smothered in Tomato Basil Cream	267	H	●	●
Salmon Burgers with Dill Sauce	268	H	●	
Crab Claws with Spicy Mustard Sauce	270	H	●	O
Easy Pickled Shrimp with Curry Mayo	271	H	●	O
Bacon-Wrapped Cod	272	H	●	O
Camarones Cucarachas (Deviled Shrimp)	274	H	●	●
Shrimp Adobo	275	H	●	●
Ahi Poke	276	H	●	O
Fish in Puttanesca Sauce	278	M	●	●

RECITES	PAGE	L M H	🌿	🥚
Garlic Lime Broiled Shrimp	279	H	●	●
Personal Salmon en Papillote	280	H	●	●
Salt-Crusted Fish	282	H	●	
Cajun Shrimp	284	H	●	●
Avocado Salmon Ceviche	285	H	●	●
Asian-Style Salmon Lettuce Cups	286	H	●	O
Yellow Curry Shrimp over Keto Fried "Rice"	287	H	●	
Super Fast Shrimp Fajitas	288	H	●	●
Simple Scallops with Garlic Sauce	289	H	●	●
Shrimp Fried "Rice"	290	H	●	
Sweet 'n' Sour Cauliflower over Vegetarian Fried "Rice"	294	M	●	
Vegetarian Curry	296	H	●	
Italian Baked Eggs	298	H	●	
Egg Roll in a Bowl	300	M	●	
Chipotle Lime Egg Salad Wraps	302	H	●	
Creamy Egg Bhurji	303	M	●	
Vegetarian Doro Watt	304	H	●	
Avocado Toast	306	H	●	
Gazpacho	308	L	●	●
Egg Masala	309	L	●	
Vegetarian Fajitas with Avocado	310	L	O	
Vegetarian Fajita Stew	312	L	●	
Grand Marnier Chocolate Candies	316	H	●	●
Sour Patch Candy	317	H	●	●
Snickerdoodle Bites	318	H	●	●
Berry Ice Pops	319	H	●	●
Personal Flourless Chocolate Tortes	320	H	●	
Mint Chocolate Chunk Gelato	322	H	O	
Mocha Fudge Mug Cakes	324	H	O	
Classic Sherbet	326	H	●	●
Dirt Cake	327	H	●	
Gummy Worms	328	H	●	●
Mexican Chocolate Mousse	329	H	O	
Banana Bread	330	H	●	
Malted Milk Push Pops	332	M	O	●
Chocolate Pudding Pops	333	H	●	
Hibiscus Strawberry Ice Lollies	334	H	●	●
Tapioca Pudding	335	H	●	
Keto Pink Squirrels	336	H		
Strawberry Hibiscus Sorbet	338	H	O	●
Keto Custard	339	H	O	
Strawberries and Cream Panna Cotta	340	H	●	●

Recipe Index

Chapter 1: Basics

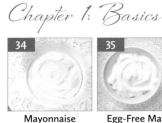
34 — Mayonnaise

35 — Egg-Free Mayo

36 — Steak Sauce

37 — Comeback Sauce

38 — Creamy Lime Sauce

39 — Cilantro Lime Dressing

40 — Tartar Sauce

41 — Béarnaise Sauce

42 — Romanesco Sauce

43 — Simple BBQ Sauce

44 — Crab Louie Dressing

45 — Creamy Ranch Dressing

46 — Greek Vinaigrette

47 — Cinnamon Syrup

48 — Lemon Syrup

Chapter 2: Break-Your-Fast

52 — Iced Green Tea Latte

54 — Cherry Almond Breakfast Shake

56 — Amazing Protein Shake

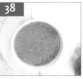
57 — Baked Eggs and Ham

58 — French Toast Cereal

59 — Breakfast Bacon Fat Bombs

60 — Lemon Minute Muffins

62 — Smoked Salmon, Egg, and Avocado

64 — Loaded Scrambled Eggs

65 — Breakfast Asparagus

66 — Spicy Fried Eggs with Chorizo

67 — Lemon Poppyseed Waffles

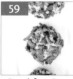
68 — Breakfast Sausage Soup with Soft-Boiled Eggs

70 — Silky Egg Breakfast Soup

72 — Snickerdoodle Mini Muffins

73 — Easy Breakfast Sandwich

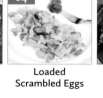

74 — Irish Breakfast

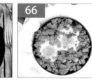

76 — Soft-Boiled Eggs with Bacon-Wrapped Asparagus Dunkers

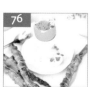
78 — Reuben Eggs Benedict

79 — Super Keto Pancakes

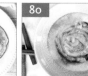
80 — French Toast Pudding

Perfect Hard-
Boiled Eggs

Chapter 3: Small Bites and Drinks

Shrimp Cocktail

Pico de Gallo

Citrus Avocado
Salsa

Guacamole

Jicana Crostini—
Two Ways

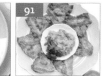
Almost Deviled
Eggs

Bacon Chips
with Dips

Amazing
Marinated Olives

Simple
Shrimp Parfait

Dry-Rubbed
Baked Wings

Devilish
Deviled Eggs

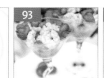
Deviled Green
Eggs and Ham

Cute Kitty
Deviled Eggs

Moroccan
Deviled Eggs

Homemade
Ginger Ale

Naked Gimlet

Virgin Strawberry
Margarita

Chapter 4: Soups and Stews

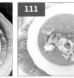
Super Fast
Bone Broth

Chinese Beef and
Broccoli Soup

Coconut Ginger
Chicken Soup

Mexican Lime
Chicken Soup

Caldo de Costilla
(Colombian
Beef Rib Broth)

Texas BBQ
Brisket Soup

Pizza Soup

Cilantro Lime
Meatball Soup

Chilled Tomato
and Ham Soup

Turkey and
"Orzo" Soup

Manhattan
Clam Chowder

Steak Fajita Soup

Smoky Spicy
Chicken Stew

Tuscan Sausage
and "Rice" Stew

126

French Onion
Meatball Soup

128

Ham and Fauxtato
Soup

129

Slow Cooker
Thai Soup

130

Chicken and
"Rice" Soup

131

Italian "Orzo" Soup

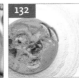
132

Thai Red Curry
Shrimp Soup

133

Salmon Soup

134

Creamy Smoked
Salmon Soup

Chapter 5: Salads and Sides

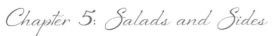

138

Asparagus
Cobb Salad with
Ranch Dressing

139

BLT Grilled
Romaine

140

Crab Louie Salad

141

Salad Kabobs

142

Chef's Salad

143

Grilled Avocado

144

Keto Brioche

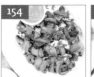
146

Brioche Croutons

147

Keto "Rice"

148

Keto Fried "Rice"

149

Cauliflower Rice

150

Keto Tortillas

152

Cabbage Pasta

153

Chow Chow

154

Bacon-Wrapped
Portobello Fries

155

Asian Coleslaw

Chapter 6: Poultry

158

Chicken Shawarma

160

BLT Chicken
Kabobs

162

Chicken Tinga
with Keto Tortillas

164

Guacamole Lovers'
Stuffed Chicken

166

Chicken and
Asparagus Curry

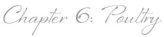
167

Curry Braised
Chicken Legs

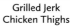
168

Grilled Jerk
Chicken Thighs

169
Easy Asian
Chicken Legs

170
Chicken and
Mushroom Kabobs

172
Chicken with
Sausage and
Greens

174
Tender Coconut
Chicken

176
Lemon Pepper
Chicken Tenders

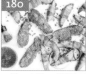
178
Bundt Pan Chicken

180
Sheet Pan BBQ
Chicken Breasts

181
Bacon-Wrapped
Chicken Fingers

182
Simple Sesame
Chicken

184
Paella

186
Greek Chicken
Thighs

188
Tender
Chicken Livers

189
Dijon Chicken

190
Curry Chicken
Meatballs

191
Grilled Chicken
and Avocado

192
Chicken Satay with
Dipping Sauce

194
Easy Chicken and
Asparagus Stir-Fry

195
Mole Chicken Legs

196
Devil Chicken

Chapter 7: Beef and Lamb

200
South of the
Border Steak

202
Spanish Spiced
Lamb Chops

204
Slow Cooker Philly
Steak Sandwiches

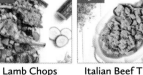
206
T-Bone Steaks
with Romanesco
Sauce

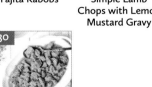
208
Easy BBQ Brisket

210
Herby Broth
Fondue

212
Curry Short Ribs

213
Simple Spaghetti

214
Saucy BBQ Wraps

216
Hungarian Goulash

217
Jamaican Jerk
Pot Roast

218
Fajita Kabobs

220
Simple Lamb
Chops with Lemon
Mustard Gravy

222
Kung Pao
Meatballs in
Lettuce Cups

224
Chinese Five-Spice
Roast Beef

225
Cowboy Steak
for Two

226
Shan Beef Stir-Fry

228
Lamb Chops
with Gyro Salad

230
Italian Beef Tips

Chapter 8: Pork

234 Citrus Pork Shoulder

236 Spring Ham Bake with Dijon Sauce

238 Easy Barbecue Ribs

239 Saucy Barbecue Pork Chops

240 Ginger Lime Pork Lettuce Cups

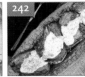
242 Pork Chops with Dijon Gravy

244 Sausage Zucchini Ravioli

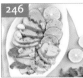
246 Juicy Pork Tenderloin

248 Thai Pulled Pork with Keto Fried "Rice"

249 30-Minute Porchetta

250 Sweet 'n' Sour Pork Meatballs

252 Deviled Ham

253 Mustard-Glazed Ham

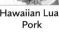
254 Hawaiian Luau Pork

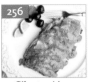
256 Cilantro Lime Slow Cooker Ribs

Chapter 9: Fish and Seafood

260 Bacon-Wrapped Scallops with Avocado Cream

262 Halibut Confit

264 Baked Sole with Zucchini

266 Pan-Fried Fish with Tartar Sauce

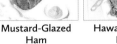
267 Halibut Smothered in Tomato Basil Cream

268 Salmon Burgers with Dill Sauce

270 Crab Claws with Spicy Mustard Sauce

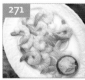
271 Easy Pickled Shrimp with Curry Mayo

272 Bacon-Wrapped Cod

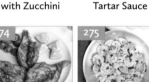
274 Camarones Cucarachas (Deviled Shrimp)

275 Shrimp Adobo

276 Ahi Poke

278 Fish in Puttanesca Sauce

279 Garlic Lime Broiled Shrimp

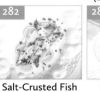
280 Personal Salmon en Papillote

282 Salt-Crusted Fish

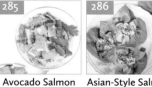
284 Cajun Shrimp

285 Avocado Salmon Ceviche

286 Asian-Style Salmon Lettuce Cups

287 Yellow Curry Shrimp over Keto Fried "Rice"

288 Super Fast Shrimp Fajitas

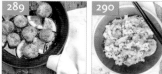

289
Simple Scallops with Garlic Sauce

290
Shrimp Fried "Rice"

Chapter 10: Vegetarian Dishes

294
Sweet 'n' Sour Cauliflower

296
Vegetarian Curry

298
Italian Baked Eggs

300
Egg Roll in a Bowl

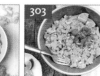
302
Chipotle Lime Egg Salad Wraps

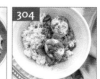
303
Creamy Egg Bhurji

304
Vegetarian Doro Watt

306
Avocado Toast

308
Gazpacho

309
Egg Masala

310
Vegetarian Fajitas with Avocado

312
Vegetarian Fajita Stew

Chapter 11: Sweet Endings

316
Grand Marnier Chocolate Candies

317
Sour Patch Candy

318
Snickerdoodle Bites

319
Berry Ice Pops

320
Personal Flourless Chocolate Tortes

322
Mint Chocolate Chunk Gelato

324
Mocha Fudge Mug Cakes

326
Classic Sherbet

327
Dirt Cake

328
Gummy Worms

329
Mexican Chocolate Mousse

330
Banana Bread

332
Malted Milk Push Pops

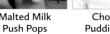
333
Chocolate Pudding Pops

334
Hibiscus Strawberry Ice Lollies

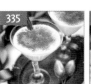
335
Tapioca Pudding

336
Keto Pink Squirrels

338
Strawberry Hibiscus Sorbet

339
Keto Custard

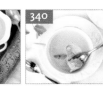
340
Strawberries and Cream Panna Cotta

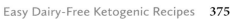
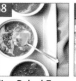
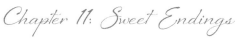
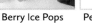

General Index

Gratitude

Like many of you, I have had some really difficult times in my life. Life is like waves of the ocean; everyone has high points as well as lows. It was during those lows that I had to stop spending money at restaurants and start cooking at home, which helped me become the healthy ketogenic cook I am today. I have learned to accept the low parts of the waves and have gratitude for the highs. These hardships have taught me amazing lifelong lessons. I struggled out of the cocoon, and it made me a butterfly with strong wings.

I am grateful to my love and best friend, Craig, who never complains, even though I often mess up the kitchen as soon as he cleans it. He has been a huge part of this book, picking up the groceries and testing recipes as well as adding all the nutritional information.

I am grateful for my boys, Micah and Kai, who love to help me in the kitchen. Even though it takes twice as long to get dinner on the table when they help, it is totally worth it. When we had to put our adoption on hold, I was devastated, but I remember my mom telling me that my children just weren't born yet. I cry as I write this because she was totally right. These two boys were meant for me!

I am also extremely grateful for Wendy and Lori, and I know you are, too! They are two of my recipe testers, and they spent numerous hours making sure my recipes tasted amazing and were worthy of inclusion in this book.

I am forever grateful for Jimmy Moore, who called me to write *The Ketogenic Cookbook* with him. Jimmy, I am so thankful for your support!

Bill and Haley, I am honored to have your photo on the cover of this book. I've always been a big fan of your photography and cookbooks. My first Victory Belt cookbook was your *Gather* book; I was in love with your artistry from the very beginning! Thank you for taking the time to make my recipes and shoot the cover. It is so lovely!

I also need to express my gratitude to the Victory Belt team. I never thought I would have the amazing support and kindness that I get from everyone at Victory Belt. I thought I was the only one who was working early in the morning on the Fourth of July, but an email from Holly came bright and early! I also had a phone call from Erich that afternoon. I am grateful for all of Victory Belt's hard work and dedication!

Holly and Pam, you played a huge part in making this book a work of art. Holly worked hard on this book even while she was visiting France on Bastille Day! I'm forever grateful for the time and dedication you both put into this book. You have such amazing ideas and attention to detail. You worked very long days and weekends to get the edits done on time, and I can't thank you enough for your amazing work!

Susan, I am grateful for your passion and how magnificently you help to endorse my books! I get a smile on my face whenever I receive an email from you. Your happiness shines through!

Lance, I can't thank you enough for helping with all my questions and creating amazingly beautiful images for promoting this lovely book!

Erich, your praise and fun outlook made this journey extraordinary and totally worth the hard work and long days of writing, editing, cooking, and photographing! I appreciate your caring phone calls just to check in on me and make sure everything was going smoothly.

Finally, I want to express my gratitude to you, the reader! I can't thank you enough for all your love and support!